AF658450

Retina and Vitreous Surgery

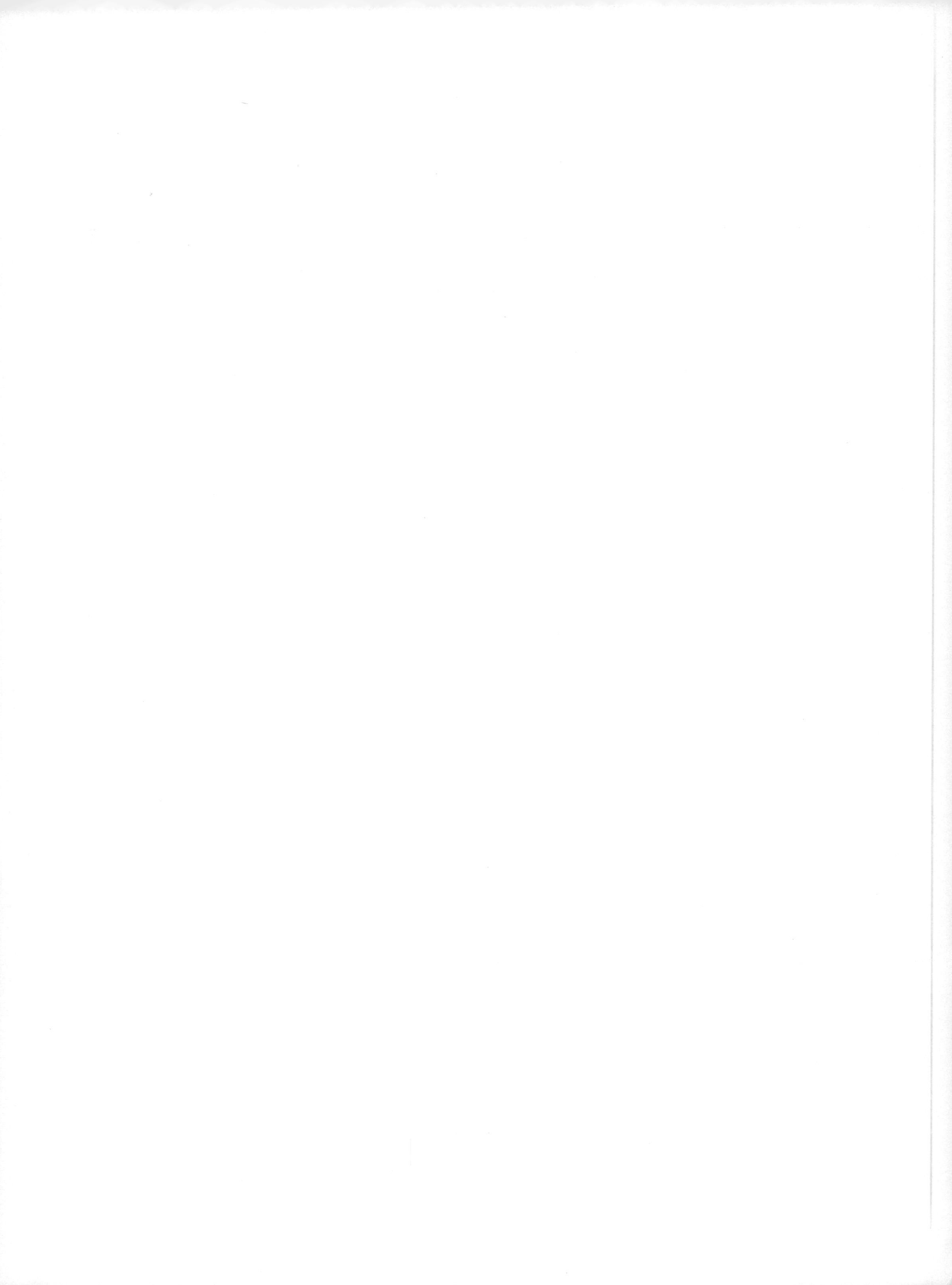

Retina and Vitreous Surgery

A Practical Guide to Theory, Practice and Management

Second Edition

Editor-in-Chief

Subhendu Kumar Boral
MD (AIIMS) DNB (Ophthalmology) FASRS (USA)
Senior Vitreoretina Consultant
Disha Eye Hospitals Pvt Ltd
Kolkata West Bengal, India

Guest Editor

Suber S Huang
MD MBA FASRS
CEO, Retina Center of Ohio, Cleveland, USA
Chair, National Eye Health Education Committee
Former President, American Society of Retina Specialists

Forewords

(Late) Hem Kumar Tewari
Suber S Huang
Lingam Gopal
Lalit Verma

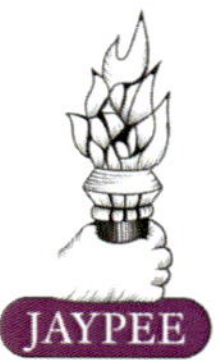

JAYPEE

JAYPEE BROTHERS MEDICAL PUBLISHERS
The Health Sciences Publisher
New Delhi | London

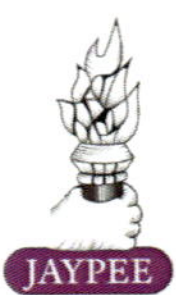

Jaypee Brothers Medical Publishers (P) Ltd

Headquarters
EMCA House, 23/23-B
Ansari Road, Daryaganj
New Delhi 110 002, India
Landline: +91-11-23272143, +91-11-23272703
+91-11-23282021, +91-11-23245672
e-mail: jaypee@jaypeebrothers.com

Corporate Office
4838/24, Ansari Road, Daryaganj
New Delhi 110 002, India
Phone: +91-11-43574357
Fax: +91-11-43574314
e-mail: jaypee@jaypeebrothers.com

Overseas Office
JP Medical Ltd.
83, Victoria Street, London
SW1H 0HW (UK)
Phone: +44-20 3170 8910
e-mail: info@jpmedpub.com

EU GPSR Authorised Representative
Logos Europe, 9 rue Nicolas Poussin
17000, La Rochelle, France
Phone: +33 (0) 6 67 93 73 78
e-mail: contact@logoseurope.eu

Website: www.jaypeebrothers.com
Website: www.jaypeedigital.com

Inquiries for bulk sales may be solicited at: jaypee@jaypeebrothers.com

Retina and Vitreous Surgery: A Practical Guide to Theory, Practice and Management

First Edition: 2016

Second Edition: 2025

Reprint: **2026**

ISBN: 978-93-6616-347-5

Printed at: Samrat Offset Pvt. Ltd.

Foreword

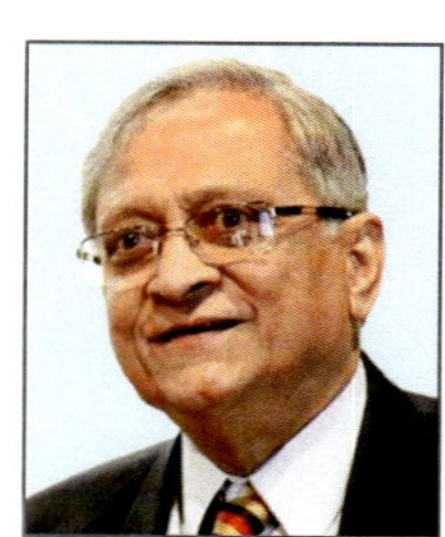

In ophthalmology, the subspecialty of retina-vitreous is ever-changing. In the last few years, there has been a revolutionary change in vitreoretinal surgical techniques and technology. Subhendu Kumar Boral's book is a kind of practical lucid book with complete text on surgical vitreoretina, practical steps with beautiful photographs, videos, and discussions on managing complications. Subhendu was my student in his residency days, and he used to assist me. My heartfelt congratulations go to him for his commendable efforts. I think this book and teaching videos will help all retina colleagues, especially fellows in retina.

(Late) Hem Kumar Tewari
MBBS MD (AIIMS)
Professor and Former Chief
RP Centre, All India Institute of Medical Sciences
New Delhi, India

Foreword

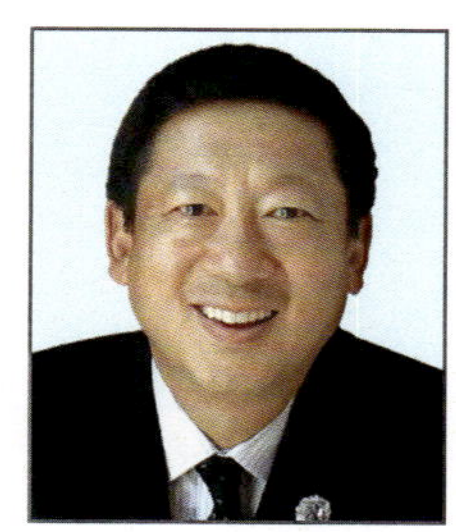

It is a pleasure to practice medicine in this extraordinary time. Rapid changes in the understanding of diseases of the retina and vitreous are reflected in new treatments and improved outcomes. Subhendu Kumar Boral's second edition, *Retina and Vitreous Surgery* textbook incorporates new organization, new surgical videos, and full online/mobile device access. Review of surgical setup, new vitrectomy instrumentation, and improved wide-angle viewing systems are thoughtfully presented. Macular surgery is a highlight of the second edition and includes surgeries for ERM, macular hole, partial- thickness macular holes, myopic foveoschisis, optic disc pit with maculopathy, macular folds, and subretinal surgery techniques. The use of internal limiting membrane, human amniotic membrane (hAM) and autologous retinal patch grafts for failed macular holes receive a detailed review. The expanded section on scleral IOL fixation with and without glue includes a new 3D animation. Whether you are an expert or novice to the surgical management of retina and vitreous disease, this textbook offers valuable insight into our most challenging conditions.

Suber S Huang
MD MBA FASRS
President, Retina Center of Ohio
President, Future Vision Foundation
Voluntary Assistant Professor
Bascom Palmer Eye Institute University of Miami
Former President, American Society of Retina Specialists
Inaugural Philip F and Elizabeth G Searle—Suber Huang MD
Professor, Case Western Reserve University School of Medicine

Foreword

Subhendu Kumar Boral is a renowned vitreoretinal surgeon from India who has established himself not only as an excellent surgeon but as an educator as well. His participation in various conferences is well appreciated because of the excellent surgical videos that he uses to support his explanation of the nuances of vitreoretinal surgery.

It is said a picture is worth a thousand words. This comparison can perhaps be extended to surgical videos as well. Dr Subhendu Kumar Boral should be congratulated for bringing out the second edition of his very practical video book on vitreoretinal surgery.

An educational video needs not only to have the required surgical steps being demonstrated but also needs to have good quality images throughout the video with logical explanatory commentary accompanying the same. I was indeed impressed by the high quality of the videos that he has collected. The contents are well-structured and include appropriate discussion on instrumentation. He has also covered a wide gamut of vitreoretinal surgeries that a novice surgeon is likely to come across.

I am sure the readers will enjoy going through these excellent surgical videos and learn from them. I deem it an honor to be asked to write a foreword for this excellent educational material that will be an asset worth possessing for people in vitreoretinal practice.

Best regards,

Lingam Gopal
Distinguished Senior Consultant
Sankara Nethralaya, Medical Research Foundation
Chennai, Tamil Nadu, India
Visiting Associate Professor
Department of Ophthalmology
National University of Singapore, Singapore

Foreword

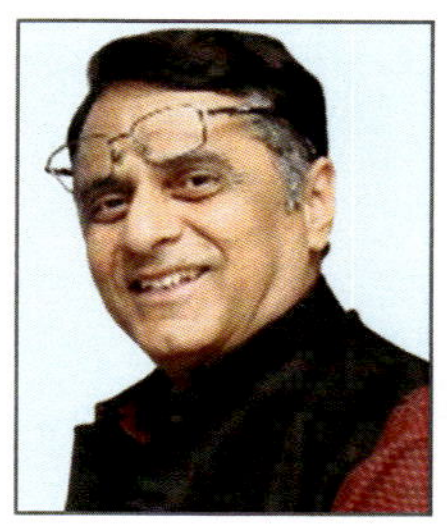

It is my proud privilege and honor to be writing forward for this beautiful masterpiece *Retina and Vitreous Surgeries: A Practical Guide to Theory, Practice and Management* by one of the finest vitreoretinal surgeons Dr Subhendu Kumar Boral.

It is a practical guide—combining theory and practical tricks for dealing with surgical vitreoretina step-by-step. It is a complete textbook on surgical vitreoretina—covering the surgical steps of each vitreoretinal procedure with illustrations, animations, and colored intraoperative photographs in 25 chapters.

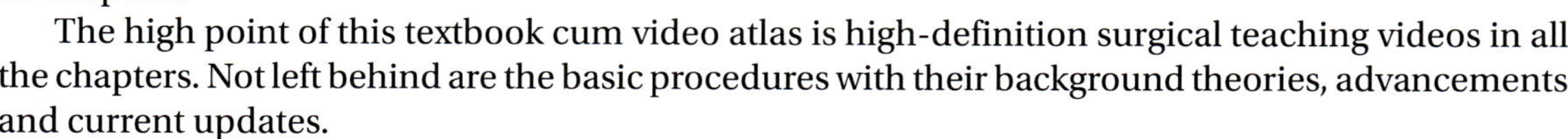

The high point of this textbook cum video atlas is high-definition surgical teaching videos in all the chapters. Not left behind are the basic procedures with their background theories, advancements and current updates.

Another notable and unique feature that makes this book worth possessing and reading is the discussion of the management of various intraoperative and postoperative complications!

It is a MUST not only for all budding and aspiring vitreoretinal surgeons but also for established and experienced colleagues.

Congratulations to Dr Subhendu, once my student but now my teacher and colleague, for bringing out this wonderful book. I know it is not an easy task!

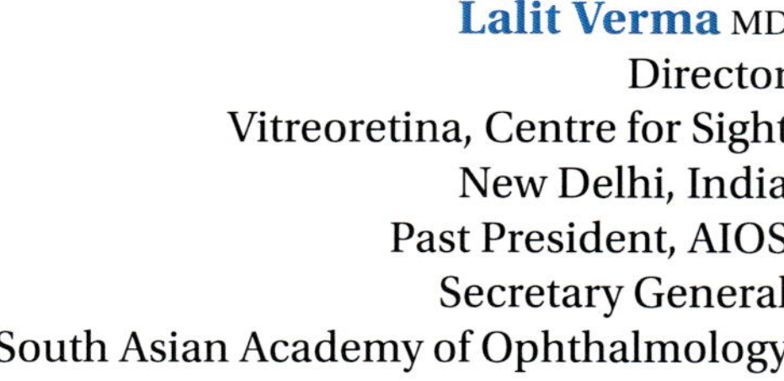

Lalit Verma MD
Director
Vitreoretina, Centre for Sight
New Delhi, India
Past President, AIOS
Secretary General
South Asian Academy of Ophthalmology

Preface to the Second Edition

Vitreoretinal procedures, surgical techniques, and technology have changed tremendously in the last 17 years since the advent of minimally invasive approaches. Newer vitrectomy machines and advanced cutter technologies have improved drastically, along with a wide-angle visualization system and enhanced endoillumination system. There was a radical shift from a 23-gauge to a 25-gauge and 27-gauge system, which finally improved the procedure's safety with negligible wound leakage, better postoperative patient comfort and better outcomes. Our first edition has already gained popularity in the last couple of years. Moreover, we have a demand to update our book and to come up with this second edition with current trends.

Our book-cum-video atlas offers a new way to combine theory with practical techniques for managing surgical vitreoretina step-by-step, featuring numerous illustrations, animations, case-based discussions, and colorful intraoperative photographs. The most compelling aspect is the discussions on managing various intraoperative and postoperative complications alongside high-definition surgical teaching videos covering all facets of vitreoretina. All videos will be accessible via a scanning QR code instead of DVDs, allowing visualization on both laptops and mobile devices. This updated edition promises to be a significantly improved version, encompassing all fundamental procedures, background theories, advancements, and current updates. I believe this effort will provide a fascinating, comprehensive guide for day-to-day practice. Hopefully, this edition will enrich vitreoretinal surgeons with the latest knowledge and inspire young professionals and fellows in this subspecialty to skillfully handle complex scenarios.

Subhendu Kumar Boral

Preface to the First Edition

Surgical Retina has changed considerably over the last ten years with the introduction of minimally invasive approach, newer vitrectomy machines with innovative cutter technologies, newer techniques, wide-angle visualization system, improved endoillumination options, changing paradigm to manage many complex surgical pathologies. Introduction of new OCT also made a revolutionary change in approaches. Conversion from 20 gauge to 23, 25 and 27 gauge. Minimally invasive vitreous surgery (MIVS) was also for better postoperative comfort and better outcome for the patients. I have discussed and highlighted the current trends in the MIVS.

The key challenges in the subspecialty of vitreoretina are that it requires dexterity, extensive surgical training as well as knowledge and sound rational reasoning during routine as well as emergency intraoperative challenges. In my residency and fellowship days, I always felt the necessity for a practical lucid book on surgical vitreoretina, especially for the students and fellows in this subspecialty. This book is a complete textbook on surgical vitreoretina with a new concept, comprising of complete texts of surgical procedures, theoretical background as well as practical surgical steps with case discussions, plenty of illustrations, animations and colored intraoperative distinct photographs of each surgical steps. It also discusses management of intra- and postoperative complications. The total unit has two parts—a textbook and 10 DVDs with high-definition surgical videos elaborately depicting almost all steps of vitreoretinal intervention. This is just an amalgamation of theories and practicals on retina and vitreous. I think this effort will provide a very complete practical guide in the day-to-day practice, with a background of theory and experiencing surgical situations in videos and to manage the complications. I hope this book will help the vitreoretinal surgeons in recapitulation of knowledge, as well as updating it, encourage and illuminate the young learning surgeons initiating in this specialty and to manage complications in more skilful manner.

Subhendu Kumar Boral

Acknowledgments

This book on surgical vitreoretina, which combines theory and practical tricks in the form of high-definition surgical videos step-by-step, is intended for students and fellows committed to mastering vitreoretina. This is an extraordinary opportunity to revise this book-cum-video atlas with all the latest updates and produce a second edition. I would like to acknowledge all my esteemed teachers from the Dr RP Centre for Ophthalmic Sciences, All India Institute of Medical Sciences, New Delhi, India, especially the late Professor HK Tewari, Dr SP Garg, Dr Lalit Verma, Dr Dinesh Talwar, and Dr Atul Kumar, who taught us vitreoretina. I am grateful to Dr Debasish Bhattacharya, Chairman of Disha Eye Hospitals Pvt Ltd, Kolkata, West Bengal, as well as Past President of the All India Ophthalmic Society, and to Dr Tushar K Sinha, Head, Department of Vitreoretina, whose constant encouragement helped me to complete this book successfully with valuable suggestions. I thank all the doctors of Disha Eye Hospitals, especially Drs Arnab Das, Debdula Chakraborty, Santanu Mandal, Santanu Mitra, Somak Majumdar, Soumen Mondol, Sumali Deb, Suchanda Sar, Abhijit Banerjee, and Arup Bhaumik for their cooperation. I am thankful to Dr Ayan Mohanta, who initiated the high-definition recording system in our hospital. I am ever grateful to Dr Sunil Parikh, whose surgical approach and immense dexterity taught me so much.

My sincere, heartfelt gratitude goes to eminent surgeon Dr Suber S Huang, CEO of Retina Center of Ohio and former President of the American Society of Retina Specialists (ASRS), who has committed himself as the 'Guest Editor' in my book as well as written the foreword for this book after going through my project. I am indebted for his constant encouragement, valuable suggestions and blessings, which have enriched my project.

Materials from many widely used books have helped me a lot. I sincerely acknowledge all the renowned authors as well as the publishers of these books and references like Gholam A Peyman's Vitreoretinal Surgical Techniques (Second edition), Stephen J Ryan's Retina (Second edition), Michaels Retinal Detachment (Second edition), Sandra F Byrne's Ultrasound of the Eye and Orbit, Claus Eckhardt's Combined Phaco-vitrectomy, Amar Agarwal's Glued Intrascleral Haptic Fixation of a PCIOL, Steve Charles's The Interface Vitrectomy Technique Retina Today, Noemi Lois & David Wong's Complications of Vitreoretinal Surgery, and many more. My sincere apologies will go to those authors whose name was not mentioned in the list of acknowledgements.

My sincere appreciation goes to Shri Jitendar P Vij (Group Chairman), Mr Ankit Vij (Managing Director), Sadhna Rajan (Development Editor), and Mr Sabyasachi Hazra (Commissioning Editor) of M/s Jaypee Brothers Medical Publishers (P) Ltd, New Delhi, India, for their constant support.

Finally, I am greatly indebted to my loving wife, Soma Boral, as, without her, this long, tiring journey could never have been completed, as well as my sons Sahoran and Sreyansh for gladly tolerating my indifference even during family time.

Video Contributors

Voice Over
Dr Jonaki Ghosh (Roy)

Editors
Sougata Burman, Subhendu Kumar Boral

3D Animation by
Sandip Jana, Sougata Burman

2D Animation and Illustrations by
Tuhin Nandy

Contributors in OT and Clinics
Sandip Jana, Kshama Chatterjee, Madhumita Mondol, Biplab Das, Atanu Dey, Asit Das, Sarmistha Sarkar, Utpal Sarkar, Pratap Dey, Soutrik Mukherjee, Janefar Romola Corraya, Nabin Dey, Suvankar Dutta, Sanatan Sau, Kaushik Acharya, and Pradip Das.

Contents

Video Contents

Steps to access the videos:
1. Scan QR code.
2. Sign up/sign in
3. Click on 'My Books'.
4. Click on the book 'Retina & Vitreous Surgery'.
5. Access the videos from chapter wise list and start learning.

Chapter 3: Endoillumination System
Video 1: Surgery with single-fiber endoillumination
Video 2: Surgery with dual-fiber endoillumination
Video 3: Surgery with Yellow filter
Video 4: Surgery with Amber filter

Chapter 4: Cryoretinopexy and Endolaser Retinopexy
Video 1: Intraoperative cryo application
Video 2: Endolaser application

Chapter 6: Perfluorocarbon Liquids
Video 1: Use of PFCL in RD
Video 2: Use of PFCL in PVR
Video 3: Use of PFCL in dropped nucleus—Animation

Chapter 7: Intravitreal Injections
Video 1: Intravitreal Triamcinolone Acetonide injection
Video 2: Intravitreal anti-VEGF injection

Chapter 9: Steps of Making Sutureless Sclerotomy Wound
Video 1: Port making in 23:25:27 gauge vitrectomy systems

Chapter 10: Vitrectomy with Recent Developments
Video 1: Vitrectomy animation
Video 2: Steps of vitrectomy in vitreous hemorrhage
Video 3: Steps to manage retro lental or retro IOL blood
Video 4: Steps to approach subhyaloid hemorrhage
Video 5: Advantages of Hypervit cutter
Video 6: Surgery with DAVS system in case of PDR and Macular Hole

Chapter 23: Interface Vitrectomy

Video 1: Interface vitrectomy under air
Video 2: Interface vitrectomy at the margin of PFCL
Video 3: Interface vitrectomy under silicone oil

Chapter 24: Managing Complications of Vitreoretinal Surgeries

Part A: Preoperative Complications

Video 1: Standard methods of ocular anesthesia and needle perforation with (Animation and Video)
Video 2: Perforation with vitreous hemorrhage (Animation and Video)
Video 3: Perforation with vitreous hemorrhage with partial retinal detachment
Video 4: Perforation with vitreous hemorrhage with total retinal detachment (Animation and Video)
Video 5: Perforation with macular break with retinal detachment (Animation and Video)
Video 6: Perforation with hemorrhagic retinal detachment with retinal incarceration

Part B: Intraoperative Complications

Video 7: Cathotomy for small palpebral fissure
Video 8: Slippage of infusion cannula
Video 9: Suprachoroidal infusion
Video 10: Subretinal infusion
Video 11: Retinal incarceration at the cannula tip
Video 12: Complications during phaco-vitrectomy—Iris prolapse during dye injection
Video 13: Complications during phaco-vitrectomy—Sudden influx of air bubbles
Video 14: Complications during PVD induction with attached retina
Video 15: Complications during PVD induction with detached retina—Inadvertent break
Video 16: Intraoperative sudden unplanned hypotony
Video 17: Intraoperative media haziness
Video 18: Stepwise approach to manage intraocular bleed—Cautery
Video 19: Stepwise approach to manage intraocular bleed—Raising IOP
Video 20: Stepwise approach to manage intraocular bleed—Start FAX in high IOP
Video 21: Stepwise approach to manage intraocular bleed—Application of triamcinolone acetonide over the bleeders
Video 22: Using heavy fluid PFCL over the posterior pole
Video 23: Intraoperative retinal break with retinal detachment
Video 24: Subretinal migration of PFCL bubbles

Part C: Postoperative Complications

Video 25: Phacoemulsification for postvitrectomy cataract
Video 26: Submacular PFCL removal
Video 27: Extraction of submacular PFCL bubbles using micro-VFC
Video 28: Managing failed macular hole with autologous retinal graft transplantation
Video 29: Failed retinal detachment—Case of missed break
Video 30: Failed retinal detachment—Case of ERM with new break
Video 31: Failed retinal detachment—Case of ERM with reopening of break
Video 32: Failed retinal detachment—Case with reopening of inferior break with inferior fixed fold with subretinal band
Video 33: Failed retinal detachment—Case with incompletely filled silicone oil with extensive ERM with subretinal silicone oil

Vitrectomy Machine, Cutter and Instrumentation

The basic equipment required for pars plana vitrectomy includes a vitrectomy machine, a visualization system, an illumination source and a microscope.

A. VITRECTOMY MACHINE, CUTTER AND INSTRUMENTATION

Since the introduction of pars plana vitrectomy by Machemer in 1971, significant revolutionary changes happened to improve the approaches, machineries and instrumentation. With the advent of closed chamber vitrectomy, vitreoretinal surgeons were able to remove media opacities and treat even complicated retinal detachments.

BASIC EQUIPMENT FOR PARS PLANA VITRECTOMY

Vitrectomy Machine

The primary aim of vitreous surgery is to remove vitreous without resulting in undue vitreous and collateral retinal damage. This balance is achieved by matching inflow and outflow system in a vitrectomy machine.

A. *Inflow system or infusion system:* This regulates the entry of fluid into the vitreous cavity. Each machine (Fig. 1.1A) is equipped with an infusion system that allows control of IOP during surgery. Infusion system can use:

i. *Gas-forced infusion (pressurized system):* A bottle of balanced salt solution (BSS) is attached to an air pump (set at a pressure of 20–30 mm Hg during normal surgery) that forces the BSS into the eye through infusion tubing (Fig. 1.1B).

Vented gas forced infusion (VGFI) is a pressurized system of controlling the infusion pressure used in Alcon Accurus machine. Here filtered pressurized gas is delivered into the infusion bottle through tubing. Rapid change in pressure can be achieved by this. This is particularly helpful to control intraocular bleed by raising the IOP without any help of the assistant.

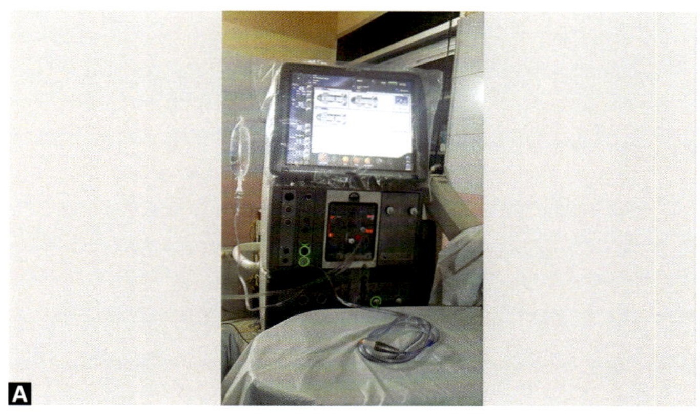

Fig. 1.1A: Shows the high-end vitrectomy machine (Constellation vision system, Alcon) with a bottle of balanced salt solution (BSS) is attached to an air pump

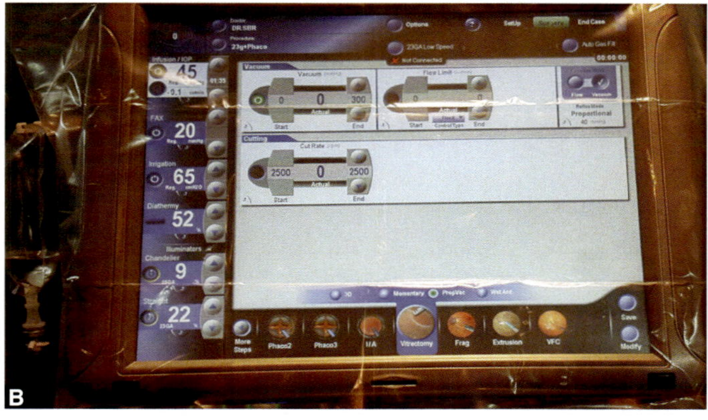

Fig. 1.1B: Modern vitrectomy panel

Alcon constellation system offers further modification into this system. Here infusion solution is pressurized within the cassette. Constellation system has inbuilt real-time IOP monitoring which track infusion cannula and tubing resistance. Moreover, presence of dual infusion chamber (where if one bottle empties, the other takes over) minimizes IOP fluctuation (Fig. 1.1B).

ii. *Gravity dependent infusion:* Depends on the height of the bottle above the patient's eye (usually 18 inch above the patient's eye level to maintain a normal IOP) to maintain IOP. It is assistant dependent and does not provide precise IOP control.

B. *Outflow system:* The vitrectomy machine pumps are the main factor to control egress of fluid from the vitreous cavity. Two types of pumps are available:

i. *Venturi pumps:* Here flow is induced by the vacuum changes within the cassette. Hence, here flow occurs as a result of vacuum and it is directly proportional to the vacuum applied for homogeneous low viscosity substances. Venturi system is controlled by surgeon's foot pedal.

ii. *Peristaltic pumps:* They are positive displacement machines. The fluid contained within a tube is forced to move into the vitreous cavity by rollers that compress it. Here, the vacuum rises only after occlusion. So flow rate can be maintained very low with peristaltic pumps and can still achieve high vacuum at occlusion.

Vitrectomy machines having both pumps: Alcon constellation, Oertli OS3, DORC Associate and Geuder Megatron S4.

Vitrectomy machines having only venturi pump: Alcon Accrus.

Vitrectomy machines having only peristaltic pump: Oertli Faros.

Other factors, controlling outflow are:

- *Gauge size:* Small/Narrow gauge vitrectomy has higher resistance to aspiration as compared to wider gauge for the same vacuum settings.
- *Port size:* It is also a limiting factor reducing the outflow. The newer 25G probes are designed with a larger port area to compensate for this deficiency. Compared with the 25-gauge vitrectomy port, the 27-gauge vitrectomy port is larger (0.079 mm^2 vs 0.066 mm^2) and closer to the cutter tip (0.211 mm vs 0.330 mm). Thus, surgeon can perform complex maneuvers such as vitrectomy-assisted membrane segmentation and delamination.
- *Duty cycle:* The duty cycle of a vitrectomy probe indicates the percentage that describes the ratio of time the port is open measured against the total time of the cut cycle. All other existing vitrectomy cutters, whether they are pneumatic or electric, have a duty cycle that cannot be adjusted. Some cutters have duty cycles that favor a more open port, while some favor a more closed port. In Constellation® Vision System, duty cycle can be adjusted to the needs and actions of the surgeon.

Constellation offers three separate duty cycle options:

i. *Core mode:* It is the maximum port-open duty cycle control. It is best suited for core vitrectomy where higher flow rates are more efficient and desirable.

ii. *Shave mode:* It is the minimum port-open duty cycle. It is best suited for delicately removing tissue in situations where lower flow rates are desirable, such as working near periphery or near detached mobile retina.

iii. *50/50 duty cycle:* It is the setting between the core and shave. This mode is for those who prefer the cutter to be open and closed for the same amount of time.
   - The added ability to vary duty cycle, as well as cut speed and aspiration rate, has an enormous impact on the safety and efficacy of the new vitrectomy probes and will likely improve our ability to treat vitreoretinal pathologies.

Advantages of Modern Vitrectomy Machines (Constellation, Alcon, USA)

1. Provision of auto infusion (infusion bottle/bag pressurization).
2. IOP control (0–120 mm Hg) set IOP and then forget-stable IOP.
3. Vacuum control (0–650 mm Hg).
4. Flow control.
5. Automated FAX (integrated airlines).

Other Advantages

1. Proportional diathermy.
2. Auto gas filling.
3. *Viscous Fluid Control (VFC):* To inject silicone oil or for extraction of silicone oil.
4. *Advanced Illumination:*
   - Dual port xenon (75 W)
   - Long bulb lifetime
   - Xenon light is less blue and it can cause less photochemical damage.
5. Embeded 532 nm purepoint laser.

Vitreous Cutter (Fig. 1.2)

Modern vitreous cutters are available in 23, 25 and 27G systems.

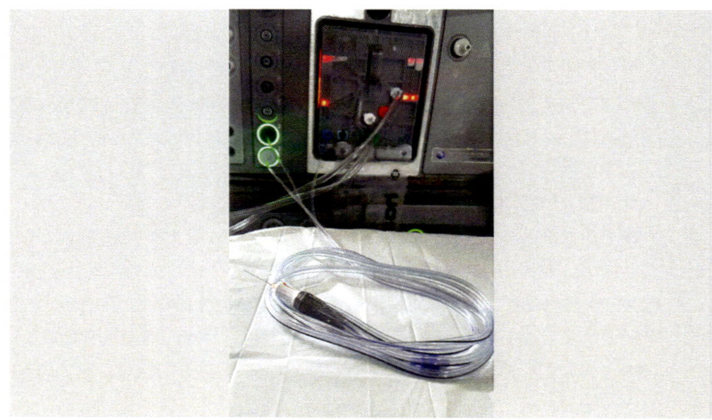

Fig. 1.2 : Shows the modern high-speed cutter with two lines

Vitreous cutters consists of a hollow inner tube surrounded by a hollow outer tube. Both tubes are arranged coaxially.

Vitreous cutter allows high-speed cutting of formed vitreous and controlled removal of the vitreous gel at low suction.

During vitrectomy, vitreous is drawn into a port near the distal end of the outer tube. Thereafter, the inner tube slides forwards, closes the port and shears off the vitreous. Finally, the cut materials are aspirated out through the inner tube.

A vitreous cutter can be of two types—rotatory and guillotine type, depending on the cutting mechanism. In the rotational type, the inner tube moves around the longitudinal axis. But in guillotine style, the inner tube moves along the longitudinal axis.

The cutter can be driven either pneumatically or electrically. Now-a-days, all cutters employ a guillotine-type of mechanism, which is driven pneumatically by vitrectomy machine. The pneumatic guillotine cutters are powered by a pneumatic drive pulse that act upon a diaphragm. When air pulses are exerted, the diaphragm is extended and the cutter tip closes, completing a cut. When air pulse is released, a spring returns the tip to the open position.

As the cut rate is increased, duration of port open time per cut decreases, while port closed time remains constant.

Another type of pneumatic drive mechanism utilizes a dual drive line system. This is used in Ultravit probe, used with the Constellation Vision System. Here, pneumatic drive pulse act upon the diaphragm, but instead of a return spring, a second pneumatic drive pulse acts against the diaphragm in the opposite direction to reopen the cutter. Thus, this unique designs makes the cutter to operate at high rate up to 7,500 cpm.

There are two setting options:

i. *Proportional setting:* Here suction is variable depending on position of foot switch but cutting rate is fixed.
ii. *3D setting:* Both cutting and suction can be independently controlled with foot switch. 3D setting enhances the safety while working closure to the retina.

Modern Ultravit 5,000 cpm cutter with duty cycle has high speed cutting as well as to modify duty cycle for flow control, independent of vacuum and cutting.

Vitreous cutter is attached to the vitrectomy machine by two lines:

i. From the cutter to the cutting drive of the machine
ii. *Aspiration line:* This line will plug into a cartridge in the machine. Vitreous cutter has to be primed in 'priming mode' before its use. For priming, the cutter tip has to be placed in a solution of fluid and 'priming command' on the vitrectomy machine has to be pressed.

Advantages of 25G+ vitrectomy probe:

1. High speed cutting from 1,500 to 7,500 cpm.
2. Higher aspiration flow rates.
3. Larger cutting port area (0.011 >0.013 in).
4. Improved duty cycle (37% > 51%).
5. Cutting port closer to end of needle.
6. Stiffer needle.
7. Higher aspiration flow rates.

Foot Pedal (Figs 1.3A and B)

Foot pedal controls the vitreous cutter, deploying suction only or both suction and cutter together.

Predetermined aspiration setting will be reached as the foot pedal is maximally depressed.

Most of the systems feature linear control of suction and sometimes linear control of cutting rate by the surgeon, as determined by the extent to which the pedal is depressed toward the floor.

Some machine allow the surgeon to click the foot pedal either to the right or to the left to switch between cutting and aspiration modes.

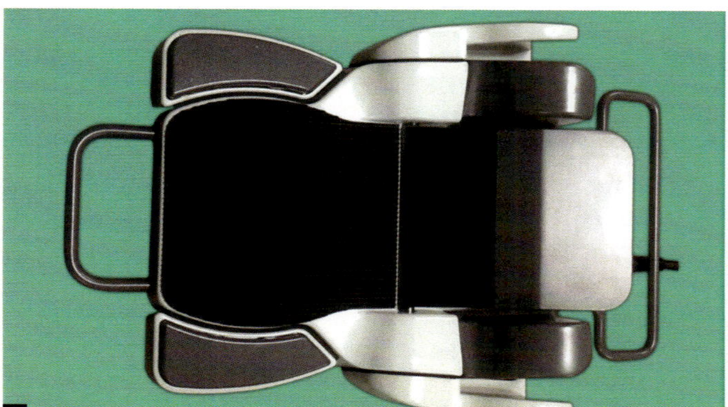

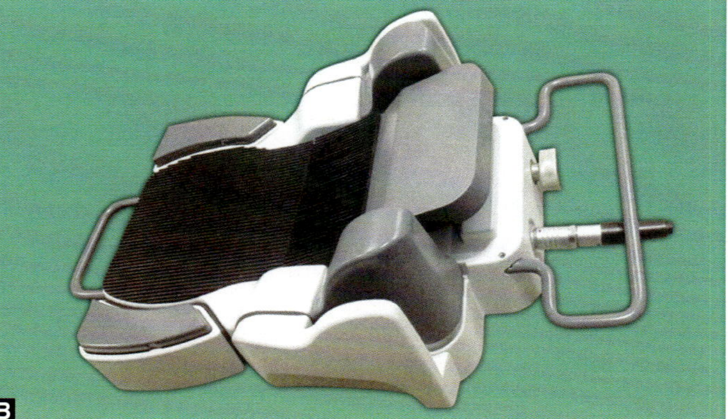

Figs 1.3A and B: Shows multitasking foot pedal

Common Additional Instruments Required for Vitreoretinal Procedures

Scleral encirclage/240 band (Fig. 1.4)—for permanent buckle indent and to support vitreous base.

Scleral Buckle (Figs 1.5 and 1.6)

i. Asymmetric scleral Buckle (275, 276)
   - Increased buckle height posteriorly
   - Decreased chance of erosion anteriorly.

ii. Symmetric scleral Buckle (277, 278, 279, 280, 281, 286, 287, 289)

Infusion cannula (Fig. 1.7): Infusion line forms the pivot of vitreous surgeries. The infusion is placed first and taken out last.

23G infusion cannula has 0.56 mm diameter.

23G infusion cannulas are available with both 4 mm and 6 mm tip. The 27G infusion line has a beveled sharp-tipped metallic tube 4 mm long, designed for single-step perpendicular insertion.

Disposable Instruments

Features of disposable instruments:

- Improved efficiency
- Better performances
- Predictable
- Saves time
- Avoid cross contamination.

Available Grieshaber and DORC Disposable Instruments:

1. *End Grasping forceps* (Fig. 1.8)
   - Fine tip enhances visualization
   - Multipurpose design
   - Available in 23G, 25G and 27G.
2. *ILM forceps* (Fig. 1.9)
   - End grasping design ideal for "maculorhexis" or other fine membrane grasping
   - Tip style improves visualization
   - Multipurpose grasping application
   - Available in 23G, 25G and 27G.
3. *Asymmetrical forceps* (Fig. 1.10)
   - Tip angle conforms to the radius curvature of the retina

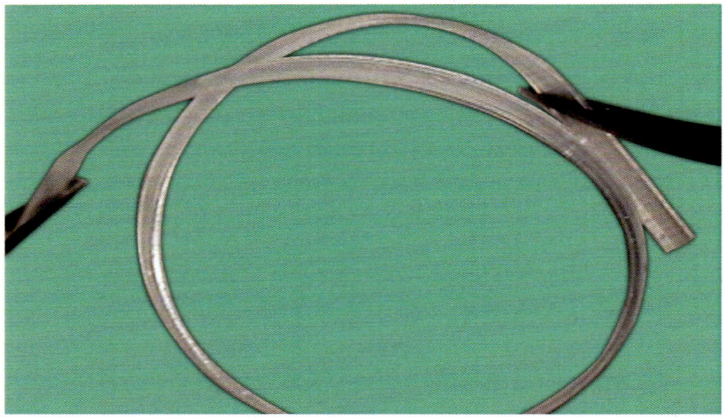

Fig. 1.4: Scleral encirclage/240 band

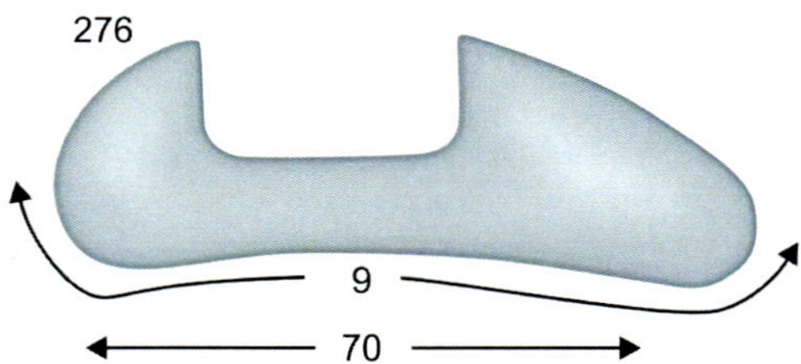

Fig. 1.5: Shows asymmetrical 276 scleral buckle

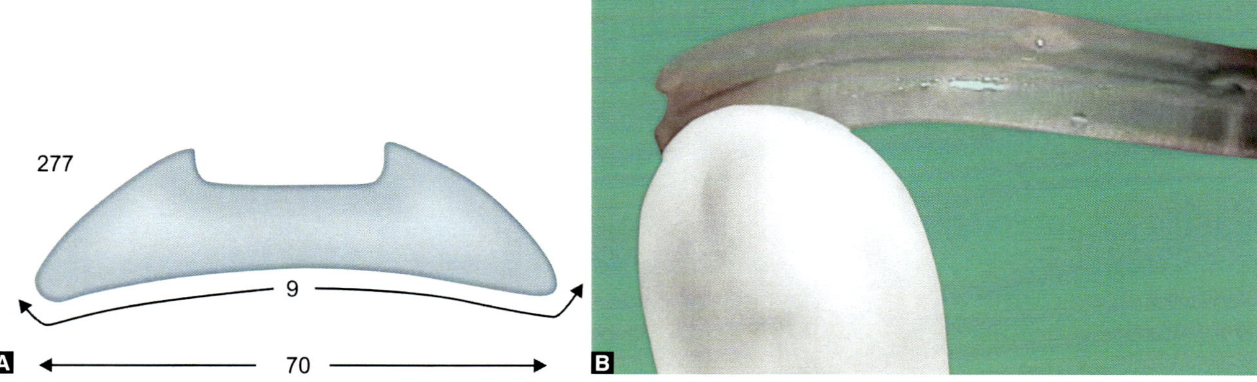

Figs 1.6A and B: Shows asymmetrical 277 scleral buckle

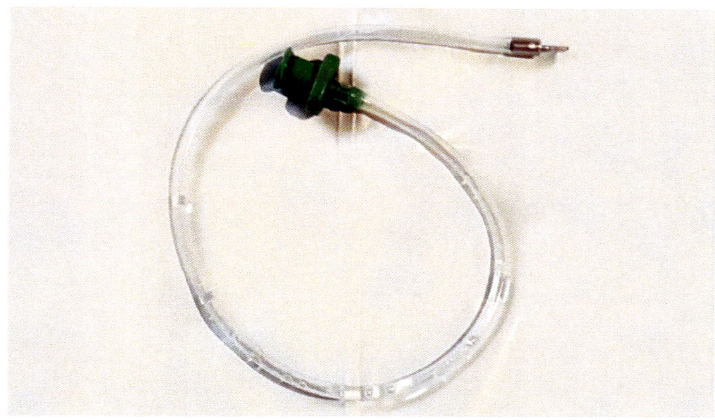

Fig. 1.7: Shows infusion cannula for intravitreal BSS infusion with 4 mm tip length

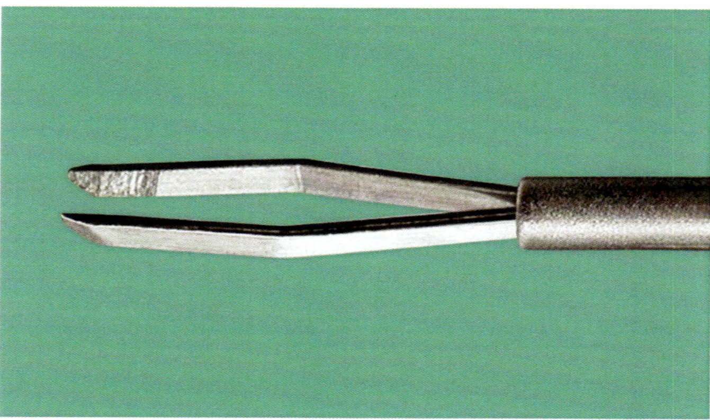

Fig. 1.8: Shows Grieshaber end grasping forceps

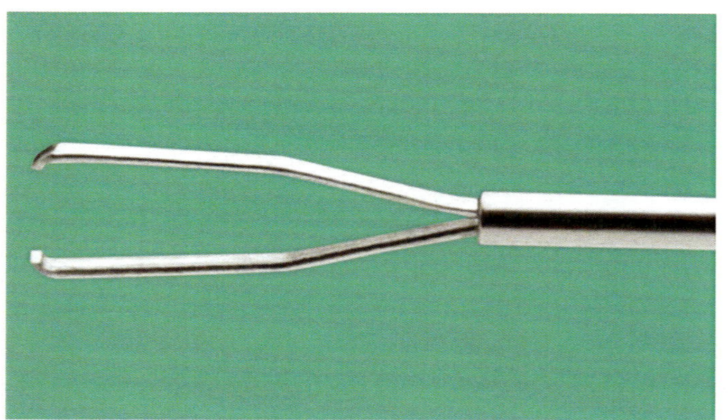

Fig. 1.9: Shows Grieshaber ILM forceps

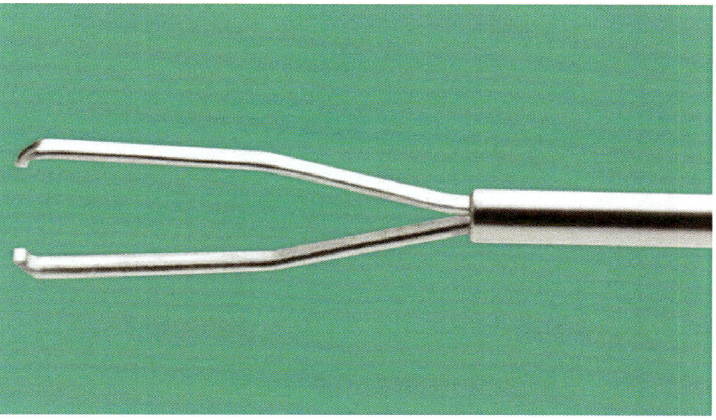

Fig. 1.10: Shows Grieshaber asymmetrical forceps

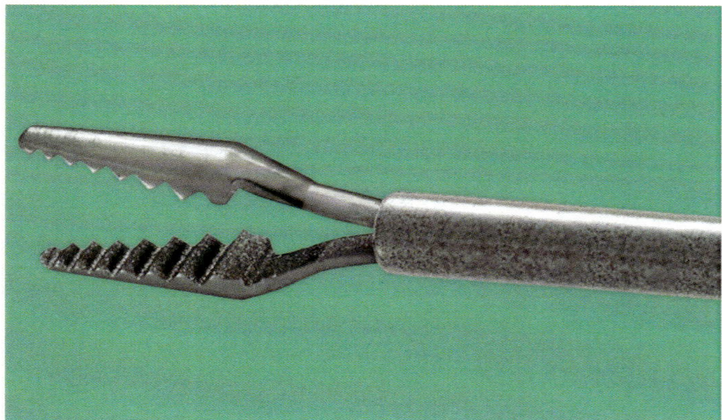

Fig. 1.11: Shows Grieshaber serrated forceps

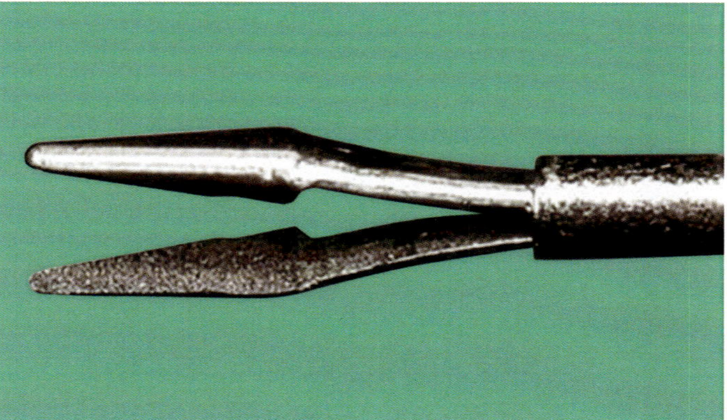

Fig. 1.12: Shows Grieshaber MAX Grip forceps

- Allows better visualization while grasping tissue
- Available in 23G and 25G.

4. *Serrated forceps* (Fig. 1.11)
   - Serrated tip allows for secure grasping of fibrous membranes
   - Blunt (slightly rounded) distal end.
5. *MAX Grip forceps* (Fig. 1.12)
   - For maximum gripping of heavy thick membrane.
6. *Intravitreal scissors* (Fig. 1.13)
   - Curved scissors
   - Fine curved blades for multipurpose cutting
   - Smooth cutting action for 40 degree curvature

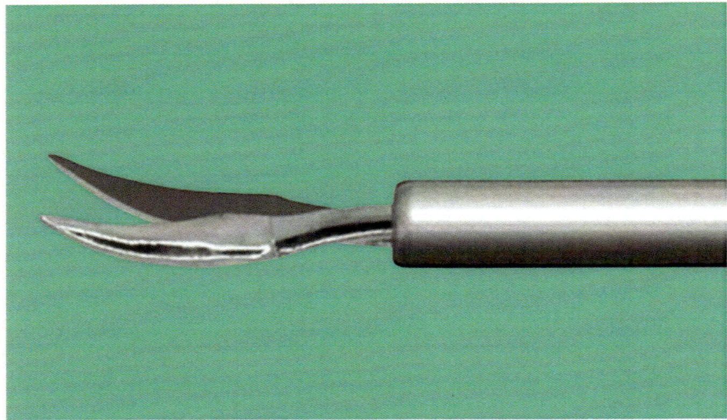

Fig. 1.13: Shows Grieshaber intravitreal scissors

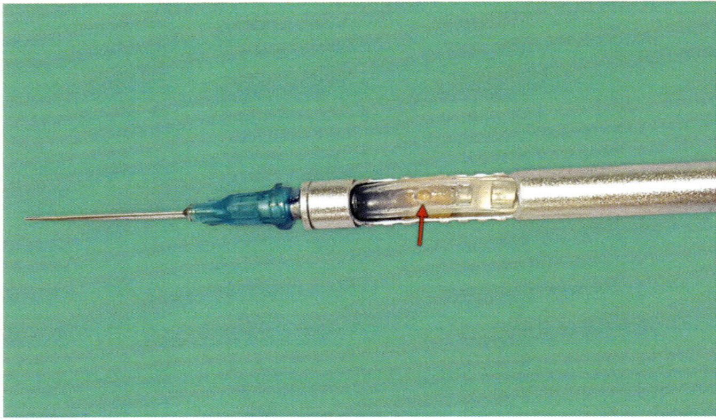

Fig. 1.14: Shows flute needle

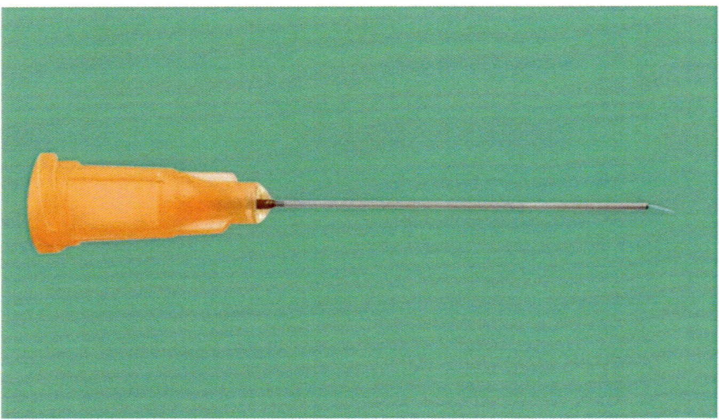

Fig. 1.15: Shows soft tip cannula

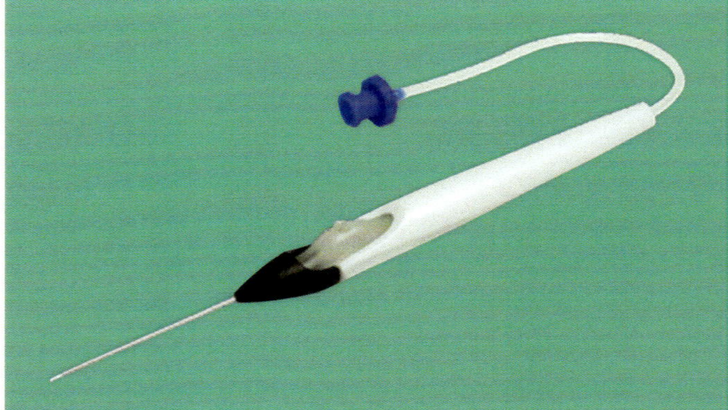

Fig. 1.16: Shows soft tip Backflush

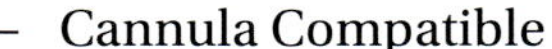

- Cannula Compatible
- Available in 23G and 25G.

7. *Flute needle* (Fig. 1.14): For vitreous lavage passively. Pressure Gradient = Intravitreal Pressure – Atmospheric Pressure
8. *Soft tip cannula* (Fig. 1.15)
   - High flow through cannula ensure efficient fluid removal
   - Teal Silicone Tip = High visibility at fluid/air meniscus and maximum color contrast to retina
   - Silicone tip length = approx. 1.5 mm
   - Available in 23G and 25G.
9. *Soft tip Backflush* (Fig. 1.16)
   - For handling tissues, hemorrhages and bleeding
   - Surgeon controlled immediate aspiration and back flush
   - Can be used as both active and passive device
   - Available in 20G, 23G and 25G.
10. *Intravitreal Tano diamond-dusted membrane scraper* (Fig. 1.17)
    - For peeling ILM, tightly adhered ERM. It is sufficient to remove membranes from the surface of the ILM and layers of the ILM without disruption of the underlying RNFL.
11. *Intravitreal spatula and membrane pic*
    - For removing ERM from detached retina.
12. *Silicone oil injector* (Fig. 1.18)
    - Both 23G and 25G viscous fluid injector/extractor are available for silicone oil injection/extraction.
13. *Finesse Flex Loop* (Fig. 1.19)
    - Available in 25G
    - It is used to create an ILM flap in case of macular hole surgery and to peel any membrane from the retinal surface. It is helpful to dissect any tightly adhered diabetic membrane and PVR membranes in cases of retinal detachment.
14. *Subretinal cannula 38G or 40G* (Figs 1.20A to D)
    - It is available as a poly-tip nonmetallic cannula or a metallic cannula for subretinal injection of any drug, such as recombinant tissue plasminogen activator, anti-VEGF agents, or Balanced Salt Solution (BSS).
      i. 38G poly-tip nonmetallic cannula subretinal cannulas have extremely thin-walled, semi-flexible tip that allows maximum flow rate in a

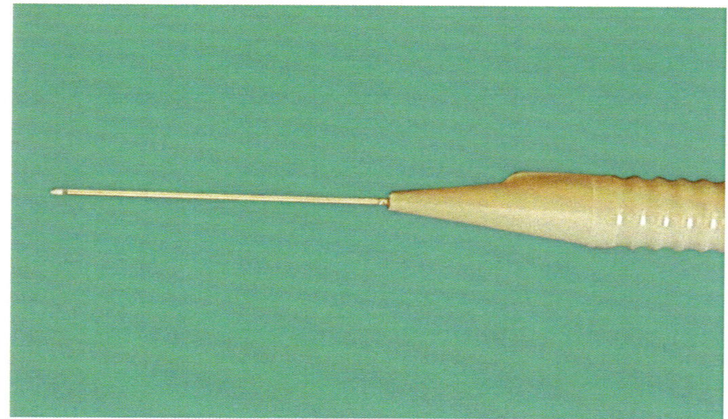

Fig. 1.17: Shows intravitreal Tano scraper

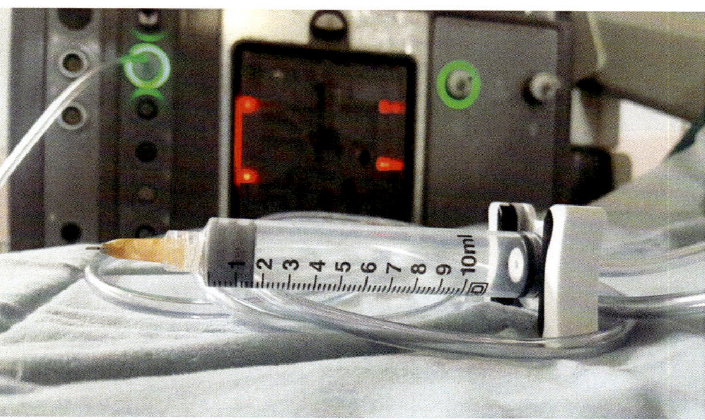

Fig. 1.18: Viscous fluid control (VFC)

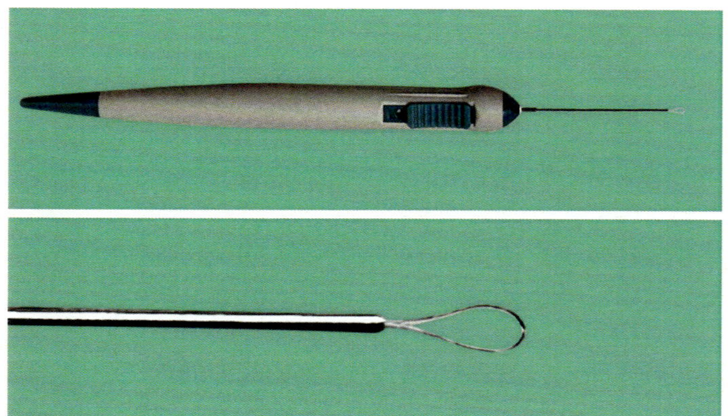

Fig. 1.19: Shows the Finesse Flex Loop

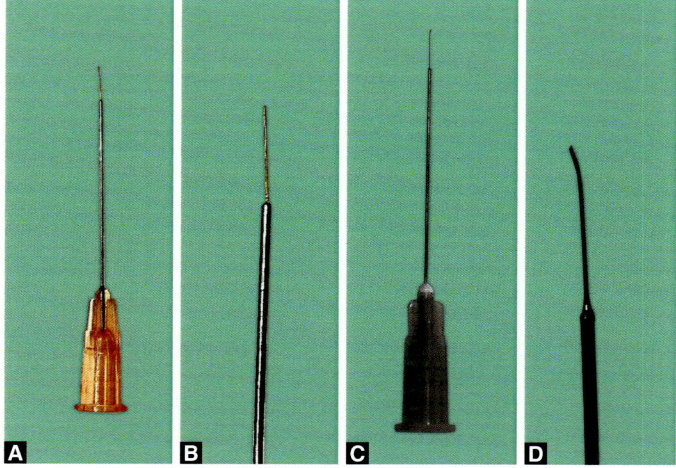

Figs 1.20A to D: Shows 38 gauge poly tip non-metallic subretinal cannula (A and B) and 40 gauge micro-tip metallic subretinal beveled-tip cannula (C and D)

small diameter cannula. They are rigid enough to penetrate the retina without creating a separate retinotomy. Its tip creates a retinal micro hole (0.12 mm in diameter), thus avoiding any need for additional laser barrage

ii. 40G subretinal metallic micro-tip straight or beveled-tip (angled) cannulas have rigid tips. Its tip creates an extremely small retinal microhole (0.10 mm in diameter)

15. *Laser probe: Curved laser probe* (Fig. 1.21) that helps to do laser near ora serrata in a phakic eye without any risk of lens touch.

B. *Viewing system*—discussed in Chapter 2

C. *Illumination system*—discussed in Chapter 3

D. *Operating microscope* (Fig. 1.22)—Purposes of operating microscope are:

   i. For clear visualization of the structures being manipulated.

   ii. Greater depth of field is required for the surgeon to focus finely.

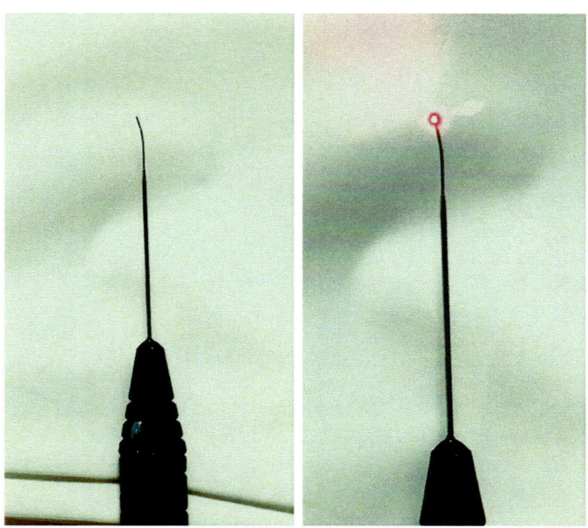

Fig. 1.21: Shows curved, flexible tip laser probe.

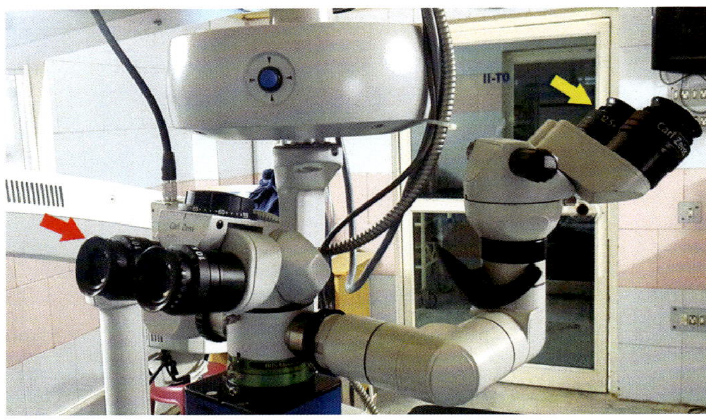

Fig. 1.22: Shows an operating microscope meant for vitreoretinal surgeries (red arrow for surgeon's view) with sideview for the assistant (yellow arrow)

It should be equipped with an assistant's scope.

A good microscope for vitreoretinal surgery should have:

- X-Y movement with respect to the patient's eye. X refers to nasal temporal movement and Y refers to superior-inferior movement
- It should have foot switch controlled zoom, on-off and fine focus
- The microscope should be fitted with the laser filter and image inverting systems.

Kindly scan the QR code below to access the online Video.

CHAPTER 2

Visualization System

The unique structure of the eyeball, with multiple refractive surfaces, including cornea and lens, prevents clear viewing of the retina without a neutralizing lens.

Following are the various viewing systems, available to facilitate the visualization of retina and vitreous cavity.

I. *Irrigating contact lens:*
   - A hand plano-concave lens to neutralize the convergence effect of corneal curvature
   - Visualization up to equator
   - Needs a skilled assistant which allows visualization during fluid-gas exchange.

II. *Sewn on retaining lens (Landers)* (Fig. 2.1)
   - Avoids absolute need of trained assistant. Biconcave lens viewing angle can be increased from 25° to 35° which allows visualization during fluid-gas exchange.
   - But
     - Not wide angle—difficult to visualize peripheral retina
     - Near absolute loss of visibility in a phakic air-filled eye.

III. *Wide angle viewing system*
   - Need stereoscopic diagonal inverter (SDI) (Spitnas and Reiver, 1987).

Noncontact Wide Angle Viewing Systems

A. *Binocular Indirect Ophthalmomicroscopy (BIOM)* (Figs 2.2 and 2.3)
Field of view—70°, 90°, 110°
Advantage—
   - Grossly assistant independent
   - No corneal trauma

There are 4 models of BIOM:

- *Model 1:* A closed cone device
- *Model 2:* An open arm device that extends from the bottom of microscope
- *Model 3:* Like model 2 but has a foot pedal-controlled motorized focusing adjustment
- *Model 4:* Up to 1300, high magnification of macula, surgery through small pupil, excellent depth of focus

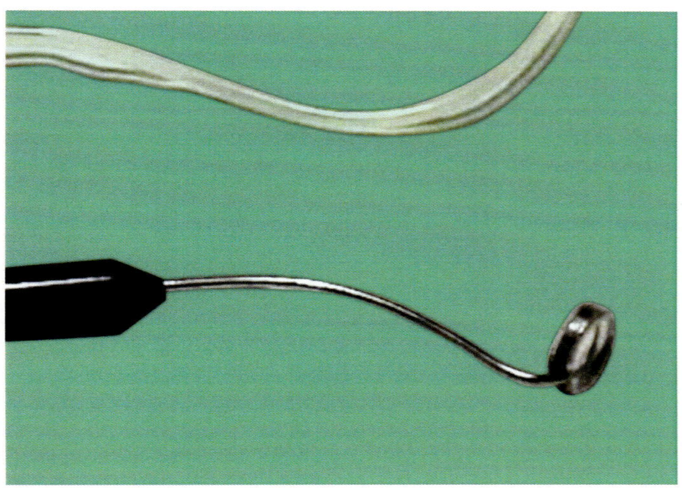

Fig. 2.1: Sewn on retaining lens (Landers)

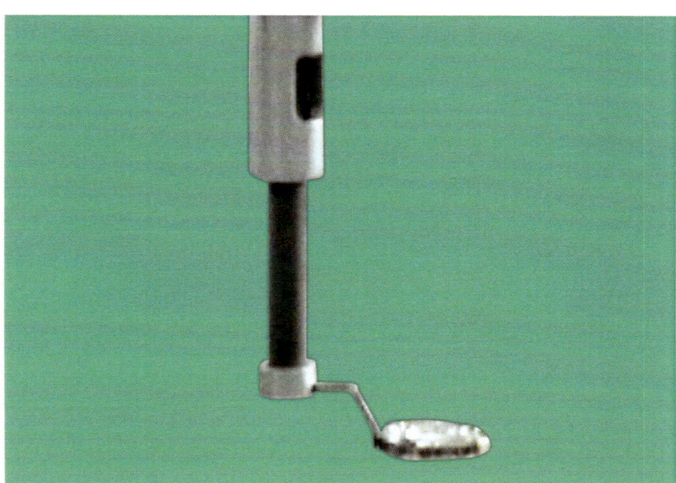

Fig. 2.2: BIOM lens

- Intermittent corneal wetting is required with a noncontact viewing system using BSS or HPMC (hydroxypropyl methyl cellulose) solution diluted with BSS.

B. *Erected Image Binocular Ophthalmoscope (EIBOS)* (Fig. 2.4)

Field of View: 100 degree with 90D and 125 degree with 60D lens

In EIBOS, the indirect and reinversion devices are consolidated and cannot be separated.

Disadvantage: It can be used with only a few microscope models.

C. *Peyman-Wessels-Landers (PWL) noncontact system* (Fig. 2.5)
   - Consists of a supporting arm and an optical portion
   - The supporting arm connects to the table or wrist rest
   - The optical portion is a sealed unit consisting of a 132D condensing lens and a reinverting prism
   - The PWL system can be used with any microscope.

Optimal distance from the bottom of optical portion to the cornea is 6 mm.

Contact Wide Angle Viewing System

A. *The Volk Reinverting Lens System (ROLS)* (Fig. 2.6).
   - Standard and self-stabilizing lens (58, 85 or 156 Diopters).

B. *The AVI inverter with miniature indirect contact lens*

C. *The iris medical contact wide angle system.*

Various Lenses of ROLS are:

Volk offers self-stabilizing vitrectomy (SSV lenses) in 3 powers (58, 85 and 156D) which reduces the need for skilled assistance (Fig. 2.7).

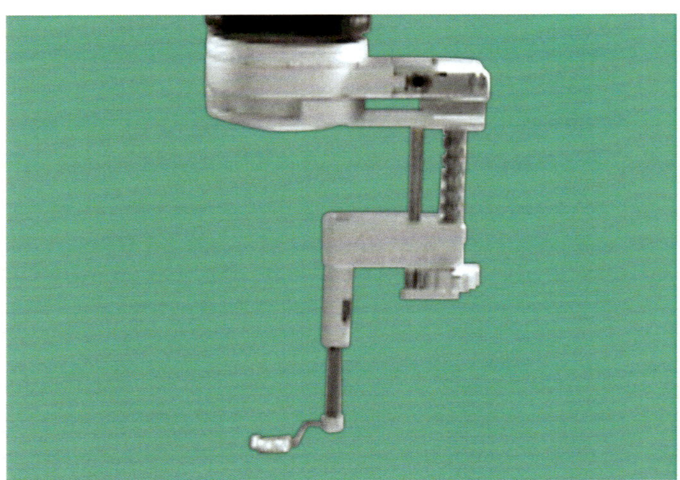

Fig. 2.3: BIOM lens with attachments

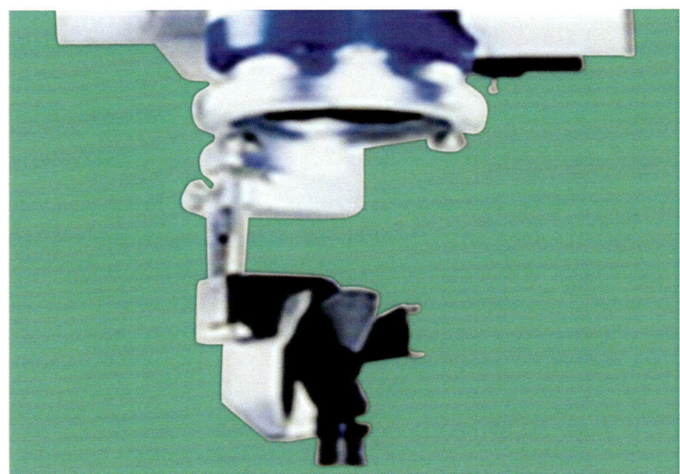

Fig. 2.4: Erected Image Binocular Ophthalmoscope (EIBOS)

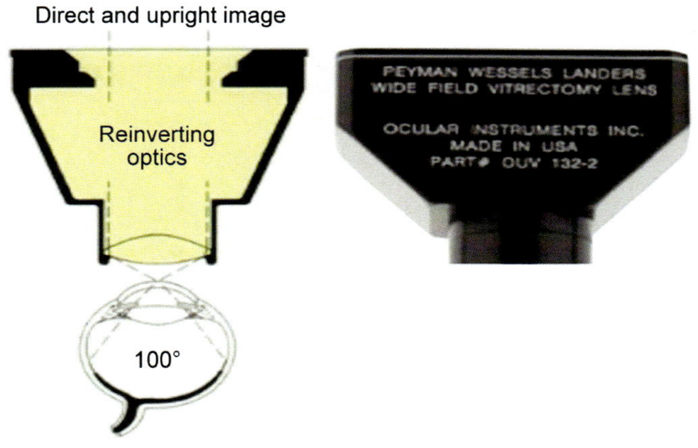

Fig. 2.5: Peyman-Wessels-Landers (PWL) noncontact system

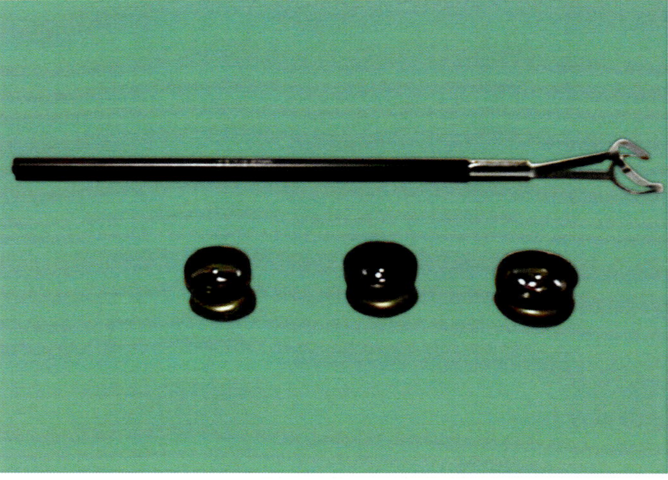

Fig. 2.6: Volk Reinverting lens system (ROLS)

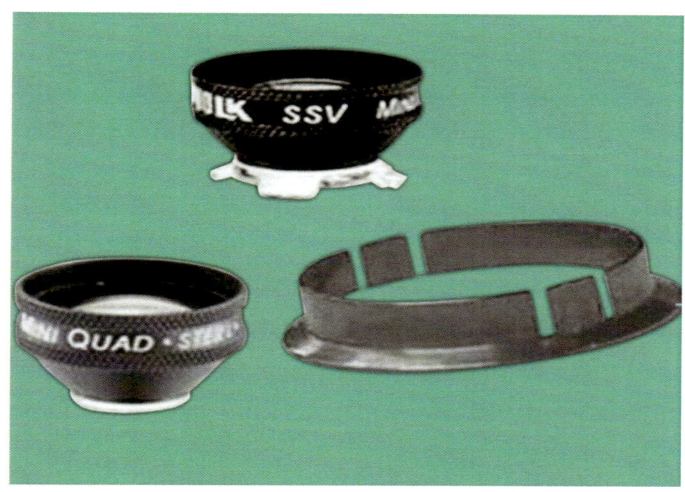

Fig. 2.7: Volk self-stabilizing vitrectomy (SSV lenses) in 3 powers (58, 85 and 156D)

Whether contact or noncontact viewing system is better?

- Contact-based wide angle visualization provides 10 degree greater field of view than noncontact systems
- Probably eliminates corneal asphericity better
- Decreases the need for ocular rotation (tool flex) to view periphery.

Kindly scan the QR code below to access the online Video.

CHAPTER 3

Endoillumination System

Source of illumination is required to illuminate the structure for manipulation and materials being removed. Most vitrectomy systems are equipped with an in-built light source, usually employing yellow light or sometimes white light.

External slit illuminator outside the eye was first used in the early 1970's.

Current style of endoillumination (optical fiber inside the eye) was first used by Gholam A Peyman in 1976.

In the 20G era, a halogen or metal halide light bulb was used as the illuminating light source.

FACTORS FOR ENDOILLUMINATION

The light pipes used for endoillumination can be of two varieties—focal or diffuse.

i. *Focal light pipes*
   - Angle of illumination—conventional "focal" light pipes with illumination fields ranging from 500 to 800 (Fig. 3.1)
   - Wide angle of illumination—offer a more than 100º field of view (Fig. 3.2)
   - Focal, specular and retroillumination increases the visibility of vitreous, ILM and ERM.

ii. *Diffuse light pipes*—used for wide-field visualization.
   - Options are torpedo, chandelier light and dual mode infusion cannula
   - Chandeliers light in 25G or 27G or 29G are available options
   - Chandelier endoillumination is the safest way to avoid retinal phototoxicity when using the same powerful light source. Increasing the working distance of the light probes from 4 mm to 8 mm from the retina can theoretically increase the retinal threshold time more than three-fold.

Currently, the gauge of choices for chandelier illumination systems:

i. *For single-fiber endoillumination (Video 1, Chapter 3)*
   - It ranges from 25G to 27G. Single-fiber chandelier endoillumination is very simple to use. Some surgeons prefer to choose larger-gauge single fibers, i.e. a 25G fiber (Figs 3.3A and B) rather than 27G fiber or smaller to obtain sufficient brightness.

     However, unlike the oblique incision technique required to insert the cannulas for vitrectomy, a vertical insertion for the 25G optic fiber directly through the sclera is required to aim the light appropriately at the posterior pole. This vertical incision may cause leakage of the wound after removal of the fiber at the end of surgery and gentle massage at the wound can stop the leakage.

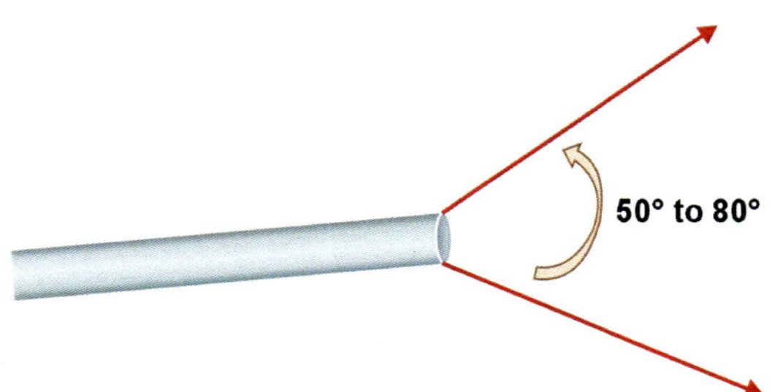

Fig. 3.1: Shows conventional "focal" light pipes with illumination fields ranging from 50° to 80°

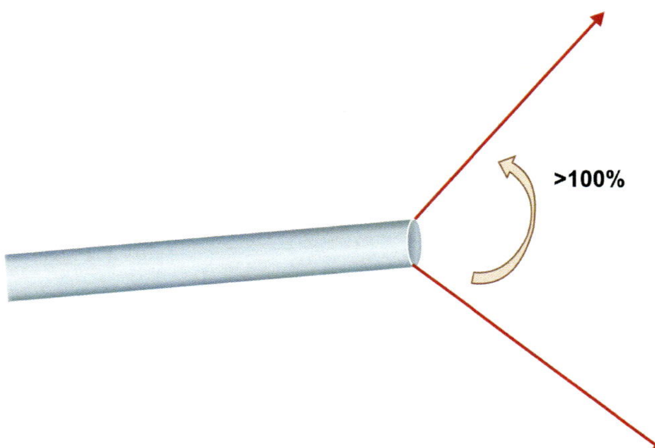

Fig. 3.2 : Shows wide angle of illumination with a more than 100° field of view

ii. *For dual-fiber systems (Video 2, Chapter 3):* Available in 27G to 29G. All fibers are designed to be self-retaining after transconjunctival insertion, with or without the use of a trocar-cannula system (Figs 3.4 and 3.5). Diffuse illumination reduces visibility of vitreous, ILM and ERM.

RETINAL PHOTOTOXICITY

It depends on—

i. *Wavelength:* UV and short wavelength visible light are more dangerous than longer wavelength light.
ii. *Exposure duration:* Longer duration of tissue handling near macula can cause more exposure and more phototoxicity.

Mechanisms of Phototoxicity

i. *Thermal damage:* Increased rate of energy deposition is faster than rate of thermal diffusion which causes temperature rise. If it is more than 10° above basal, thermal damage occurs.
ii. *Mechanical damage:* If light energy deposited faster than mechanical, relaxation can occur, it produces thermoelastic pressure wave which can cause tissue disruption by shear forces/by cavitation.
iii. *Photochemical damage:* Chemical (oxidative) reactions induced by absorption of energetic photons.

ILLUMINATION SOURCES FOR SMALL-GAUGE VITRECTOMY

Efficiency vs Safety

In a small-gauge optic fiber with a conventional halogen light source, only 50% or less of the brightness found with the 20G system is obtained.

Xenon Light Illumination

- Luminous efficacy is 277–355 lumens/watt
- The increased lumens of xenon light sources are substantial, even with 25G optic fibers or smaller

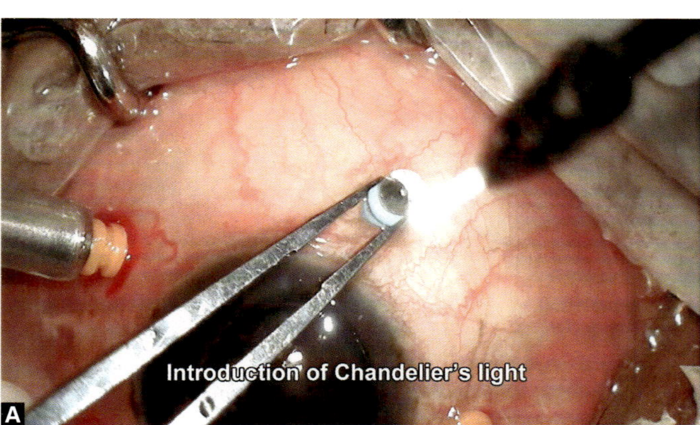

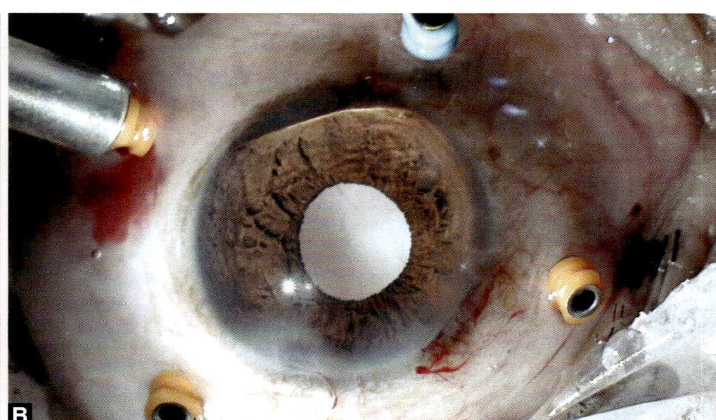

Figs 3.3A and B: (A) Surgery under 25G single-fiber endoillumination system; (B) Three 23G ports and a 25G single-fiber chandelier endoillumination system

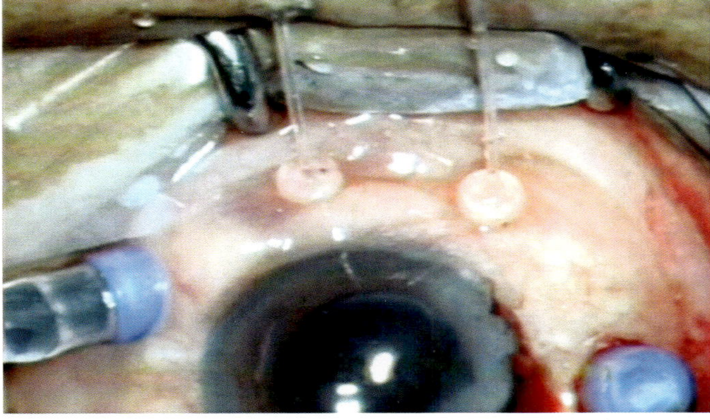

Fig. 3.4: Surgery under 27G dual-fiber endoillumination

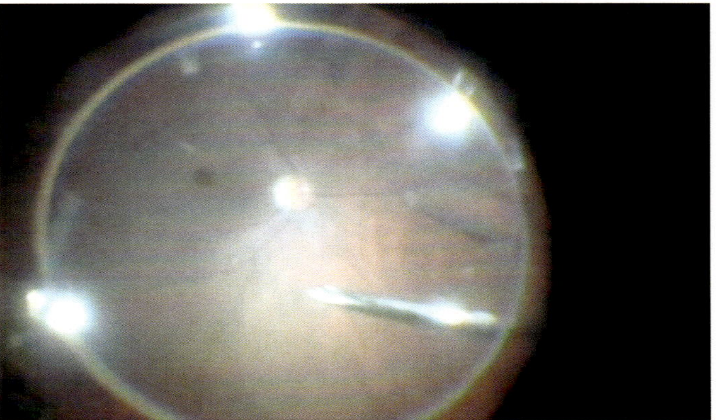

Fig. 3.5: Surgical field under 27G dual-fiber endoillumination

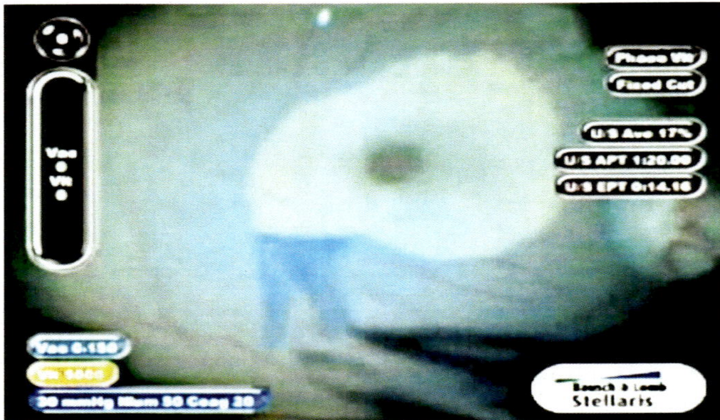

Fig. 3.6: Surgery with yellow filter during ILM peeling

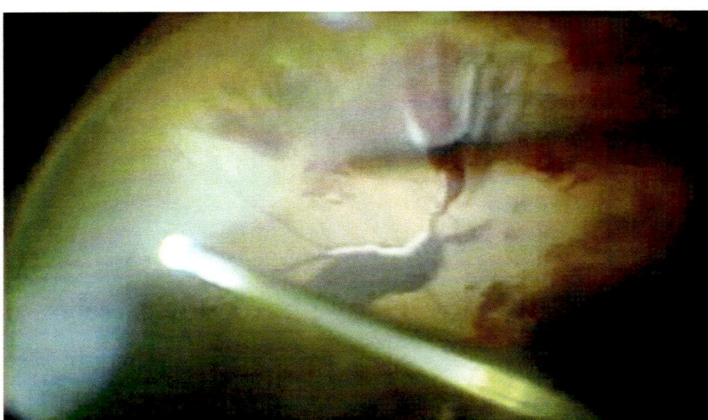

Fig. 3.7: Surgery with amber filter during peripheral vitrectomy

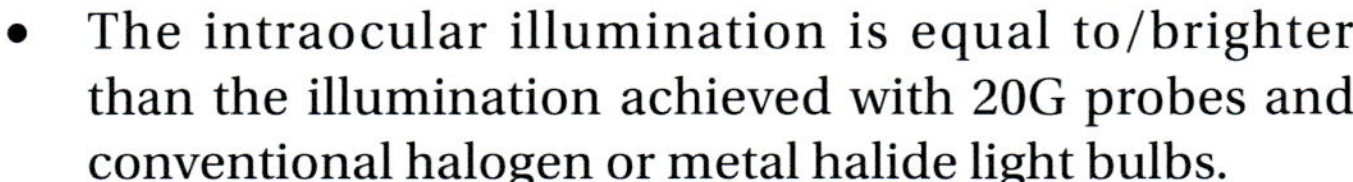

- The intraocular illumination is equal to/brighter than the illumination achieved with 20G probes and conventional halogen or metal halide light bulbs.

Currently available xenon illuminators have lower wavelength filters (at least <420 nm), cutting off ultraviolet and blue light to reduce phototoxicity with higher hazard efficiency.

Commercially available Xenon light sources:

- Accurus High Brightness Illuminator (AHBI, Alcon)
- *Photon (Synergetics):* An adapter with a 485 nm filter with improved safety
- Bright Star (DORC)
- Constellation Vision System (Less blue-Alcon)
- The Stellaris PC (B+ L).

Mercury Vapor Light Illumination

- More powerful illumination source with minimal photo toxicity
- *Luminous efficacy:* 402 lumens/watt
- 435 nm cut off filter to reduce exposure to UV and blue light
- Mercury vapor bulb is green-yellow which produces a less dazzling reflection from the fundus, and thus may be comfortable to the surgeon's eyes
- Can provide clear contrast during peeling ILM, stained with brilliant blue G dye.

Stellaris PC—have dual bulb, both xenon white and mercury vapor bulb

- *Yellow filter:* Avoiding UV & blue light
- *Green filter:* Enhance contrast
- *Amber filter:* For better peripheral vitreous dissection.

Surgery with Yellow Filter *(Video 3, Chapter 3)*

- Yellow filter is important to increase the contrast during dye-assisted membrane peeling especially during the macular hole surgery
- Yellow filter increases the difference in color contrast between already peeled and stained nonpeeled areas of ILM that helps the surgeon to work more precisely (Fig. 3.6).

Surgery with Amber Filter *(Video 4, Chapter 3)*

Amber colored filter is important to work in periphery, as peripheral uncut vitreous will be more distinctly visible (Fig. 3.7) and peripheral tissue dissection will be easier.

Kindly scan the QR code below to access the online Video.

CHAPTER 4

Cryoretinopexy and Endolaser Retinopexy

CRYORETINOPEXY

Cooling effect of cryotherapy is due to expansion of nitrous oxide gas in the probe tip (Joule-Thompson effect).

- Temperature at the tip varies from - 30° to - 60° C.
- Diameter of tip of cryoprobe - 2 to 2.5 mm.
- Temperature of nitrous oxide cylinder = - 89°C

The whole unit comprises of (Fig. 4.1) the following:

1. Cryo machine
2. Cryo probe
3. Nitrous oxide cylinder

Reactions

Mild cryopexy: Seen clinically as a yellow subretinal glow with unsharp edges.

Medium cryopexy: Appears white with sharp edges and as ice in retina.

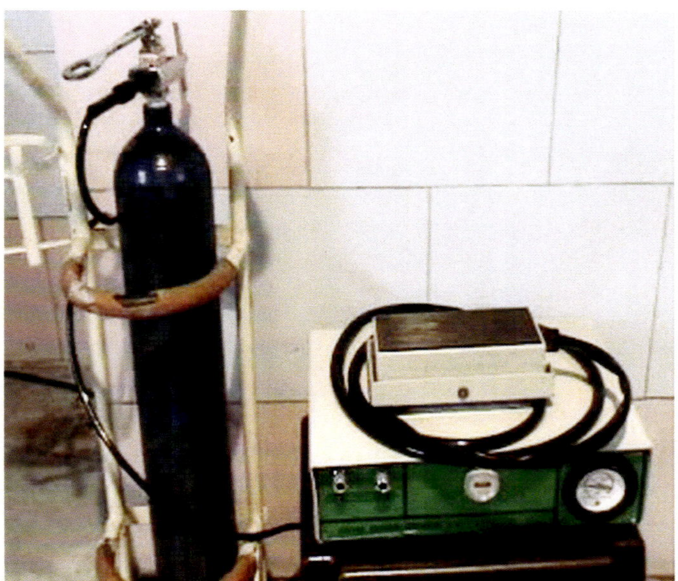

Fig. 4.1: Unit for cryoretinopexy

Heavy cryopexy: Occurs when the white ice ball in the retina is allowed to grow for several seconds.

Indications of transconjunctival cryoretinopexy: For anterior retinal breaks or lattice degenerations and to supplement a PRP.

Precautions during Cryoretinopexy

1. Freezing, snowball formation (Fig. 4.2) and thawing effect (Fig. 4.3) should be checked before application of cryotherapy.
2. The conjunctiva and fornices should be kept dry (Fig. 4.4), otherwise the freezing effect is absorbed by the lake of fluid surrounding the probe *(Video 1, Chapter 4).*
3. During cryopexy, it is important not to move the probe until the ice ball is fully thawed to prevent further tear formation in retina.

Method

Only tip of cryo probe should touch the sclera and indirect ophthalmoscope-guided or under microscope, medium cryo (sustained freezing until the retina first turns white) should be applied (Fig. 4.5). Interrupted cryopexy spots should be applied around the retinal break in an overlapping fashion.

Mechanism

Cryosurgery produce inflammatory reaction that can cause retinal adhesion by—

- Interdigitation of newly formed rods with villi of RPE
- Desmosomal connection between Müller cells and smooth surface of new RPE (strong adhesion)
- Infiltrative chorioretinal adhesion in which processes of Müller cells infiltrate the lamellae of Bruch's membrane (very strong adhesion).

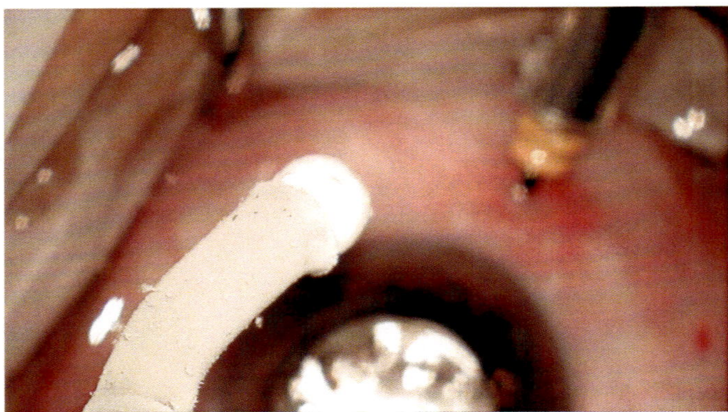

Fig. 4.2: Snowball formation in tip of cryo probe

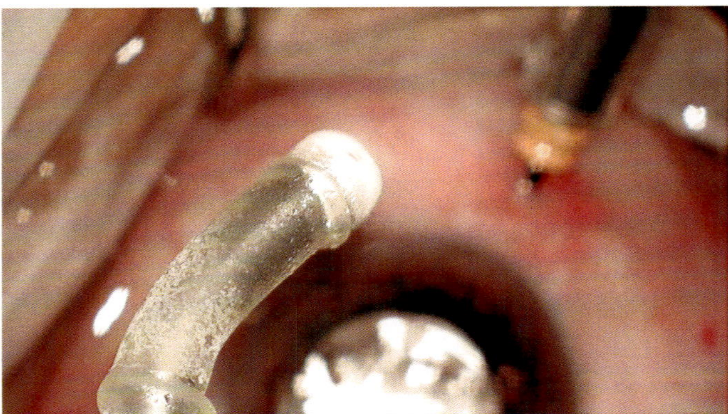

Fig. 4.3: Thawing effect in tip of cryo probe

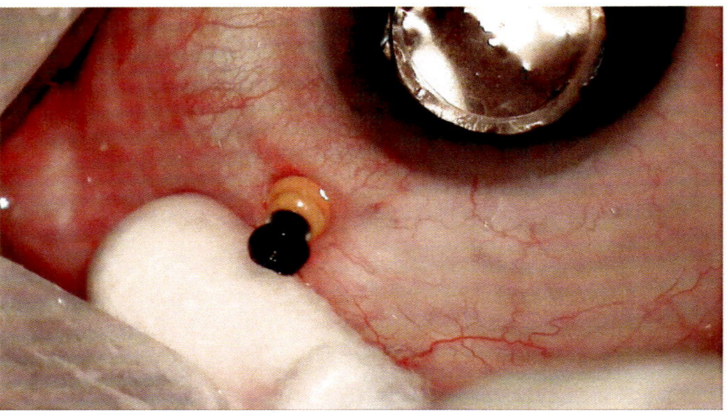

Fig. 4.4: Conjunctiva and fornices should be kept dry during cryopexy

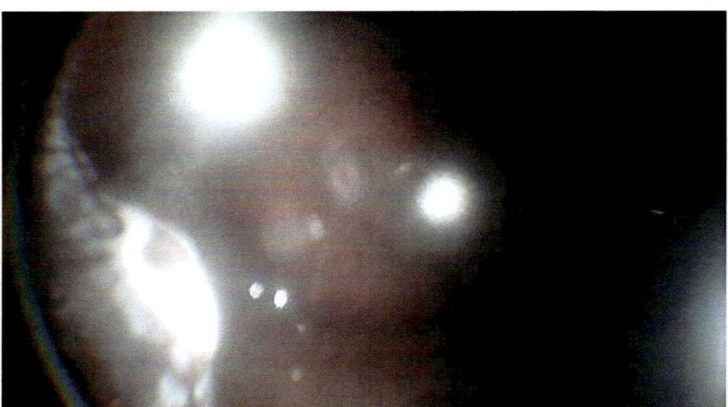

Fig. 4.5: Medium cryo reaction during treating a horse-shoe tear

Complications

The complications are rare.

1. Probe can perforate thin sclera (blue sclera). This is an effect of pressure, not freezing.
2. Excessive freezing can cause breakdown of blood-aqueous barrier and dispersion of RPE and cause vitreous haze.
3. Macular proliferative membrane formation and macular pucker as a result of release of RPE cells through the breaks.
4. Cystoid macular edema and rarely.
5. Exudative retinal detachment.

A study showed that cryosurgical adhesion gained strength after the 2nd day and maximum adhesive strength by 12th day.

ENDOLASER RETINOPEXY

It produces photocoagulative response, as light is absorbed by the tissue pigments and increase the temperature (10–20°C), resulting in protein denaturation (clinically whitening).

The first photocoagulation probe for vitreoretinal surgery was developed by Charles in 1979 using a portable xenon arc coagulator. But xenon arc light was not ideal for vitreoretinal surgery, as it generates heat which prohibit rapid firing application.

Payman and associates developed an endolaser probe for the argon laser.

The advantages of the argon laser over the xenon are:

- Smaller angle of divergence, which facilitates a more comfortable and safe working distance, a finer spot size
- Laser probe tip withstands rapid laser application
- Can be fired through air/gas.

Prerequisites

1. Proper endolaser filter positioning is important to protect both the operating surgeon as well as the assistant from the laser flash.
2. *Intensity of laser burn:* The intensity of laser burn depends upon—
   - The duration and the power settings of the laser
   - Degree of underlying pigmentation

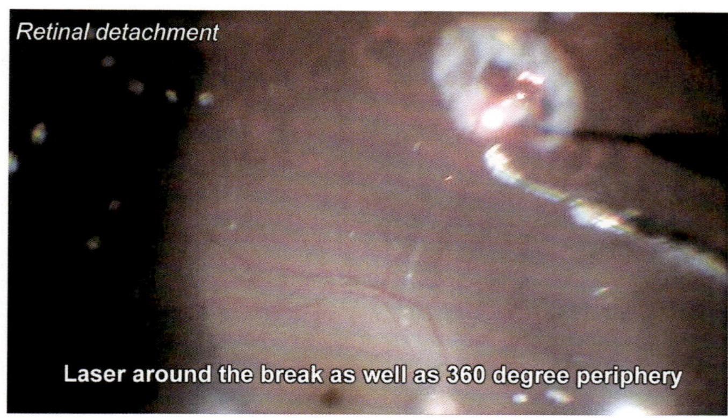

Fig. 4.6: Endolaser around the retinal hole

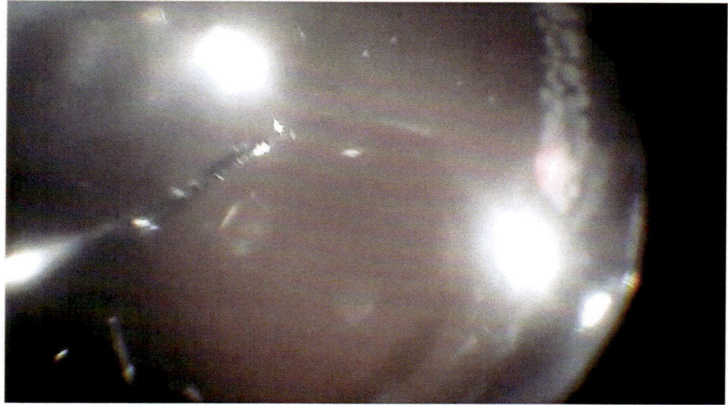

Fig. 4.7: Endolaser surrounding the margin of GRT

- The working distance from the probe tip to retinal surface. Longer duration, higher power settings, more pigmented RPE-choroid and decreased working distance result in more intense laser uptake.

3. Surgeon's hand should be supported firmly over the wrist rest.
4. The endolaser tip should be perpendicular to the retinal surface to create a round uniform spot.
5. *Settings:* The initial settings of the argon laser:
   - Duration—0.1-0.2 second
   - Power—200-600 mW

The power should be adjusted incrementally (in 30-50 mW steps) until a light gray-white spot is achieved.

Both straight and curved and lighted endorser probes are available in 23, 25 and 27G system.

Indications of endolaser in vitreoretinal procedures *(Video 2, Chapter 3)* are as follows:

- To create a laser barricade around the retinal holes (2-3 rows—there must be no SRF around the hole as SRF insulates RPE from the laser) (Fig. 4.6)
- Surrounding the retinectomy edges or giant retinal tear margins (under air or PFCL) (Fig. 4.7)
- To deliver scatter retinal photocoagulation (more peripheral retina is accessible with eyeball tilt or viewing lens tilt) (Fig. 4.8)
- To do retinal vessel photocoagulation (for new vessels to minimize retinal bleeding).

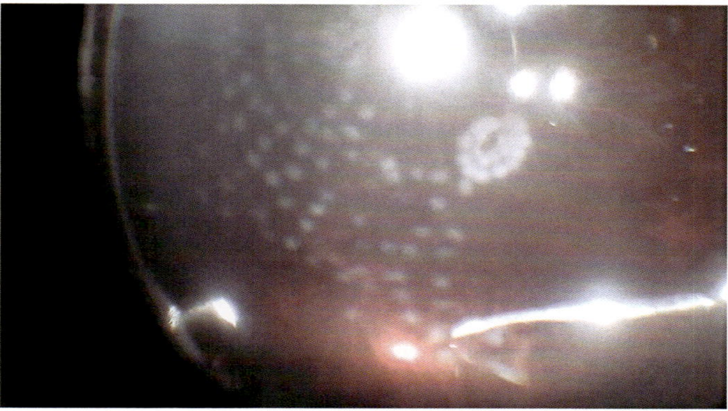

Fig. 4.8: Endolaser for scatter retinal photocoagulation in PDR

Both silicone oil and PFCL liquid creates a hyperopic shift in the eye's refraction, thus increasing the laser beam spot size. But air and gas cause a myopic shift, thus decreasing the laser beam spot size. Moreover, they do not absorb heat of laser energy. Thus, the power setting should be kept low.

Complications of Laser

1. Retinal necrosis.
2. Choroidal neovascularization.
3. Tear formation from intense laser burn or direct contact and adhesion of laser probe tip to retinal surface.

Kindly scan the QR code below to access the online Video.

CHAPTER 5

Intravitreal Tamponading Agents

INTRAVITREAL GAS

Use of intravitreal gas for the treatment of retinal detachment was first reported by Ohm in 1911. Rosengren first founded the concept of internal tamponade by air after Gonnin's discovery of the importance of localizing and sealing of retinal breaks in the treatment of retinal detachment.

Their clinical use depends on their expansile ability and intraocular longevity:

1. ***Nonexpansile gases***—Air (simplest tamponade), Xenon (heaviest rare earth gas).
2. ***Expansile gases***—
   - Sulfur hexafloride (SF_6)—Nontoxic, 5 times heavier than air.
     Expansion—1.9–2 times, Longevity—10–14 days, Nonexpansile concentration—18%, Maximum expansion by 24–48 hours.
   - Perfluorocarbon gases—Perfluoropropane (C_3F_8)
     Expansion—6 times, Longevity—55–65 days, Non-expansile concentration—14% Maximum expansion by 72–96 hours. Highest surface tension.

Functional Role

1. If gas bubble is larger than the retinal break, the surface tension of gas prevents it from passing through the retinal break and when gas bubble is positioned against break, the fluid passage from vitreous into subretinal space is blocked.
2. Intravitreal gas injection create gas-fluid interface and thus the gases have highest surface tension of any presently available vitreous replacements, approximately 70 dynes/cm.
3. Gas-fluid interface is inert and thus the proliferating cells cannot attach onto the surface.
4. It exerts a buoyant force (which is 10 times greater than silicone oil) that pushes the retina against the RPE, smooth out retinal folds around the margin of retinal tear and in case of properly positioned head posture, as it is maximum at the apex of gas bubble, it has role in postoperative prone positioning after macular hole surgery.
5. It is less soluble than nitrogen and water, thus the gases from the surrounding tissue-fluid diffuse into the injected gas bubble and expand it until the partial pressure equilibrate between two compartments and a stage of nitrogen equilibration (i.e., the rate of nitrogen diffusing into the bubble is equal to the diffusion of expanding gas into the surrounding tissue fluid) reached. The most rapid rate of volume increase occurs within first 6–8 hours.

Preparation of Intraocular Gas Injection

Intraocular gas gases are usually marketed either disposable or reusable cylinders with two-stage regulator valve, which prevents gas leakage from the cylinder and contamination entering the cylinder. Pure gas of desired volume is withdrawn in a syringe, which is attached to the outer end of the regulator valve with two 0.22 micrometer millipore filters. The syringe is initially flushed two or three times to remove gas mixed with air from the "dead space" of the tubing and connections. Pure gas of the desired volume is then withdrawn into the syringe. For achieving a nonexpansile concentration of gas, the syringe with desired volume of pure gas is disconnected from the regulator valve along with the distal filter. Atmospheric air is withdrawn through the distal filter into the syringe to obtain the desired concentration of gas-air mixture.

Technique of Intravitreal Gas Injection

Once the fluid-air exchange is complete, specific concentration of gas-air mixture is prepared. The infusion line is clamped with a hemostat and disconnected from the airpump, the 50 mL syringe is quickly connected to the infusion line. The hemostat is removed. A 27-gauge needle connected to an empty tuberculin syringe without the plunger or a vent is introduced through the valved 23- or 25-gauge cannula and placed inside the vitreous cavity. This allows the air from the vitreous cavity to escape. The nonexpansile gas mixture in the 50 mL syringe is injected to flush the vitreous cavity as air escapes through the 27-gauge needle. Injecting the gas slow enough to match the rate of air exit can prevent IOP rise. When the last 10 mL of gas is left in the syringe, the 27-gauge needle or the vent is withdrawn. The valved cannulas are removed by sliding them over the light pipes placed through them. The light pipe is then removed in the similar direction as the cannula was introduced, pressure over the sclerotomy is applied with a cotton-tipped applicator. The cannula with infusion line is removed and pressure over the sclerotomy is applied in a similar manner. If there is any gas leakage, the sclerotomy is sutured with a single, radial, transconjunctival 8-0 vicryl suture.

In case of hypotony, further gas injection is given.

IOP is assessed digitally or using the Barraquer tonometer.

Another method is to remove both superior valved cannulas. A 27-gauge needle connected to an empty tuberculin syringe is introduced through the sclera at 3.5–4.0 mm from limbus to allow the air to escape.

Another approach is to inject gas-air mixture directly into the eye through the sclera with 30-gauge needle or sclerotomy, and allow the air to exit via the infusion line, which is open to the atmosphere at the other end.

Precautions to be Taken While Using Intraocular Gas

1. Rapid decompression of atmospheric pressure during air travel can cause increase in gas volume in postoperative patient, resulting in rapid increase in IOP, which in turn may compromise intraocular blood flow through central retinal artery. It has been seen air travel can be done safely with gas volume 1.0 cc or less (5% or less volume) with normal outflow facility.
2. Nitrous oxide anesthesia should be avoided during retinal surgery where intraocular gas has been used for tamponade as dissolved nitrous oxide is very soluble in the vitreous cavity and it's entry into intraocular gas bubble leads to marked increase in IOP within 10–15 minutes of sclerotomy closure. That's why nitrous oxide anesthesia should be discontinued (if at all has to use) 15–30 minutes before the gas is instilled into the eye.

Arc of Contact and Sector Angle

Parver and Lincoff measured the arc of bubble-retinal contact by its sector angle for different volume.

0.3 cc of gas would tamponade 90° of arc, but 1.0 cc will cover only 126° of arc.

Better to Avoid Intravitreal Gas Tamponade for

- Multiple breaks scenarios
- Breaks in inferior four clock hours
- PVR C onwards
- Uncontrolled glaucoma cases.

Complications

1. Elevated IOP may cause more than 30 mm Hg. Usually it is transient, aggravated by poor compliance for prone positioning. Mainly angle closure episodes precipitates. Treatment
   - Topical and systemic aqueous suppressants (Beta-blocker, prostaglandin analogs, alpha agonist and carbonic anhydrase inhibitor.
   - Improvement of prone positioning help to decrease angle-closure episodes.
   - Anterior chamber reformation with viscoelastic between cornea and anterior iris in case of flat anterior chamber help to open the angle.
   - Laser peripheral iridotomy help in immediate reformation of anterior chamber.
   - Rarely removal of some amount of intraocular gas is necessary where maximum antiglaucoma therapy fails.
2. Bullous keratopathy.
3. Lens opacity and cataract formation (most common in phakic patient).
4. Subretinal and suprachoroidal gas—These are very rare complications in cases of anterior PVR with anterior vitreous contraction or detachment of pars plana.
5. New or enlarged break.

SILICONE OILS

A polymer of dimethyl siloxane with transparency, refractive index viscoelasticity similar to vitreous.

In 1962, Cibis et al. successfully used silicone oil for intravitreal use.

Types

Clinically, three types of silicone oil are present. These are:

1. Lighter than water—Polydimethyl siloxane, most commonly used.
2. Heavier than water—Polytrifluropropyl methyl siloxane.
3. Heavier than water—Polyphenyl methyl siloxane (High-tech bike oil).

Characteristics

- Polydimethyl siloxane—
  Refractive index = 1.40
  Specific gravity = 0.97
  Surface tension = 21.2–21.5.
- Polytrifluoropropyl methyl siloxane—
  Refractive index = 1.38
  Specific gravity = 1.28–1.30
  Surface tension = 26–29.

Mechanism of Action

1. Tamponade effect—As SO is immiscible with water, there is an interface between two liquids causing surface tension along the SO bubble which is responsible for the tamponade effect.

   Surface tension at water gas interface is due to—a) van der walls force and, b) strong polar binding forces between adjacent water molecules.

   Surface tension at SO aqueous interface is lower because SO is a nonpolar substance and less attractive forces between its molecules. So, silicone oil has less effective tamponade than gas. But its tamponade effect is enhanced by the previous fluid gas exchange to flatten retina.
2. Floatation force—
   - It is small in SO, as its density is slightly less than water.
   - Floatation force at each point of retinal surface is proportional to height of SO bubble at that point and the difference of density between water and SO. As this density difference is small in case of SO and high in case of gas bubble, a gas bubble of equal height exerts 32 times of floatation force than SO.
3. Hydraulic space occupying property.

Refractive Change

In phakic eyes—As RI of SO is greater than vitreous, refractive power of posterior surface of lens is reduced and there is a hyperopic shift of 5-7 Dsph.

In aphakic eyes—Anterior surface of SO globule acts as a converging lens and reduces aphakic hyperopia by 4-6 Dsph.

Heavy Silicone Oil

- As temporary tamponade (maximum 3 months)
- For Inferior complex retinal detachment, GRT, PDR with RD
- Not for superior retinal detachments.

Densiron-68 (Fluron Co, Neu-Ulm, Germany)

- A solution of perfluorohexyloctane (F6H8) and 5000cST silicone oil
- Specific gravity—1.06, i.e. higher than water.

Oxane-HD (Bausch and Lomb, Toulouse, France)

- A mixture of silicone oil and a fluorinated and hydrocarbonated olefin (RMN3)
- Specific gravity—1.02.

Complications

Anterior Segment Complications

1. Emulsification—Its incidence varies from 5 to 100% and is the result of fragmentation of the oil globule into multiple micelle. It occurs due to—
   - Increase in number of low molecular weight silicone oil polymer chains (as impurities)
   - Any mixing with biologically active substances like fibrinogen, fibrin, globulin and balanced salt solution.

   Emulsified silicone oil particles may block trabecular meshwork and cause rise in IOP, that warrants removal of silicone oil.
2. Keratopathy—Due to its contact with endothelium, causing loss of endothelial cells. Stromal edema may lead to bulls keratopathy changes.
3. Glaucoma—Its incidence varies from 2-40% and it occurs due to acute pupillary block in absence of inferior iridectomy in aphakic eyes or chronic closed angle glaucoma (due to peripheral anterior synechia formation) or open angle glaucoma (due to damage of trabecular meshwork).
4. Cataract formation—Posterior subcapsular cataract in young and nuclear sclerosis in older patients. It is most common complication in phakic eyes as it causes squamous metaplasia of lens epithelium and prevent metabolic exchange across the posterior lens capsule.
5. Hypotony—In approximately 20% of cases due to toxic effect or ischemic effect on ciliary process.
6. Chronic inflammation.

Posterior Segment Complications

1. Ineffective tamponade—Due to inadequate size or distorted globe due to buckle.
2. Secondary retinal break formation.

3. Recurrent ERM formation. Especially in long standing silicone oil-filled eyes with advanced emulsification.
4. Direct retinal toxicity—Experimental studies shows SO derived toxic phospholipid complexes within retinal tissues.
5. Decreased ERG response—Due to electrical insulating effect of silicone oil on photoreceptors. Decreased *a* and *b* wave amplitude are seen in ERG and this depressed response is reversible after silicone oil removal.
6. Endophthalmitis—Rare.

Kindly scan the QR code below to access the online Video.

CHAPTER

6 Perfluorocarbon Liquids

Perfluorocarbon liquids (PFCL), originally introduced by Clark and Gollan as high oxygen-content blood substitutes. Haidt et al. first inject PFCL inside the vitreous cavity in animal model.

PFCL are fluorinated synthetic liquids containing carbon-fluorine bonds.

Physical Properties of PFCL

1. They are optically clear, heavier than and immiscible with water. Any hydrokinetic manipulation of retina can be done under PFCL.
2. With specific gravity 1.7–2.03, the PFCL is denser than water, allowing hydrokinetic manipulation of retina under PFCL. Heavy liquid fills the eye in posterior to anterior fashion, hydrokinetically tamponading the posterior retina against the underlying RPE. SRF is steam-rolled out through an anterior retinal break into the vitreous cavity. The intravitreal fluid then egress though the sclerotomy cannulas as the PFCL level rises.
3. It has lower viscosity than silicone oil, so that it can be injected through the small bore needle.
4. The high surface tension of PFCL (same as silicone oil) in water creates an effective internal tamponading effect and prevents any substance from passing through the anterior retinal break into subretinal space.

Injection and Removal Techniques

Perfluorocarbon liquid (PFCL) is to be injected after vitrectomy and posterior vitreous detachment (PVD) induction from the disc/macula. Approximately 5 mL of PFCL is drawn up in a sterile fashion with a 20–27 gauge needle attached to a lure-lock syringe to prevent inadvertent injection of PFCL into the eye. PFCL injection requires a 20–30 gauge cannula. For removal, active aspiration via an extrusion needle or a silicone-tipped cannula can be used by starting air-PFCL exchange.

If surgeon is not sure about the complete removal of PFCL, a few drops of balanced salt solution (BSS) plus fluid can be added following FAX to visualize PFCL bubbles and then after few minutes, the remaining fluid should be removed.

Indications

1. *Rhegmatogenous retinal detachment (Video 1, Chapter 6):* In case of retinal detachment, after PVD induction from the posterior pole, this PVD is to be extended peripherally. During this process, central retina can be damaged due to inadvertent touch by the cutter. PFCL injection can stabilize posterior pole from posterior to anterior fashion due to it's high specific gravity as well as added gravity. This will facilitate to carry forward the separation of posterior hyaloid from the detached peripheral retina up to vitreous base and then complete vitreous base excision by external scleral depression. PFCL is to be injected up to the posterior margin of the breaks or up to the level of sclerotomies (SRF is steamrollered out through the anterior retinal breaks) (Fig. 6.1). In first situation, fluid air exchange is to be started to remove remaining peripheral somatotropin-releasing factor (SRF) through the peripheral retinal breaks. Once all the SRF has removed, one can start peripheral laser.

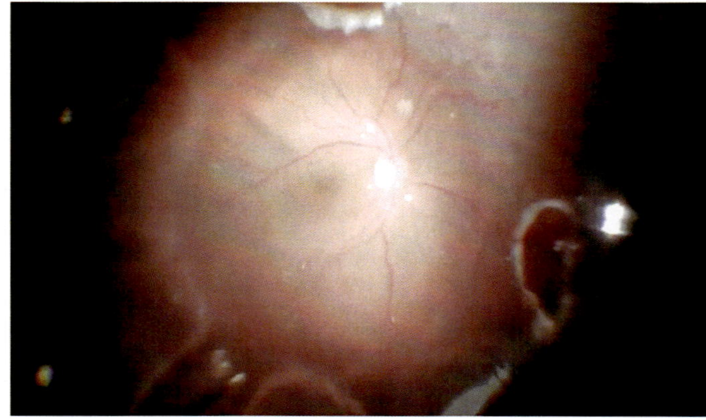

Fig. 6.1: PFCL is to be injected up to the posterior margin of the breaks in a case of rhegmatogenous retinal detachment

2. *Giant Retinal Tear:* In this type of complicated retinal detachment with giant retinal tear, PFCL is injected over the posterior pole, filling the eye in posterior to anterior direction, sometimes directing beneath the inverted flap (if present) to unfold it as the PFCL bubble enlarges. The SRF is forced anteriorly as the retina is hydrokinetically repositioned against the RPE. The force of PFCL is enough to prevent slippage of retina. PFCL is to be injected till the bubble level reaches the edge of the GRT. Anterior retinal flap as well as vitreous base has to be trimmed at this stage with external scleral depression. Endolaser or cryotherapy or both are then applied to the edges of tear. In presence of PVR changes, membrane dissection has to be carried out to remove residual traction, necessitating further membranectomy sometimes more retinectomy.
3. *Proliferative vitreoretinopathy (Video 2, Chapter 6)*: Conventional approach is to tackle anterior pulmonary vascular resistance (PVR) first then posterior PVR. But use of PFCL has reversed the approach—posterior to anterior in a more controlled fashion. An edge is to be created from the membrane and PFCL has to be injected over the disc and posterior pole under the membrane edge so that posterior pole will be flat and membrane removal can be carried out safely (Fig. 6.2). Even advanced closing/closed funnel PVR can be opened in a similar fashion. After membrane dissection more PFCL is to be injected to notice persistent RD or foreshortening of retina (Fig. 6.3).
4. *Dislocated crystalline lens and dislocated IOL (Video animation 3, Chapter 6)*: Both crystalline lens and IOLs are lighter than the PFCL and thus can float on the surface of a PFCL bubble. During phacofragmentation of dislocated lens over the PFCL, this PFCL bubble protects retina from chattering effect of emulsified lens materials (Fig. 6.4). Care should be taken to reposition the floating dropped crystalline lens as it can move towards periphery due to convex superior surface of PFCL bubble. In case of dislocated IOL, PFCL bubbles prevent the development of retinal break, detachment and hemorrhage. IOL can be removed through the limbal route holding it by an end-grasping forceps.
5. *Ocular trauma:* PFCL will confine and control the bleeding from retinal vessels in a severely traumatized eyes due it's immiscibility with blood.
6. *Massive suprachoroidal hemorrhage:* To drain suprachoroidal blood, PFCL can be injected inside the vitreous cavity and it evacuates suprachoroidal blood from posterior to anterior fashion with the blood exiting through the anteriorly placed sclerotomies.
7. *Retinal detachment with macular hole:* ILM peeling in detached retina is challenging and difficult. As PFCL provide the counteraction and ILM peeling under the PFCL is relatively easier as PFCL keeps the detached posterior pole flat.

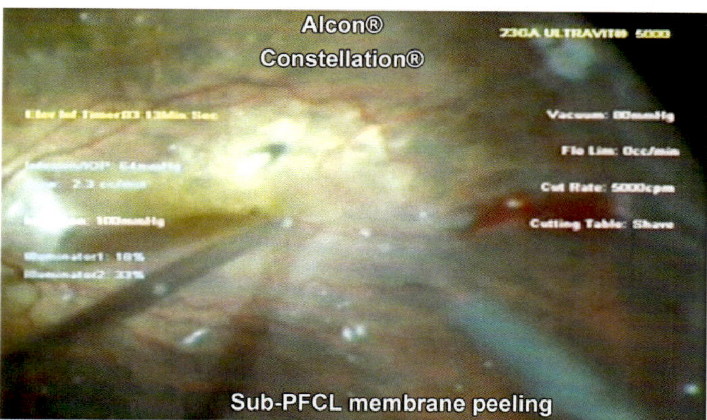

Fig. 6.2: Sub-PFCL membrane peeling to release residual fixed folds

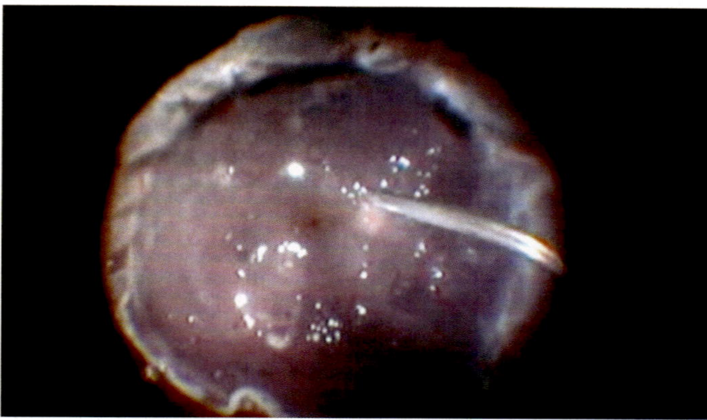

Fig. 6.3: More PFCL is to be injected to notice persistent RD or foreshortening of retina after releasing fixed folds

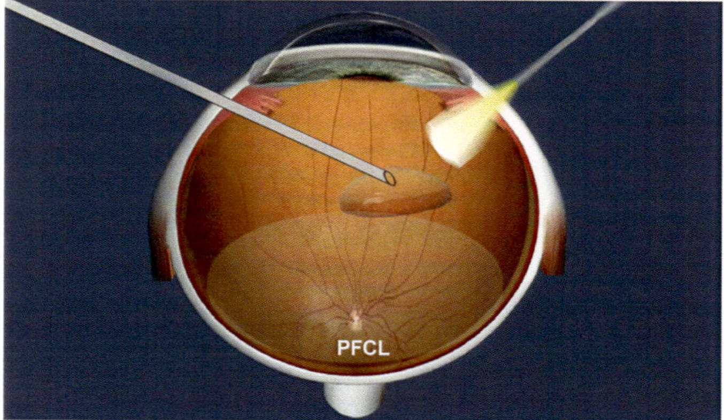

Fig. 6.4: Phacofragmentation of dislocated cataract over the surface of PFCL

8. *Other complicated retinal detachments:*
   - In stage IV/V ROP surgery, PFCL facilitates membrane dissection and in opening of the funnel- shaped PVR
   - In macular translocation surgery, some people routinely use PFCL
   - To manage complicated combined tractional-rhegmatogenous retinal detachments
   - To control intraoperative bleeding as PFCL may sequester the clot at the site of bleeding.
   - For repair of retinoschisis-related retinal detachment
   - For removal of submacular hemorrhage with tissue plasminogen activator
   - To remove subretinal gas
   - During removal of submacular neovascular membrane to control hemorrhagic complications.

Kindly scan the QR code below to access the online Video.

CHAPTER 7

Intravitreal Anti-VEGF and Steroid Injections

Intravitreal Anti-VEGF Injections (Bevacizumab, Ranibizumab, Pegaptanib Sodium)

Indications

1. Choroidal neovascular membrane (CNVM) from any etiology.
2. Proliferative vascular diseases [like in diabetics (PDR), branch retinal vein occlusion (BRVO), central retinal vein occlusion (CRVO)] in absence of tractional retinal detachment.
3. Macular edema from vascular pathology (diabetics, BRVO, CRVO, periphlebitis).

Technique (Video 1, Chapter 7)

- Pupil should be mid-dilated to visualize tip of the needle to avoid lens touch, retinal injury or suprachoroidal injection
- Preoperative antibiotic application should be started 3 days prior to intravitreal injection
- Ocular surface is thoroughly washed with saline
- 5% povidone iodine is applied
- Intravitreal anti-VEGF injection is taken in an 1 mL tuberculin syringe
- In phakic case, it is introduced through pars plana area 4 mm away from the limbus
- Tip of the 30G needle should be well visualized with beveled tip up directed towards the center of the vitreous cavity (Fig. 7.1)
- The injection is pushed inside the vitreous cavity drop-by-drop
- Then the needle is taken out
- Paracentesis can be done to normalize the IOP.

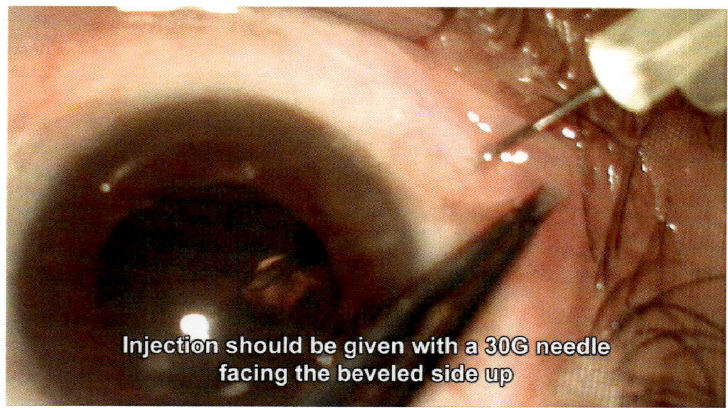

Fig. 7.1: Intravitreal anti-VEGF injection with a 30G needle facing beveled tip up

Intravitreal Triamcinolone Acetonide Injection

Indications

1. Diabetic macular edema.
2. Macular edema secondary to vascular occlusion.
3. Cystoid macular edema after cataract surgery or secondary to uveitis.

Technique (Video 2, Chapter 7)

The technique is same as in intravitreal anti-VEGF injection.

- Pupil should be mid-dilated to visualize tip of the needle to avoid lens touch, retinal injury or suprachoroidal injection
- Preoperative antibiotic application should be started 3 days prior to intravitreal injection
- Thorough wash of ocular surface is done with saline
- 5% povidone iodine is applied
- Intravitreal triamcinolone acetonide injection is taken in a 1 mL tuberculin syringe with 26G needle

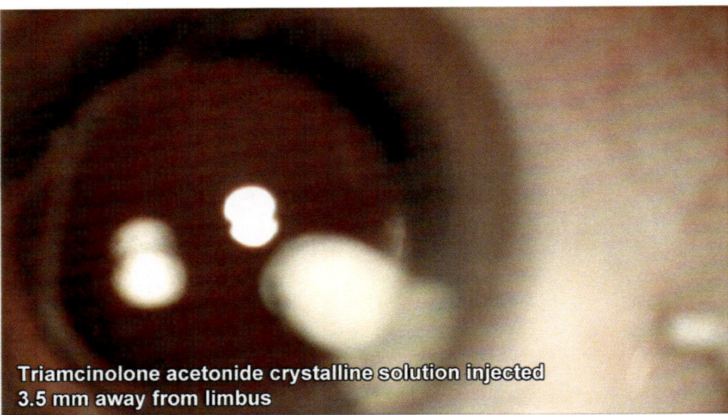

Fig. 7.2: Intravitreal triamcinolone acetonide injection with a 26G needle facing beveled tip up

- In phakic case, it is introduced through pars plana area 4 mm away from the limbus
- Tip of the 26G needle should be well-visualized with beveled tip up directed towards the center of the vitreous cavity (Fig. 7.2)
- The injection is pushed inside the vitreous cavity drop by drop
- Then the needle is taken out
- Paracentesis can be done to normalize the IOP.

INTRAVITREAL ANTI-VEGF DRUGS AND STEROID INJECTIONS

Comparative analysis of available intravitreal anti-VEGF agents have been highlighted in Table 7.1. Dexamethasone, Triamcinolone acetonide and Fluocinolone acetonide all three compounds are lyophilic. The lipophilicity is maximum with Fluocinolone acetonide and minimum with dexamethasone. Thus, triamcinolone has more affinity for depositing in the trabecular meshwork and causing aqueous outflow obstruction. That's why triamcinolone acetonide has more propensity to cause IOP rise than dexamethasone (Table 7.2).

Complications after intravitreal injections:

The risk of vision-threatening complications after intravitreal injections (anti-VEGF/steroid) is fortunately quite low, and adherence to good technique should reduce this risk even further.

During the informed consent process, the patient should be made aware of all possible complications. Patients should be instructed about possible nonserious complications as well as rare but serious vision-threatening complications.

I. Ocular complications:

A. Nonserious complications:
   i. *Foreign body sensation:* It is almost a normal consequence following an injection and may not start for several hours after the anesthetic begins to wear off. It may also occur secondary to conjunctival irritation and povidone-iodine-induced superficial punctuate keratopathy.
   ii. *Subconjunctival hemorrhage:* It can also occur and may exacerbate foreign body sensation.
   iii. *Floaters:* Especially in cases involving triamcinolone acetonide and occasionally with dexamethasone implants, patients may see the medication suspended within the vitreous cavity. It is important to warn patients about this "coagulum" of medication and advise them to sleep with the head of the bed elevated for 1 or 2 days to allow the "coagulum" to move out of the visual axis. Patients should be reassured that these medication "floaters" are harmless. However, caution is advised if there are any occurrences of flashing lights or peripheral scotomata, as these could indicate a retinal tear and/or retinal detachment.

B. Serious complications:
   i. *Inadvertent wrong site selection:* If the selected site is beyond the pars plana, specifically more than 4.5 mm, the introduction of a 26G or 30G needle can inadvertently cause retinal dialysis or retinal perforation.
   ii *Wrong direction of needle tip:* If the direction of the needle tip is not towards the center of a vitreous cavity or the optic disk, but rather a flat entry, the needle tip can strip off the posterior capsule or more severe kind of lens injury in phakic eyes.
   iii. *Vitreous prolapse:* Although it is uncommon with a 30 G needle, injection with a wider bore needle can cause a vitreous wick at the wound just after its withdrawal.
   iv. *Rise of intraocular pressure (IOP):* IOP rise is a common sequela after any intravitreal injection. But this rise is immediate and does not last for long. But one may do paracentesis to correct this immediate rise, especially in cases of compromised optic disk in diabetics or advanced glaucoma patients.
   v. *Cataract formation:* Cataractous changes can happen after any intravitreal injection in phakic eyes. Rarely it is due to direct injury by the needle tip due to faulty direction. Cataract formation is an uncommon acute complication following intravitreal triamcinolone injection but is a common longer-term complication. Cataract progression following IV triamcinolone acetonide does occur for nuclear sclerotic, cortical, and posterior subcapsular types. With repeated administration, the rate of progression of nuclear and cortical cataracts is also increased; however, this effect is rare with posterior subcapsular cataracts.

TABLE 7.1: Comparative analysis of available intravitreal anti-VEGF agents.

Intravitreal anti-VEGF injections	*Format*	*Mode of action*	*Molecular wight*	*Rate of retinal penetration*	*Vitreous half-life (in human)*	*Clinical dose*
Pegaptanib sodium	Single-stranded RNA aptamer	Anti-VEGF 165	50 kDa	24 hours	10 ± 4 days	0.3 mg in 90 μL
Bevacizumab	Full antibody IgG1	Anti-VEGF-A	147 kDa	24 hours	6,7 days	1.25 mg/0.05 mL
Ranibizumab	Fab fragment	Anti-VEGF-A	48 kDa	>6 hours	7.2 days	0.5 mg/0.05 mL
Aflibercept	VEGFR1/ 2-Fc fusion	Anti-VEGF-A , B and PlGF	97–115 kDa	6–24 hours	5.65 days	2 mg/0.05 mL
Brolucizumab	Single-chain antibody fragments - scFv	Anti-VEGF-A	26 kDa	1–6 hours	7.43 days	6 mg/0.05 mL
Faricimab	Both anti-VEGF and anti-angiopoietin	Both anti-VEGF-A and anti-angiopoietin 2	150 kDa	24 hours	7.5 days	6 mg/0.05 mL

TABLE 7.2: Comparative analysis of available intravitreal steroid agents.

Intravitreal steroid injections	*Size*	*Duration*	*Lipophilicity*	*Mode of action*	*Molecular weight*	*Clinical dose*	*Complications*
Triamcinolone acetonide	Particle size—mostly <50 microns	2–4 months	Moderate	Anti-inflammatory	434 Da	2 mg/ 0.05 mL	• Cataract (54%) and glaucoma (44%) • Glaucoma surgery in 5.9%
Dexamethasone implant	Implant size—6 mm × 0.46 mm	4–6 months	Minimum	• Anti-inflammatory • Stabilizes blood-retinal barrier • Suppress the VEGF production	392.46 Da	0.7 mg intravitreal implant	• Cataract (64.1–67.9%) • Glaucoma surgery in 0.3–0.6%
Fluocinolone acetonide implant	Implant size—3.5 mm × 0.37 mm	3 years (release rate 0.2 μg/day)	Maximum	• Anti-inflammatory, binding with glucocorticoid receptor • Inhibit phospholipase A2 • Anti-VEGF	452.49 Da	0.19 mg intravitreal implant	• Cataract (80–87.2%) • Glaucoma surgery in 4.8–8.1%

vi. *Endophthalmitis after intravitreal injection:* If the needle tip touches the eyelashes in cases where the eyelashes are not properly covered by a sterile drape, the needle tip may carry the pathogens to the vitreous cavity. However, if the conjunctival and scleral prick are in the same site, the external pathogens can enter intravitreally. Recent studies reported that endophthalmitis caused by *Streptococcus* species was significantly more frequent after intravitreal injection than after intraocular surgery. *Streptococcus* species comprise at least 41% culturable adult salivary flora, and probable etiology has been attributed to the contamination of the injection field by aerosolization or droplet spread. In multicenter clinical trials with anti-VEGF therapy, the incidence of endophthalmitis per patient has been reported to range from 0.019 to 1.6%. Prophylactic and postinjection antibiotics are frequently used to reduce the likelihood of endophthalmitis. Prophylactic antibiotics may reduce ocular flora. However, povidone-iodine preparation is considered more effective. Preoperative as well as postoperative application of povidone-iodine is very effective.

vii. *Pseudoendophthalmitis:* In patients receiving triamcinolone acetonide, sometimes triamcinolone acetonide particles may appear in the anterior chamber and stimulate inflammatory reactions. The same kind of inflammatory reaction happens in the vitreous also. One should rule out true endophthalmitis from these cases by its response to the topical steroid-cycloplegic treatment.

viii. *Sterile endophthalmitis:* This condition should be reserved for patients who present with intense inflammation, possibly due to the preservatives or vehicles within the solution. It has been seen that the use of a preservative-free solution or flushing the vehicle from the triamcinolone acetonide and resuspending it in a sterile saline solution can reduce its incidence.

ix. *Retinal tear or retinal detachment:* Although very rare, the incidence of retinal tears and retinal detachment after any intravitreal injection is a known complication. The overall incidence of rhegmatogenous retinal detachment (RRD) after intravitreal injection of anti-VEGF agents is low (0 to 0.67%). In the VEGF Inhibition Study in Ocular Neovascularization (VISION) trial, only 4 RRDs developed over 7545 injections (0.05% per injection).
   - The mechanism for the development of an RRD is vitreoretinal traction, usually in the vitreous base, producing a retinal tear with subsequent retinal detachment. Sometimes, wrong site measurement by calipers or sometimes due to anterior insertion of ora serrata, retinal dialysis at ora or even direct perforation of retina at the periphery can happen.
   - If a patient complains about floaters, flashing of light, or loss of peripheral field of vision, a prompt evaluation of the retina is necessary because early recognition and treatment of retinal tears and retinal detachment can prevent further macular involvement and therefore further vision loss.

   Prevention:
   a. The use of small-gauge needles reduces the chance of vitreous traction at the vitreous base.
   b. Careful measurement of the injection site with a calliper is mandatory. By performing this step, one can further reduce the risk of RRD.

x. *Intraocular inflammation (IOI):* Anterior chamber reaction can occur after any intravitreal injection, which can be minimal to severe. With Brolucizumab, sometimes, this IOI may present as retinal vasculitis or central retinal artery occlusion (CRAO)-like occlusive retinal vasculitis as a type III antigen-antibody hypersensitivity reaction. Anterior chamber reaction mostly responds in treatment with topical steroids and cycloplegic drugs. However, cases with retinal vasculitis need systemic steroids with extremely poor visual prognosis.

II. Systemic toxicity:

Systemic hypertension, arterial thromboembolic events (ATEs), or serious hemorrhagic events have been reported in patients receiving pan-VEGF inhibitors intravitreally. There is a concern that intravitreal anti-VEGF therapy may increase the risk of an adverse event. In large, randomized, prospective multicenter studies, neither pegaptanib sodium nor ranibizumab is associated with an increased risk of ATE in patients with neovascular AMD compared to control groups. As all of the intravitreal anti-VEGF agents have been reported to be associated with detectable levels in the systemic circulation that may significantly suppress systemic VEGF levels, there is a scientific rationale for the occurrence of potential systemic adverse events. Reported nonocular hemorrhagic events to include ecchymosis, gastrointestinal hemorrhages, hematoma, vaginal hemorrhages, hemorrhagic stroke, and subdural hematomas.

The rates of any cause of death, myocardial infarctions, and cerebrovascular events were not significantly increased. Different studies reported in the recent head-to-head trials and meta-analyses, the higher risk of all-cause mortality with anti-VEGF injections.

Specific adverse events following intravitreal anti-VEGF injections considering specific diseases:

A. Diabetic retinopathy and retinal vascular occlusions
   i. Development or progression of tractional retinal detachment (TRD) after intravitreal injection of anti-VEGF before vitrectomy for advanced proliferative diabetic retinopathy (PDR). TRDs developed or progressed at 5–7 days after the injection (average 13 days, range 3–31 days). In eyes with active

PDR with extensive new vessels, there is a risk for progression of TRD to involve the fovea. Moreover, delay in further vitrectomy can lead to secondary break formation at the base of new vessels due to traction from shrinkage of vascular polyps at the apex of TRDs and ultimately formation of combined rhegmatogenous-tractional retinal detachments.

ii. Ghost cell glaucoma has been reported following the use of bevacizumab as an adjunct to vitrectomy for PDR. It is rare.

iii. Decreases in retrobulbar blood flow parameters, retinal arteriolar vasoconstriction, and worsening of macular ischemia have been reported after intravitreal injection of anti-VEGF agents. It is also very rare.

B. *Age-related macular degeneration:* Retinal pigment epithelium (RPE) tears may occur spontaneously or after intravitreal injection of an anti-VEGF agent in patients with neovascular AMD. The reported incidence of RPE tear after anti-VEGF therapy varies from 0.06 to 27%. Pre-existing RPE detachment (PED) or fibrovascular PED is considered the major risk factor for RPE tear. Large diameter and vertical height of PED on OCT increase the risk of RPE tear.

Kindly scan the QR code below to access the online Video.

CHAPTER 8

Ophthalmic Ultrasonography

Ultrasonography was first used in ophthalmology in 1956 by Mundt and Hughes.

The first standard A scan was developed by Ossoinig in 1960s. Later, he further expanded his diagnostic method by adding the use of a contact B scan to evolve standard echography for accurate detection and differentiation of intraocular and orbital disorders.

Physics

- Ultrasound is an acoustic wave that consists of oscillation of particles within a medium
- Ultrasound waves have frequencies greater than 20 KHz (i.e. 20,000 oscillations/sec), which are inaudible to humans (frequencies of less than 20 KHz are audible)
- Frequencies of diagnostic ophthalmic ultrasound varies from 8 to 10 MHz (1 megahertz = 10,00,000 cycles/sec) with short-wavelength (this allow resolution of minute ocular and orbital structure)

[For large structures of abdomen and pelvic region, USG frequencies used is 1–5 MHz]

- Velocity of ultrasound wave is dependent on the medium through which it passes. As water is very compressible, sound waves are transmitted through water at a slower velocity than through more solid media. Thus, sound travels faster through a solid lens than it does through liquid vitreous.

Sound Wave Velocities (Table 8.1)

- Acoustic interfaces are created at the junction of two medias that have different acoustic impedances and reflected longitudinal waves from these interfaces towards the source of emitted energy (i.e transducer/probe) is called an echo
- Angle of the sound beam has importance—longitudinal (perpendicular probe) angle of sound beam produces stronger echoes than oblique ones
- Absorption—higher frequency sound waves have higher absorption by tissues than lower frequencies.

TABLE 8.1: Sound wave velocities in various medium

Medium	*Velocities (meter/sec)*
Water	1480
Aqueous/Vitreous	1532
Soft tissue	1550
Crystalline lens	1641
Bone	3500

Thus, 20–50 MHz frequency probe can detect anterior segment structures only, but 8–10 MHz frequency probe can detect posterior segment pathologies.

Ultrasound Unit

It has four components:

- Pulser
- Transducer
- Receiver
- Display screen.

Transducer/Probe (Figs 8.1A and B)

The key component is a piezoelectric crystal (a quartz or ceramic), located near the face of the probe, undergoes a mechanical vibration when stimulated by electrical energy. This vibration produces a longitudinal sound wave that passes through the media. Reflected energy produces another mechanical vibration which produces an electrical signal that is transmitted to the receiver and display screen. This whole cycle is repeated a thousand or more times per second to produce a 'real-time' display.

- Probe has a marker (a dot/line/logo) which indicate the side of the probe that is represented on the upper portion of the B scan screen display.

Another component is the damping material, that is attached to the back of the crystal, that can limit the vibration of crystal, thus shortening the pulses.

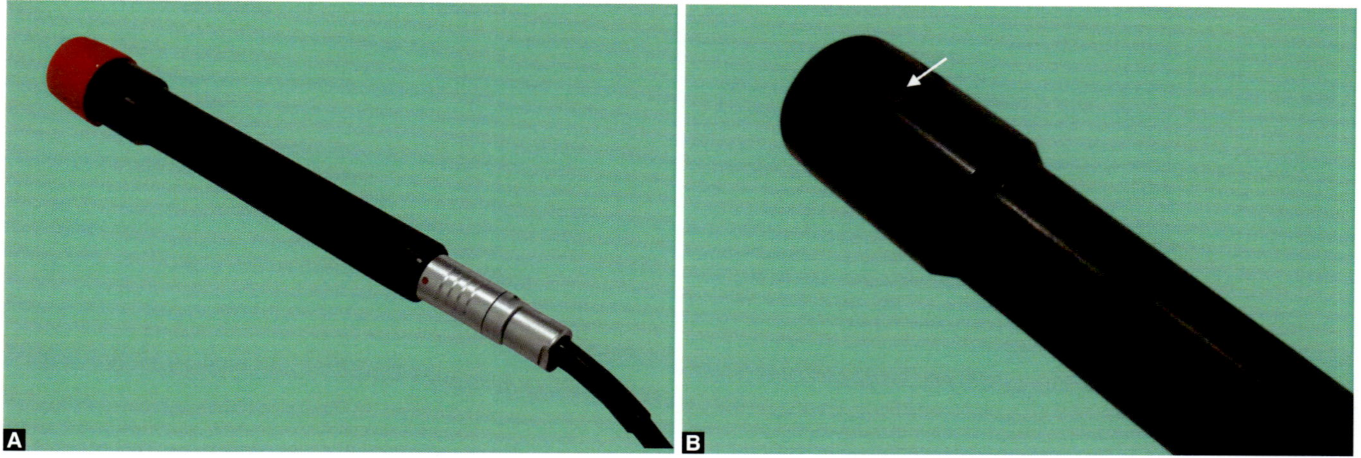

Figs 8.1A and B: 10 MHz transducer for ophthalmic ultrasonography with the marker (white arrow).

Sector Angle of the Transducer

Varies from 45° to 60° which means the area of the eye and orbit that can be imaged on echogram at any one time.

Types of Ultrasound Display System (Figs 8.2A and B)

A Scan

- One-dimensional acoustic display
- Echoes are represented as vertical spikes from a baseline
- Spacing between two spikes indicate distance
- Height of the displayed spikes indicate the strength of the echoes
- Primarily used for measuring axial length.

B Scan

- Two-dimensional (vertical and horizontal) acoustic display
- An echo is represented as a dot on the screen and brightness of the dot indicate strength. Coalescence of multiple dots form a two-dimensional representation of the examined tissue section
- Indicate configuration and location
- B scan transducers operate at 10 MHz frequency
- B scan probe produces multiple slices through a tissue in each second, called frame rate (varies 10–60 frames/second).

Gain

It represents relative units of ultrasound intensity and measured in decibels (db).

Adjusting gain means adjusting the intensity of the returning echo that is displayed on the screen. Higher the gain level, greater the ability of the instrument to display weaker echoes (i.e vitreous opacities). In lower gain, only the stronger echoes will continue to be displayed (i.e retina and sclera).

Examination Techniques

- The patient is in reclined position
- Methylcellulose (a coupling medium) is applied on the face of the B scan probe.
- Examination through open eye (under topical anesthesia)-probe has to place directly over cornea or conjunctiva or through the closed lids (disadvantages are sound attenuation can occur by lid tissue and globe position is not certain).

B Scan Probe Orientation

Transverse, longitudinal and axial.

- In transverse and longitudinal scans, probe is placed on conjunctiva, thus sound beam bypasses the lens, allowing better sound beam penetration
- In axial scan, patient's eye is in primary gaze and probe is placed on the center of the cornea.

Anatomic reference point is optic nerve which is echographically considered as the center of posterior fundus (not macula, which is the true anatomic center)

Diagnostic ophthalmic ultrasonography is most useful in following situations:

- In the presence of opaque ocular media caused by corneal opacities, anterior chamber opacities, cataracts, vitreous hemorrhage, or inflammatory opacities
- Also valuable in the presence of clear media and for evaluation of the iris, lens, ciliary body, and orbital structures.

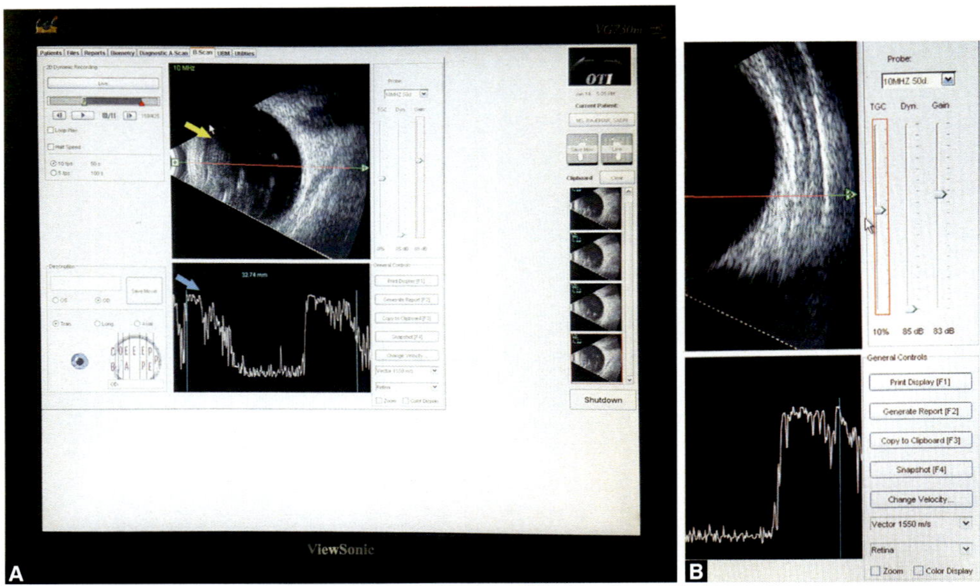

Figs 8.2A and B: (A) Ultrasound display system with B scan (yellow arrow) and A scan (blue arrow); (B) Ultrasound display system with gain column

Characteristic Ultrasonographic Features of Posterior Segment Pathologies

Normal Posterior Segment

Vitreous cavity (Fig. 8.3)

- Clear jelly-like vitreous (in young) produces no echoes
- Scattered vitreous opacities (in aged)—Very low reflectivity.

Asteroid hyalosis (Figs 8.4A and B)

- Typically bright, point-like echo sources on B scan—Diffuse or focal and medium to high reflectivity in A scan which is persisting with low gain also
- An area of clear vitreous is normally present between posterior boundary of opacities and the posterior hyaloid.

Normal vitreous attachments

- Retina—Mainly at macula, periphery and around the blood vessels
- Optic nerve.

Posterior Vitreous Detachment (PVD)

- PVD may occur in the normal aging eye, or it may be associated with vitreous hemorrhage or inflammation
- In a normal eye, PVD manifest as a very thin smooth line on B scan and as a very low-reflective spike on A scan
- When blood or inflammatory debris is layered on the surface of PVD, B scan show thickened line especially inferiorly and posteriorly

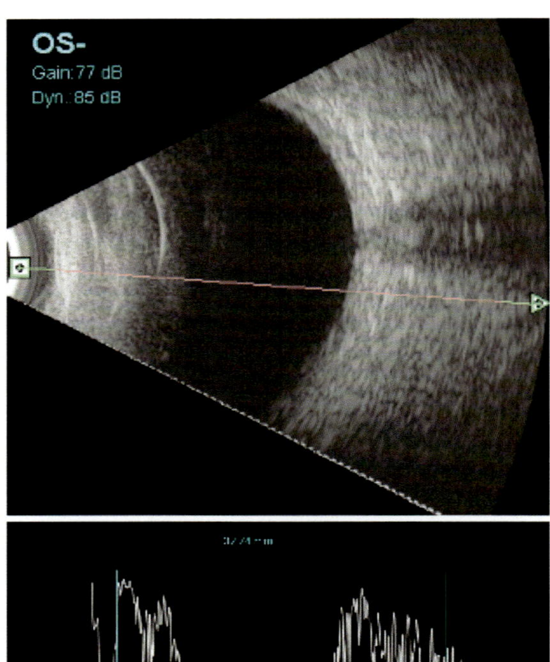

Fig. 8.3: Anechoic vitreous cavity and on retina in a normal posterior segment ultrasound

- In some challenging situations, thick PVD may be difficult to differentiate from retinal detachment.

Kinetic echography shows undulating after movement of PVD. It can be incomplete/focal or complete.

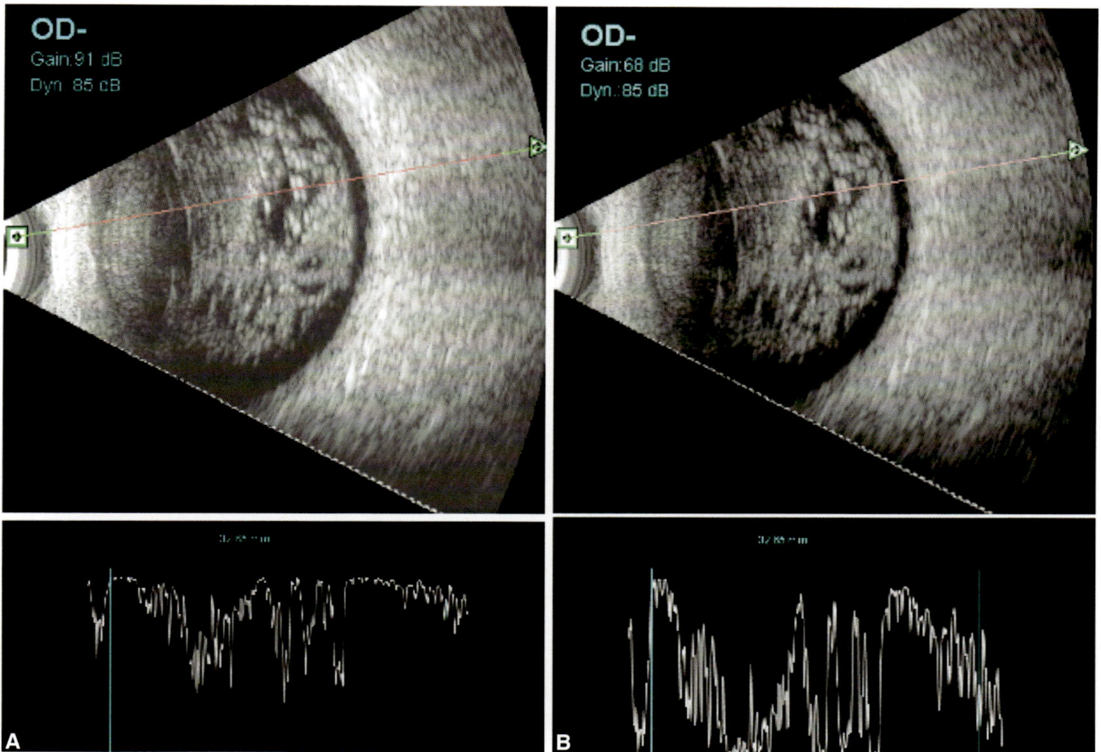

Figs 8.4A and B: USG shows diffusely distributed bright, point-like echoes in B scan with medium to high reflectivity in A scan with high-gain (A) and persistence of moderate to high amplitude spikes in A scan low gain; (B) Suggestive of asteroid hyalosis

When incomplete

- It may attached to the disc (Fig. 8.5)—Funnel-shaped configuration
- It may attach to the areas of neovascularizations
- May be attached to the areas other than optic disc-like at the site of retinal tear or at the site of retinal injury in penetrating trauma or macula (Fig. 8.6).

When complete

Vitreous is completely separated from the optic nerve head and present as Weiss ring. This appears on B scan as two closely packed opacities at the level of PVD (Fig. 8.7).

Vitreous Hemorrhage

- Common etiologies are proliferative diabetic retinopathy, trauma, venous occlusion, wet type of age-related macular degeneration (AMD) and retinal tear
- Ultrasonography is a useful adjunct to clinical examination to assess the density and associated findings of vitreous hemorrhage as well as its etiology.

Fresh Vitreous Hemorrhage (Fig. 8.8)

Dots and short lines on B scan a chain of low amplitude spikes on A scan. More dense hemorrhage appear as greater number of opacities and higher reflectivity.

Old Organized Vitreous Hemorrhage (Fig. 8.9)

- Formation of membranous surfaces results in larger interfaces with higher reflectivity on A scan
- Gravity may cause the layer inferiorly forming a pseudomembrane which sometimes mimic retinal detachment. It can be differentiated from the retinal detachment by noting its thinness superiorly and it's insertion into vitreous gel (not into fundus like partial RD) (Fig. 8.10).

Subhyaloid Hemorrhage (Fig. 8.11)

- Hemorrhage in subhyaloid or subvitreal space can occur with or without vitreous hemorrhage
- Subhyaloid hemorrhage typically does not clot; therefore, it remains low-reflective and mobile, even in long-standing cases
- Multiple low-amplitude spikes on A scan under PVD with medium to high-reflective spikes is the standard picture.

Sometimes cellular component of subhyaloid blood may settle and layer like hyphema in anterior chamber. This appear as dense smooth membrane on B scan, mimicking RD and called 'posterior hyphema'.

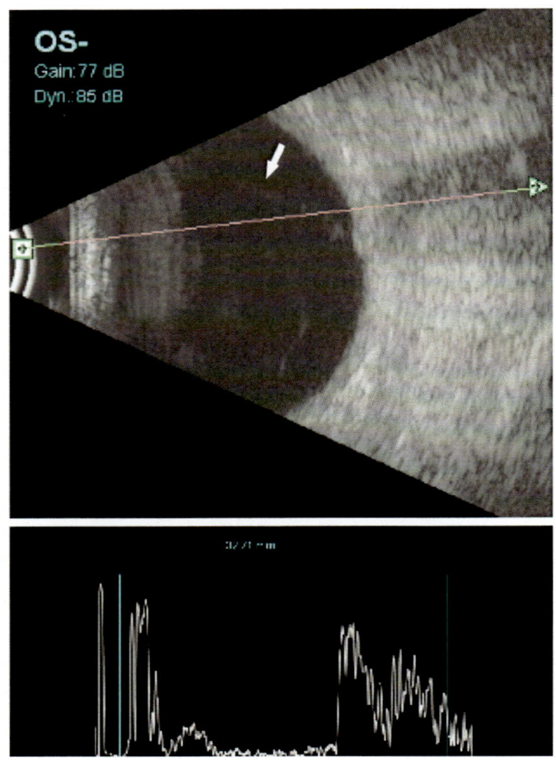

Fig. 8.5: Incomplete PVD with very thin smooth line (white arrow) on B scan and very low reflective spikes on A scan

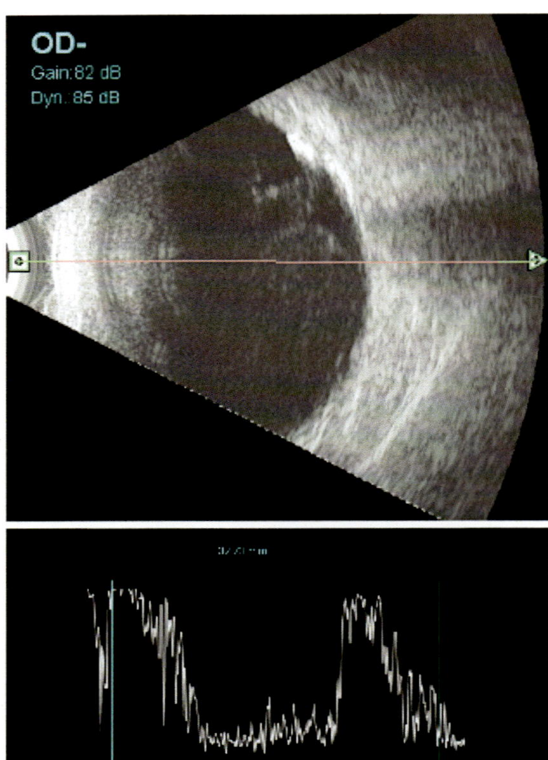

Fig. 8.6: Vitreous hemorrhage with incomplete PVD attached to macula

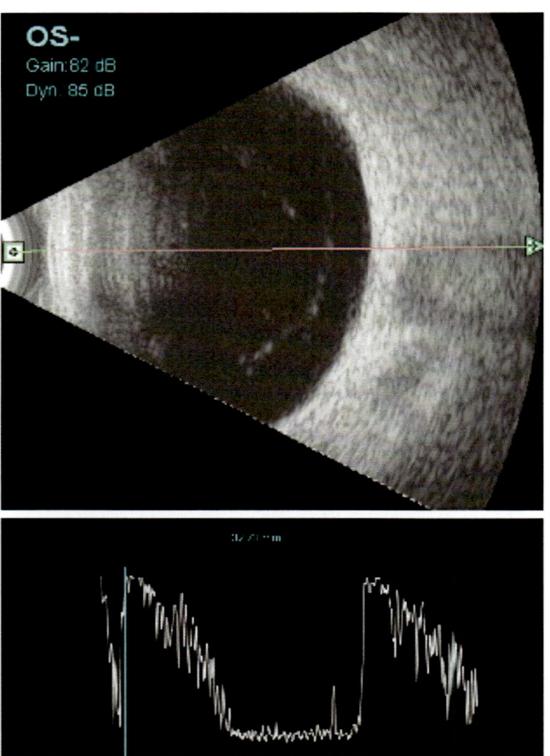

Fig. 8.7: Complete posterior vitreous detachment

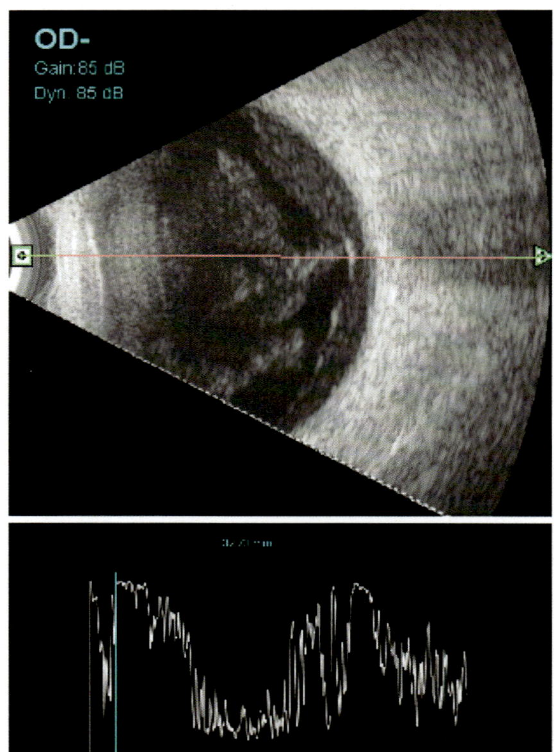

Fig. 8.8: Fresh vitreous hemorrhage—dots and short lines on B scan a chain of low-amplitude spikes on A scan along (vitreous hemorrhage) with a thin membrane (Incomplete PVD) with weak dots underneath it (subhyaloid hemorrhage)

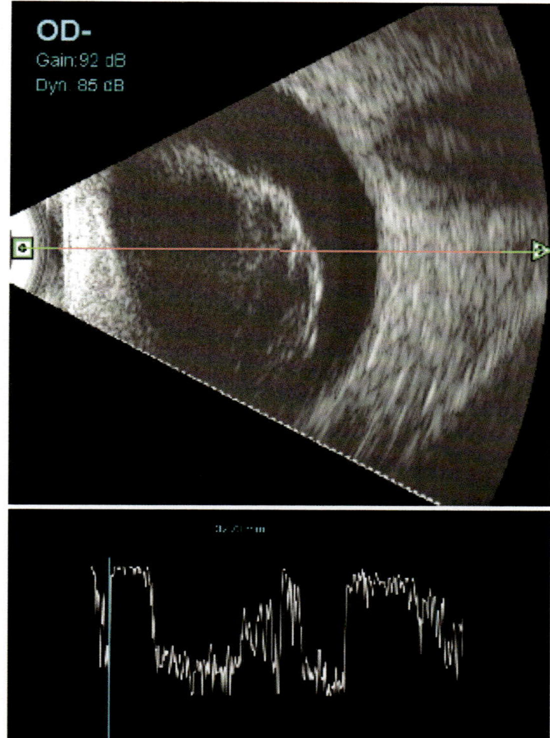

Fig. 8.9: Old vitreous hemorrhage—dots and short lines on B scan a chain of low-amplitude spikes on A scan with complete posterior vitreous detachment

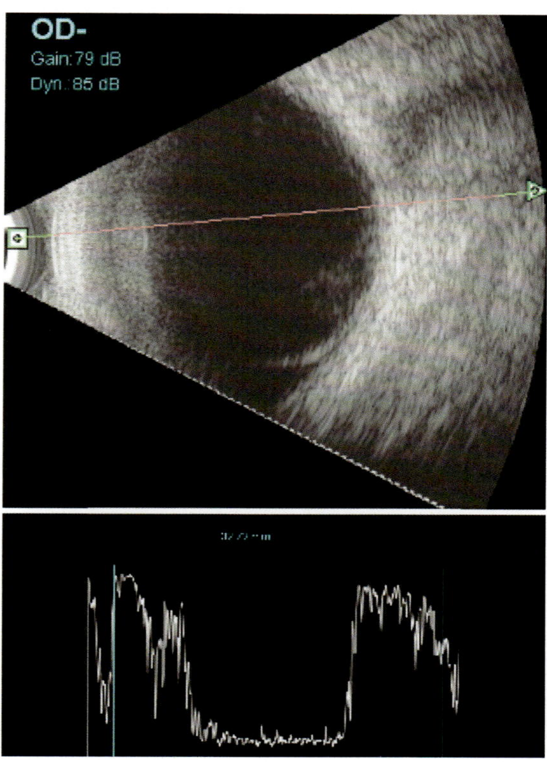

Fig. 8.10: Inferior organized vitreous hemorrhage mimicking retinal detachment

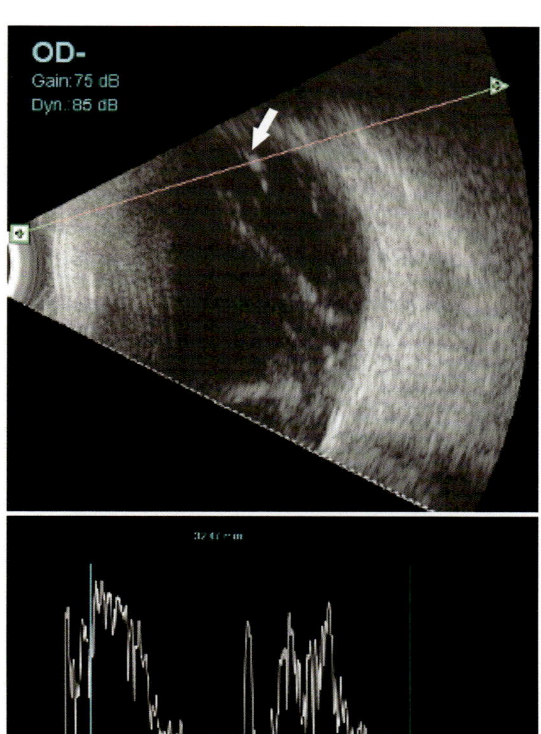

Fig. 8.11: Multiple low-amplitude spikes on A scan under PVD with medium to high-reflective spikes is the standard picture, suggestive of subhyaloid hemorrhage along with vitreous hemorrhage with flap tear (white arrow) at temporal periphery

Subretinal Hemorrhage (Fig. 8.12)

- It typically does not clot.
- Mild subretinal hemorrhage need high-gain setting for detection.

Suprachoroidal Hemorrhage (Figs 8.13 and 8.14)

- It usually produces solid clots
- It may present in single (Fig. 8.13) or multiple quadrants as hemorrhagic choroidal detachments after cataract surgery or after sever trauma with globe rupture
- On B scan, there are large dome shaped membranes can be seen to adhere to one another in the central portion of the eye 360° choroidal detachment sometimes produces appositional configuration, called "kissing choroidals" (Fig. 8.14)
- After a few weeks, many of these choroidal detachment decrease in size, but RDs may become echographically apparent
- Ultrasound helps to determine the timings and site for drainage.

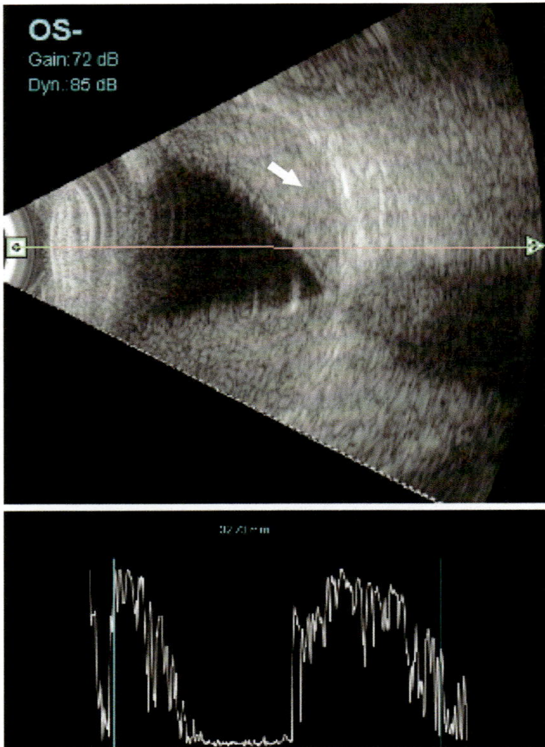

Fig. 8.12: Subretinal thick blood layer (white arrow) with moderate to high-amplitude spikes on A scan

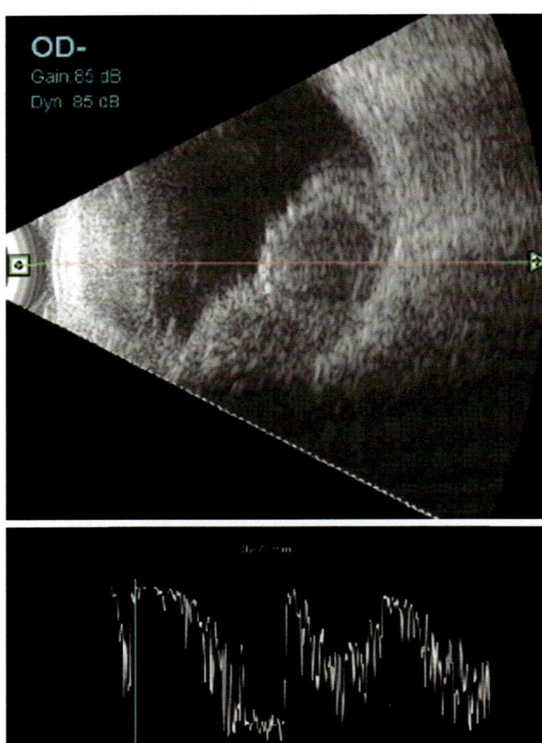

Fig. 8.13: Suprachoroidal hemorrhage with large dome-shaped membranes with high-reflectivity on A scan, confined to one quadrant

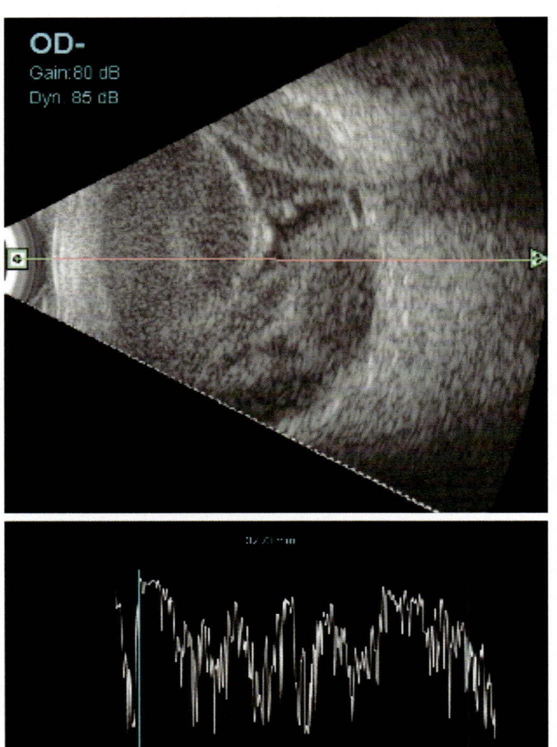

Fig. 8.14: Suprachoroidal hemorrhage with large dome-shaped membranes with high reflectivity on A scan, adhered to one another in the central portion of the eye with an appositional configuration, called "kissing choroidals"

Retinal Detachment

Rhegmatogenous Retinal Detachment

- A bright, somewhat folded membrane on B scan with its insertion at optic disc and ora serrata and highly reflective spike on A scan. When RD is partial, it may not extend to the optic disc or ora serrata (Fig. 8.15). Total retinal detachment shows the attachment at disc and ora serrata (Fig. 8.16)
- RD typically exhibit a tethered, restricted after movement that contrast with the highly mobile, undulating movement of PVD
- PVR changes can be noted as the V-shaped configuration, which indicate old RD (Fig. 8.17)
- Closed funnel RD will be revealed as T-shaped configuration with the stalk attached at the optic nerve head (Fig. 8.18).

Exudative Retinal Detachment

Show greater shifting of the subretinal fluid than do rhegmatogenous RD (Fig. 8.19).

Tractional Retinal Detachment

Tent-like elevated retina with high reflectivity along the attachments of PVD (Fig. 8.20).

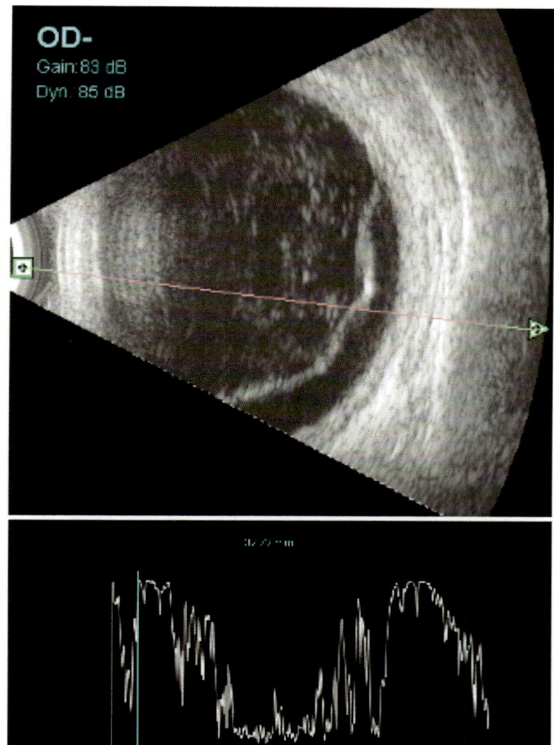

Fig. 8.15: A bright membrane on B scan and moderate to high-amplitude spikes on A scan and from ora serrata it may or may not extend upto optic nerve head, suggestive of partial inferior retinal detachment along with vitreous hemorrhage with low amplitude spikes on A scan

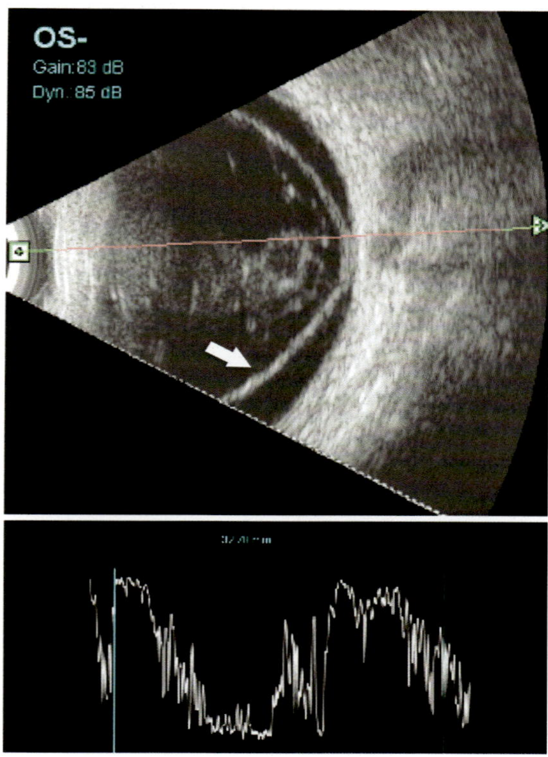

Fig. 8.16: A bright membrane on B scan (white arrow) and moderate to high-reflective spikes on A scan with it's insertions both at optic disc and ora serrata, suggestive of total retinal detachment along with vitreous hemorrhage

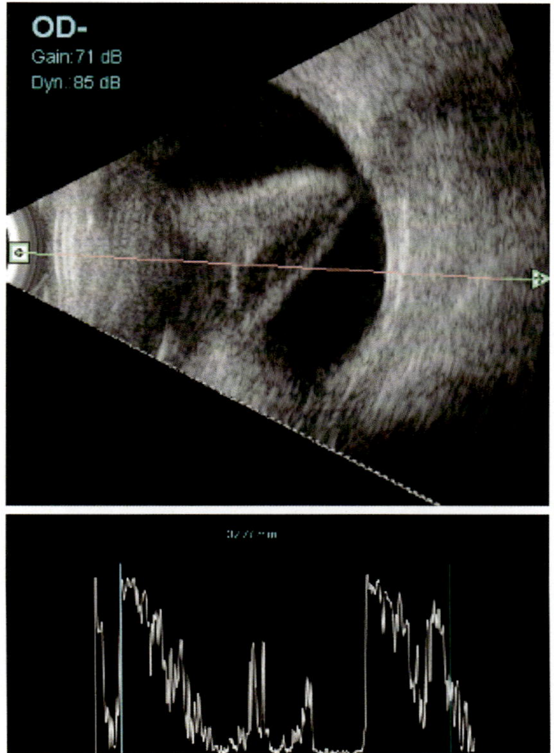

Fig. 8.17: Total old 'V-shaped' retinal detachment with closing funnel PVR

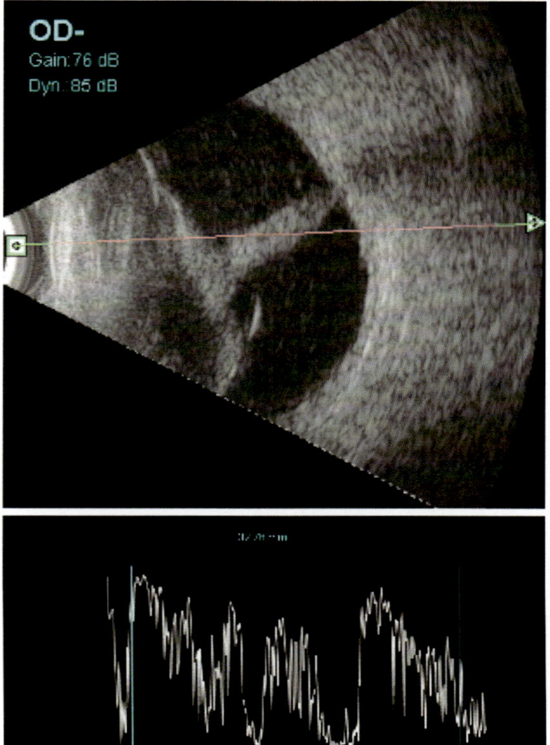

Fig. 8.18: Total old RD with 'T-shaped' closed funnel PVR with thick subretinal fluid with moderately high-amplitude spikes on A scan

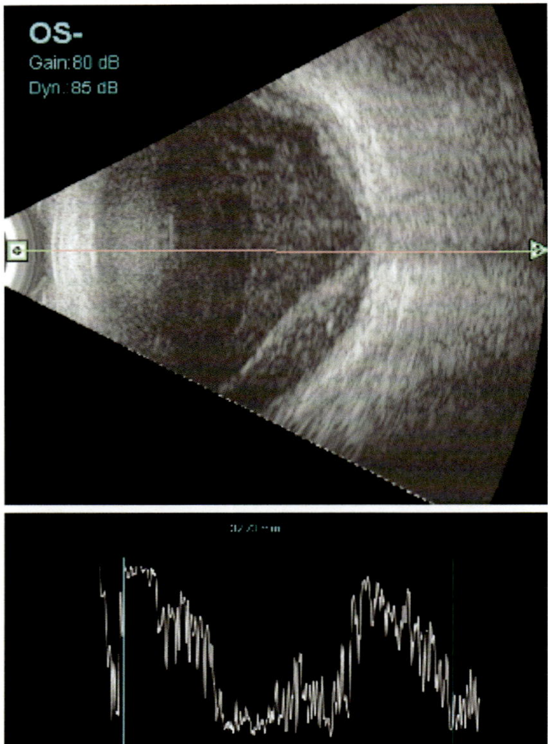

Fig. 8.19: Total exudative retinal detachment with moderate-to-high reflectivity on A scan and thick subretinal shifting fluid with low to medium reflectivity on A scan

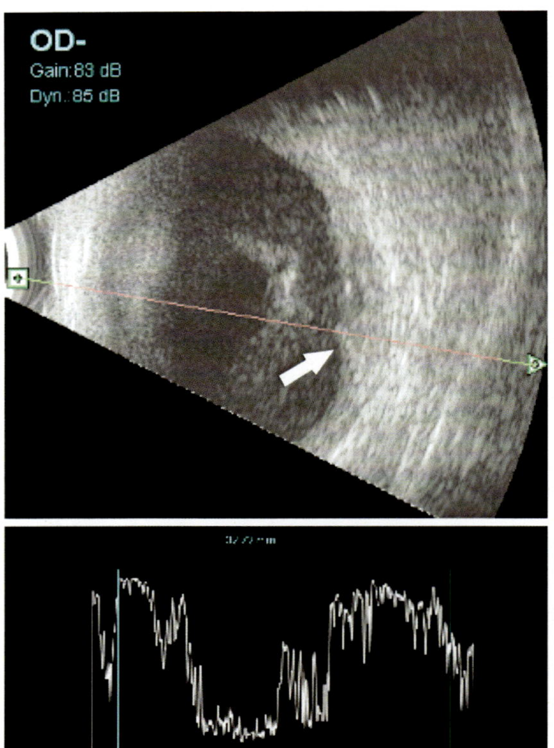

Fig. 8.20: Subhyaloid hemorrhage with 'tent-like' elevated tractional retinal detachment

Retinoschisis (Fig. 8.21)

- Most often in inferotemporal peripheral fundus
- Bilateral
- Smooth, thin, sharply demarcated, dome-shaped non-mobile membrane in B scan
- Nearly 100% high single-peaked spike on A scan
- It differs from RD in its more localized, smooth, thin character and lack of mobility on B scan.

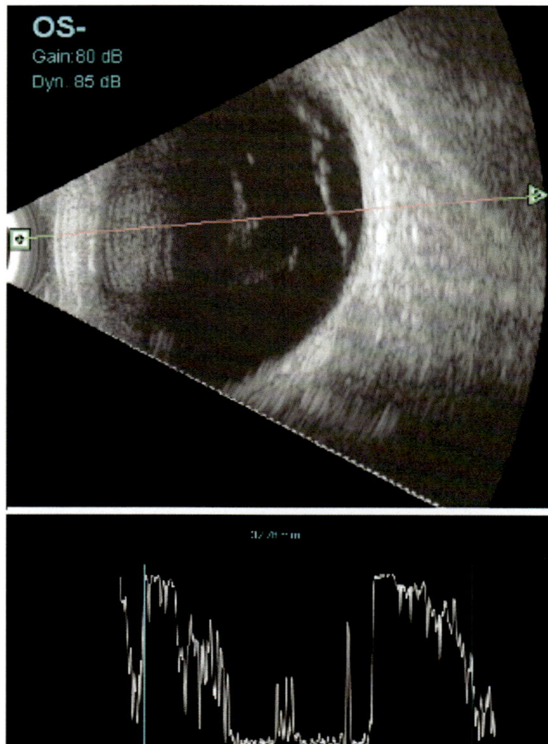

Fig. 8.21: Smooth, thin, sharply demarcated, dome-shaped nonmobile membrane in B scan with nearly 100% high single-peaked spike on A scan

Choroidal Coloboma

A full thickness defect in retinochoroidal layer with intact scleral coat, especially confined inferiorly (Fig. 8.22). It may be associated retinal detachment (Fig. 8.23).

Dislocated Crystalline Lens

- Normal lens appears as a very well outlined, oval, echo lucent structure on B scan and very low internal reflectivity on A scan with distinct echoes from anterior and posterior capsules. The cataractous lens exhibits varying degrees of echo density on B scan and internal spikes of differing amplitude on A scan
- Dislocated cataractous lens during surgery generally gives irregular shape (oval if nucleus) swollen lens with

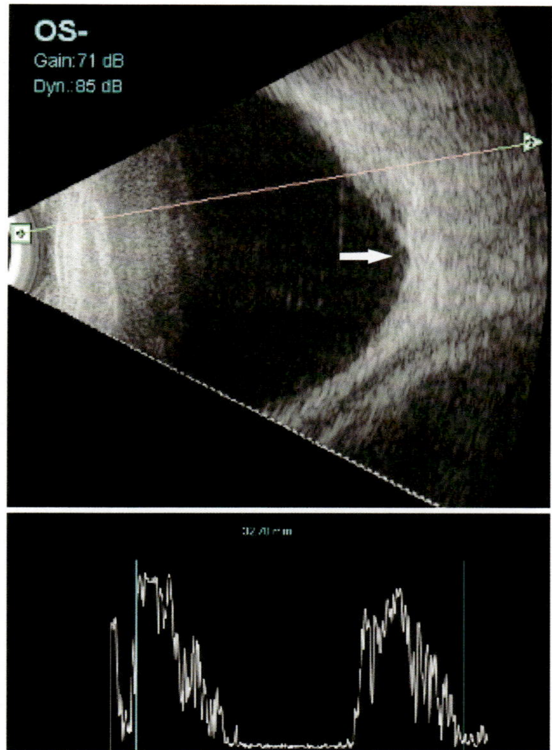

Fig. 8.22: Retinochoroidal coloboma (white arrow)

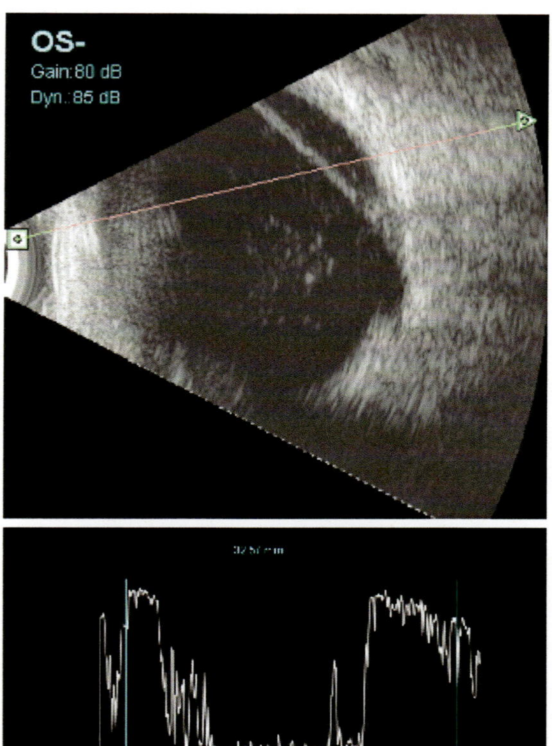

Fig. 8.23: Choroidal coloboma with retinal detachment

varying degrees of echo density on B scan (depending on the density of cataract) with moderate-to-high amplitude spikes on A scan (Figs 8.24 to 8.26).

Dislocated Intraocular Lens (IOL) (Fig. 8.27)

- It appears as a large intraocular foreign body like structure inside the vitreous cavity
- Bright echoes in B scan and moderate-to-high amplitude spikes in A scan from optic and haptics
- Dislocated IOL in anterior vitreous and a normally placed posterior chamber IOL will produces multiple signals that can hinder visualization of the vitreous cavity. Reverberations in B scan can occur because some of sound energy passes back to the transducer, producing a series of echo signals of decreasing amplitude that appear to the right of the IOL echo
- There is shadowing effect of IOL when it is over the surface of retina.

Retained Intraocular Foreign Body (RIOFB)

Metallic RIOFB (Fig. 8.28)

- Very echo dense signal that persists at low gain settings in B scan

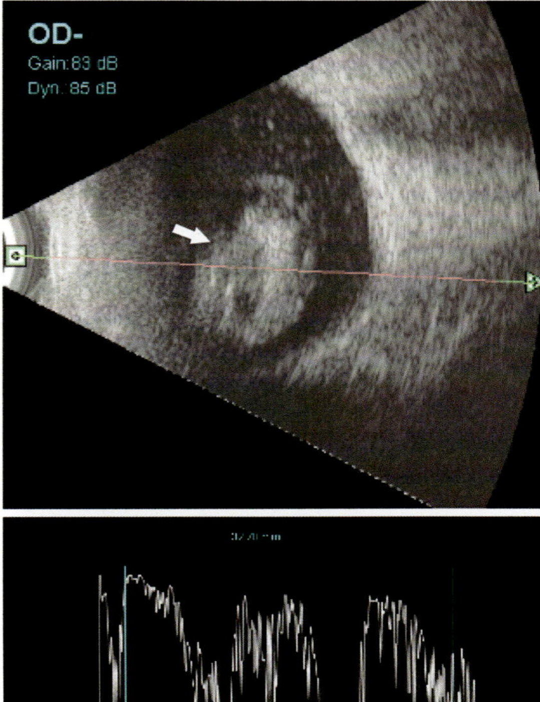

Fig. 8.24: Oval-shaped dropped swollen intravitreal nucleus with varying degrees of echo density on B scan (white arrow) with moderate-to-high amplitude spikes on A scan

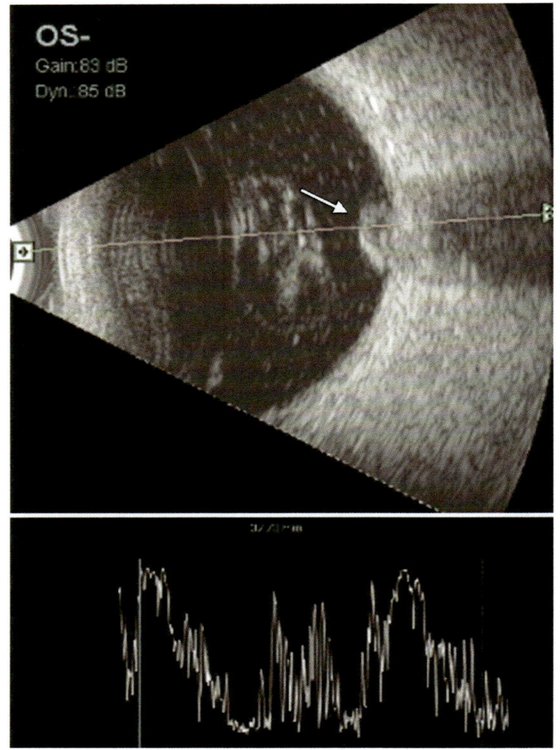

Fig. 8.25: Dropped epinuclear fragment (white arrow) with lens cortex

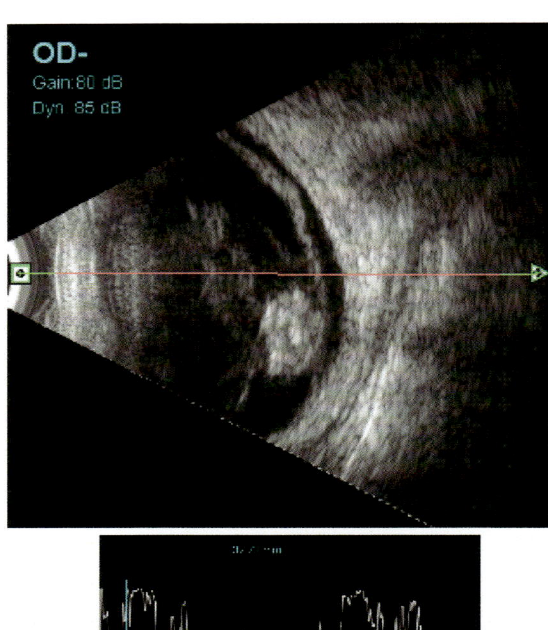

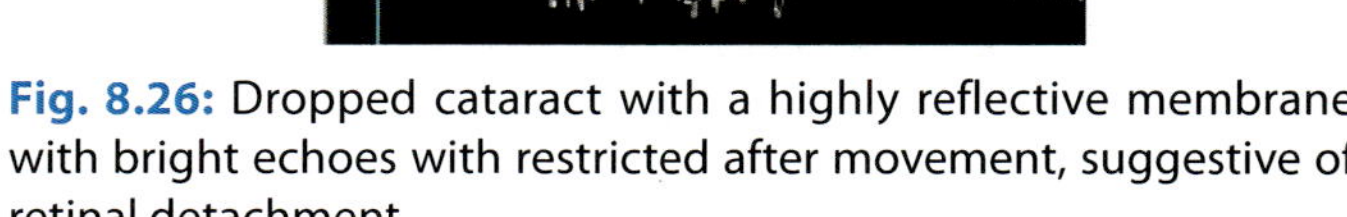

Fig. 8.26: Dropped cataract with a highly reflective membrane with bright echoes with restricted after movement, suggestive of retinal detachment

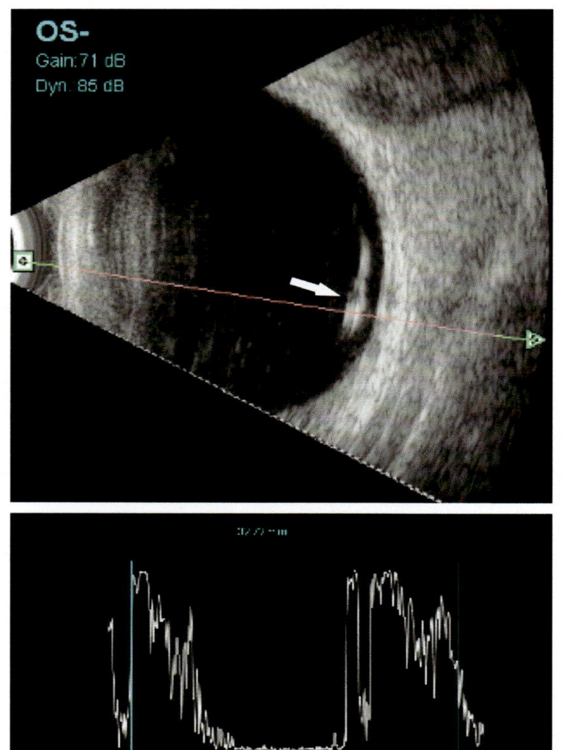

Fig. 8.27: Dropped IOL with bright echoes on B scan (white arrow) and high amplitude spikes on A scan

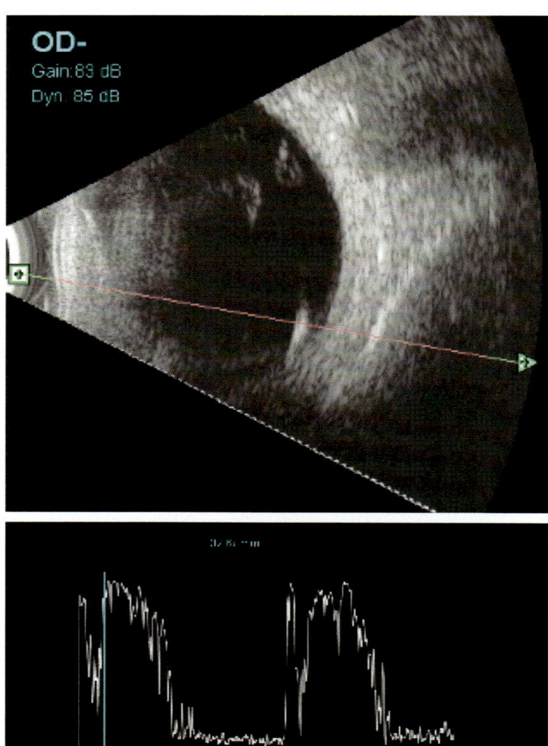

Fig. 8.28: Retained intraocular foreign body with echo dense signal embedded in inferior retina with vitreous hemorrhage

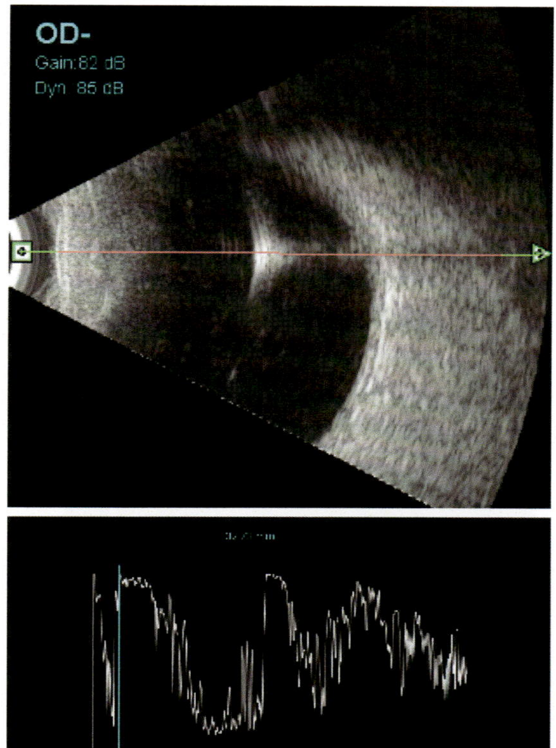

Fig. 8.29: Presence of glass RIOFB (for more than 11 years) intravitreally with very echo dense signal on B scan without any reaction

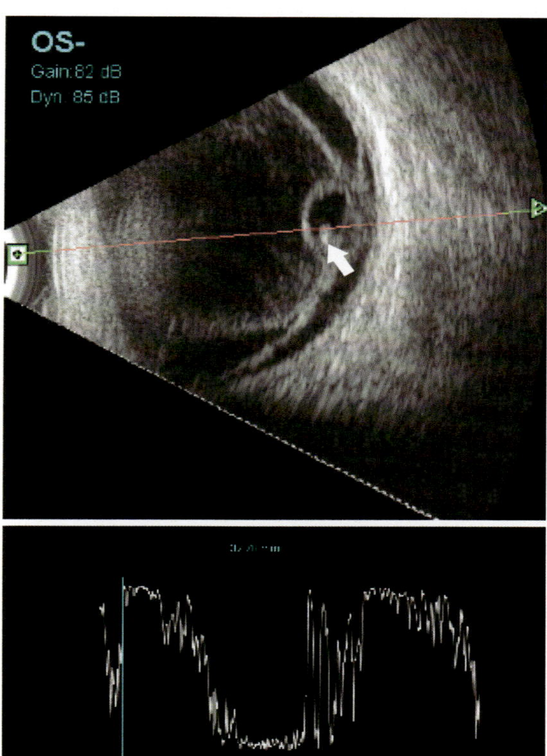

Fig. 8.30: Subretinal cysticercosis with scolex with old retinal detachment

- Marked shadowing of ocular and orbital structure just posterior to the RIOFB
- Very high reflectivity on A scan.

Spherical RIOFB

When sound waves pass through a spherical metallic RIOFB (like gunshot pellet), a portion of the sound waves reverberates within the objects. Reverberations in B scan can occur because some of sound energy passes back to the transducer, producing a series of echo signals of decreasing amplitude that appear to the right of the RIOFB echo.

Glass RIOFB

In most cases, glass enters in the eye as silver. If sound beam strikes long smooth surface of glass silver obliquely, the sound is reflected away from the probe, resulting in a weak echo that can be mistaken as small RIOFB. But if sound beam strikes perpendicularly, then very echo dense signal will be produced (Fig. 8.29).

Wood and vegetable materials—Initially RIOFBs are highly reflective, but over time their reflectivity decreases.

Intraocular (Intravitreal/Subretinal) Cyst

Cysticercosis (Fig. 8.30)

- One or multiple well-outlined, oval-shaped cysts located within vitreous cavity and/or subretinal space
- The scolex appears as a very highly reflective echo dense nodule attached to the inner wall of the cyst
- May show movement during kinetic evaluation.

Endophthalmitis (Fig. 8.31)

Endophthalmitis with dense vitreous exudates with low to moderate amplitude spikes on A scan. In chronic case, vitreous membranes can form.

Postsurgical Findings

Scleral Buckle (Fig. 8.32)

- Produces scleral indentation
- A broad solid silicone buckle have a very highly reflective surface that is indistinguishable from the sclera
- Produces sound attenuation and orbital shadowing.

Vitreous Shirt (Fig. 8.33)

- Postoperative peripheral residual vitreous skirt often can be confused with peripheral RD

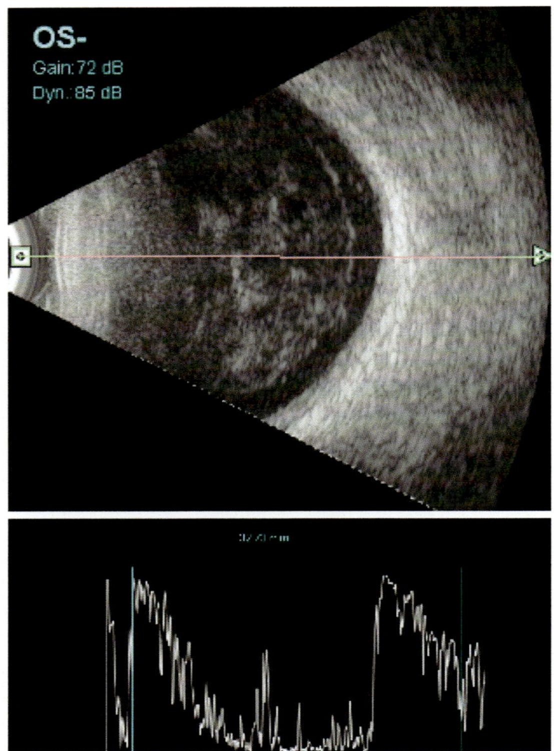

Fig. 8.31: Postoperative endophthalmitis with dense vitreous exudates with low to moderate amplitude spikes on A scan

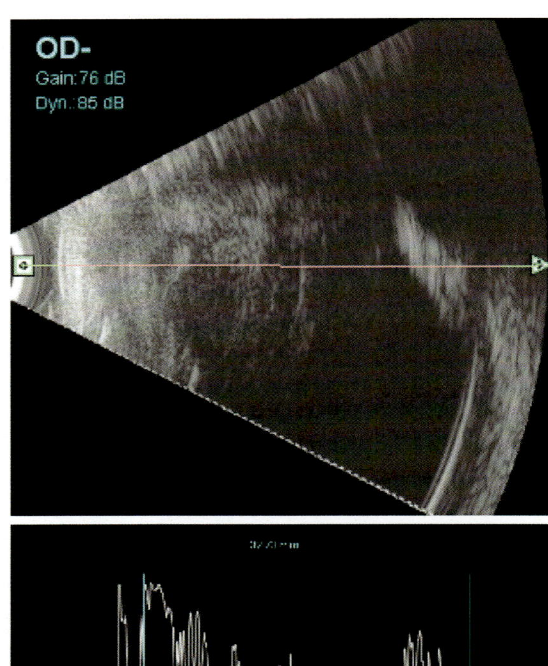

Fig. 8.32: Buckle shadow in a silicone oil filled eye

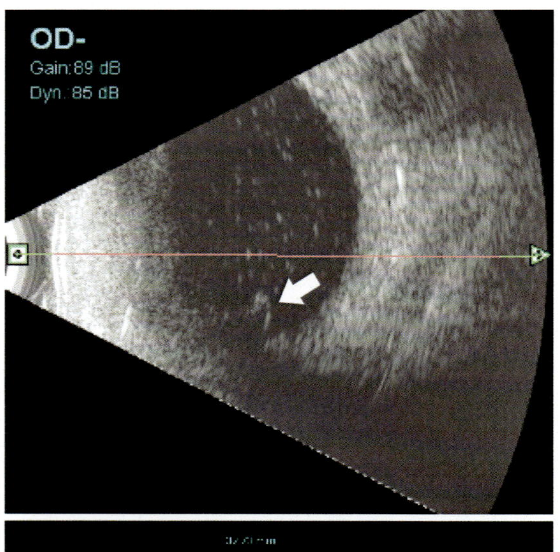

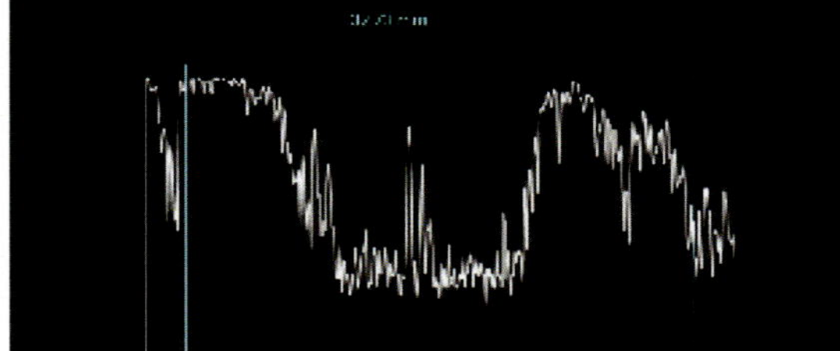

Fig. 8.33: Postvitrectomy peripheral uncut vitreous (white arrow)

- A transverse B scan through the far periphery of the globe typically shows circumferential configuration of the vitreous skirt.

Postoperative Vitreous Hemorrhage (Fig. 8.34)

Postoperative diffuse vitreous hemorrhage produces very weak echoes, because blood remains in a liquified state and does not in clotted state as it does in vitreous gel.

Intraocular Gas/Air (Fig. 8.35)

- Large gas/air bubble in the vitreous cavity hinder echo graphic examination of the posterior segment
- Gas or air bubble strongly reflects the sound waves and thus prevents imaging of any structure posterior to the bubble
- Small gas does not hinder the posterior segment evaluation
- Multiple signals typically present
- Sometimes, it is necessary to have the patient in upright or with head tilt to shift the air/gas bubble from the central axis.

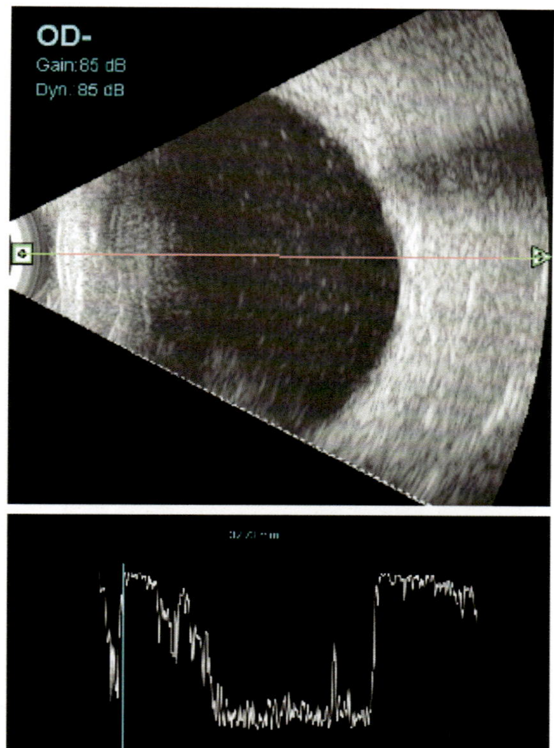

Fig. 8.34: Postoperative intravitreal dispersed dot-like echoes with low-amplitude spikes suggestive of recurrent vitreous hemorrhage

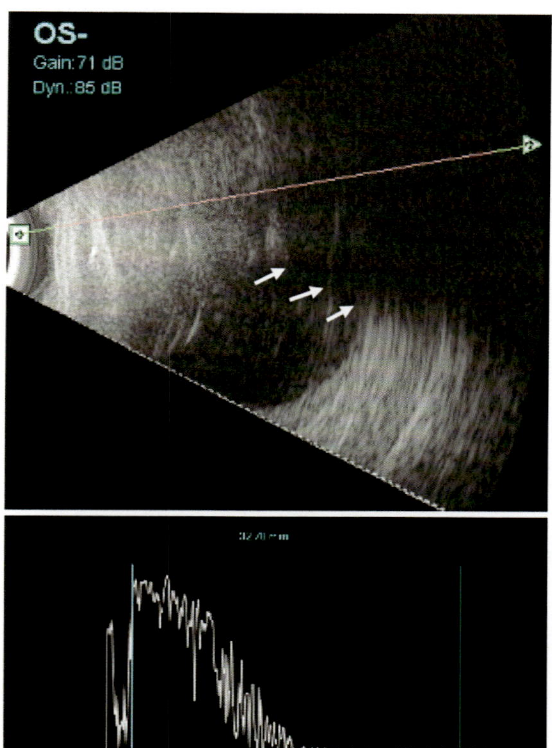

Fig. 8.35: Gas-filled eye creating shadowing effects (white arrows)

Residual PFCL Bubble (Figs 8.36 and 8.37)

Residual PFCL bubble appear as small bright echoes followed by a chain of multiple signals as these bubbles have a tendency to adhere to the retinal surface.

Intravitreal Silicone Oil (Figs 8.38 and 8.39)

- The sound velocity of silicone oil is much slower than that of normal ocular tissue. Thus, silicone oil-filled eyes appear typically larger than normal
- Detection of RD in a silicone oil-filled eye is quiet difficult.

Macular Lesions

Macular Edema (Fig. 8.40)

- Elevated dome-shaped lesion temporal to the optic nerve shadow
- Small elevation does not show any internal reflectivity
- Moderately elevated lesion show medium-to-high internal reflectivity
- Differential diagnosis are AMD, epiretinal membrane, macular hole or small macular tumor-like choroidal hemangioma, nevus, melanoma or metastasis.

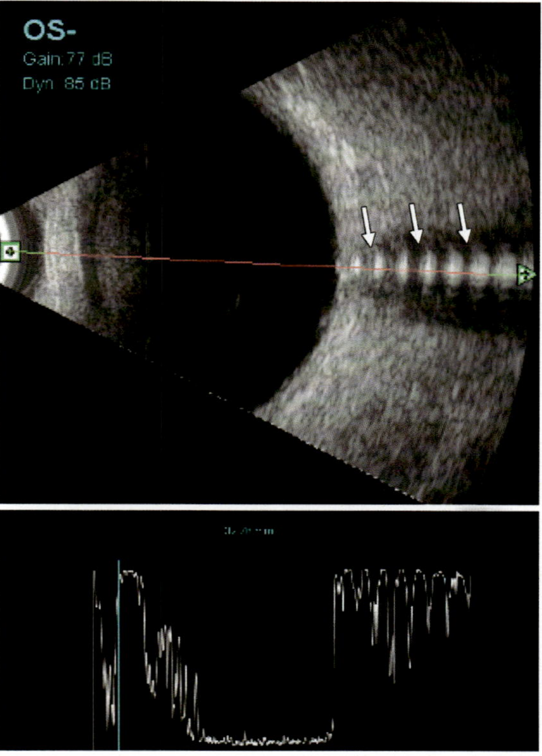

Fig. 8.36: Preretinal PFCL bubble over the disc creating series of multiple shadowing effect posterior to the bubble (white arrows)

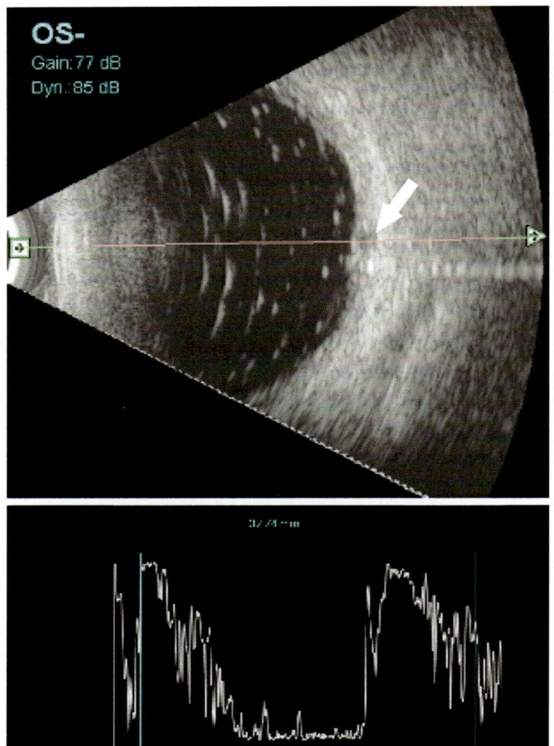

Fig. 8.37: Submacular PFCL bubble (white arrow) creating series of multiple shadowing effects posterior to the bubble after silicone oil removal

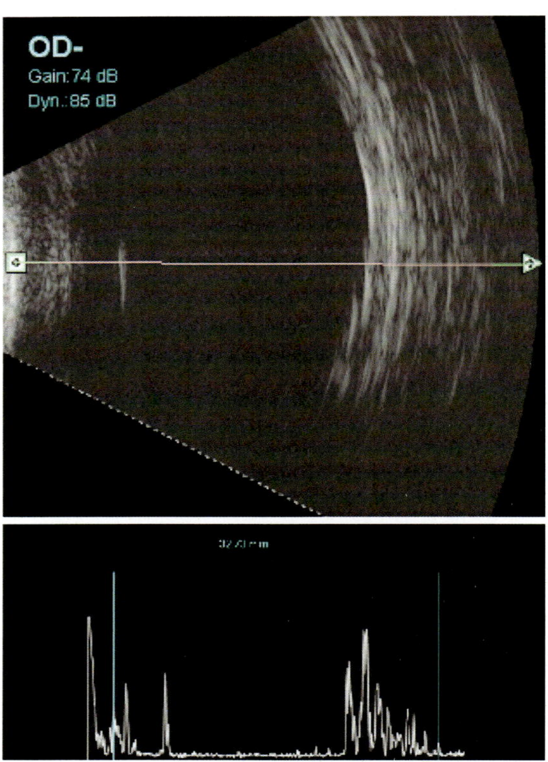

Fig. 8.38: A silicone oil-filled eye (retina on) appeared to be large sized eyeball

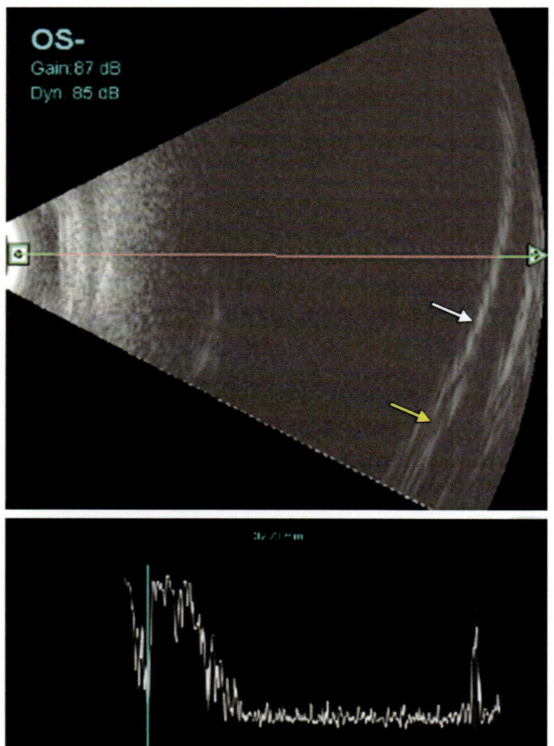

Fig. 8.39: A silicone oil-filled eye with retinal detachment (white arrow) with silicone oil reflection (yellow arrow)

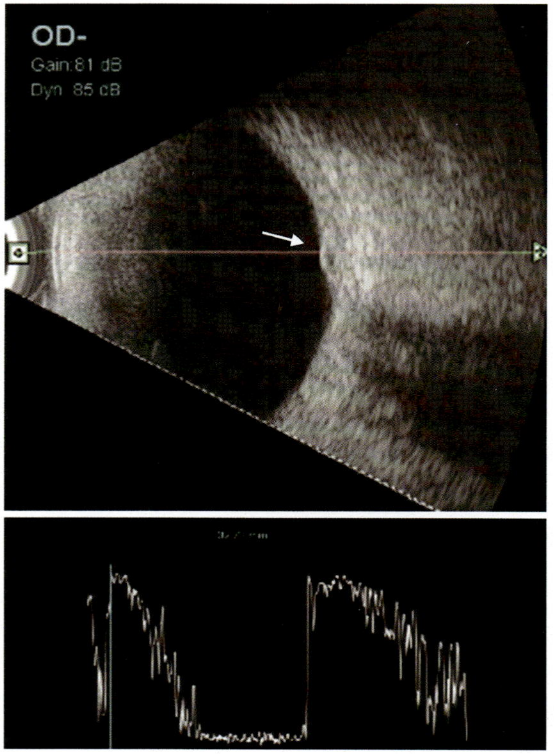

Fig. 8.40: Elevated lesion at macula (white arrow) suggestive of presence of macular edema

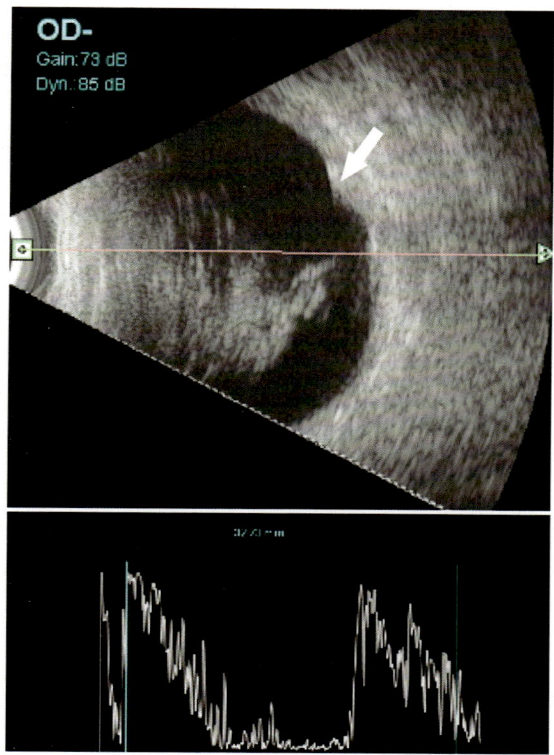

Fig. 8.41: Submacular disciform scar (white arrow) with high internal reflectivity with old vitreous hemorrhage

Fig. 8.42: Submacular hemorrhagic retinal pigment epithelial detachment with smooth, dome-shaped configuration in B scan with thin highly reflective surface spikes and very moderate-to- high internal reflectivity on A scan

AMD Lesions

a. Disciform scar (Fig. 8.41)—Generally mild-to-moderately elevated dome-shaped heterogenous lesion on B scan and few highly reflective spikes on A scan

b. Submacular hemorrhagic retinal pigment epithelial detachment (Fig. 8.42)—Smooth, dome-shaped configuration in B scan with thin highly reflective surface spikes and very low internal reflectivity on A scan.

Kindly scan the QR code below to access the online Video.

CHAPTER 9

Steps of Making Sutureless Sclerotomy Wound

Length of Scleral Entry Wounds

Vitreoretinal interventions by 20G, length of scleral entry wound—0.9 mm.

- In MIVS by 23G—The length of each scleral entry wound is 0.7 mm
- In MIVS by 25G or 25G+—The length of each scleral entry wound is 0.5 mm
- In MIVS by 27G—The length of each scleral entry wound are 20% smaller than 25G, i.e. 0.4 mm.

Scleral ports in phakic cases, it is 4 mm, for pseudophakic eyes 3.5 mm and for aphakic eyes, it should be 3 mm away from the limbus (Fig. 9.1).

Superior two pars plana ports are to be made at superotemporal and superonasal quadrant with 160° angle between each other (Fig. 9.2).

Wound Construction *(Video 1, Chapter 9)*

- Scleral fibers are arranged in a concentric manner around the limbus
- In case of oblique perpendicular entry, scleral tunnel will cut these concentric fibers and produce less stable wound
- But if we make oblique parallel entry, scleral tunnel will not cut these concentric scleral fibers; thereby the scleral wound will be resistant to stretching and tearing (Fig. 9.3A)
- Fixation of globe is necessary before insertion of trocar-cannula
- Then conjunctival displacement is necessary prior to insertion of trocar-cannula (Fig. 9.3B). Holding anterior to the site of incision helps in exerting the counter pressure while introducing the trocar and prevents the torsion of the globe. Alternatively, a pressure plate can be used
- The ideal way is oblique insertion of trocar-cannula system through the sclera at 15–30° angle or even less (Fig. 9.3C) until bevel of the trocar blade is no longer visible, then redirect trocar-cannula (Fig. 9.3D) towards the center of the vitreous cavity or towards the optic disc (Fig. 9.3E). This is the accepted one-step entry. Both 23G and 25G trocar-cannula system are to be introduced by this one-step entry
- For more smaller gauge like 27-gauge, both oblique as well as direct perpendicular one-step entry is acceptable (Fig. 9.4)
- Tip of infusion cannula is to be checked before turning infusion on (Fig. 9.5).

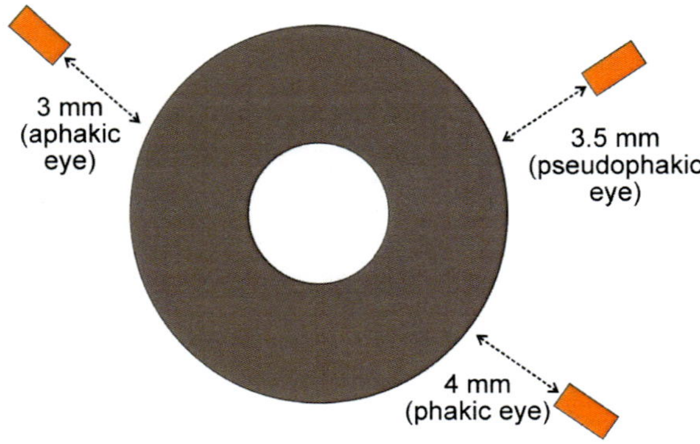

Fig. 9.1: Distance of scleral ports from limbus in phakic, pseudophakic and aphakic eyes

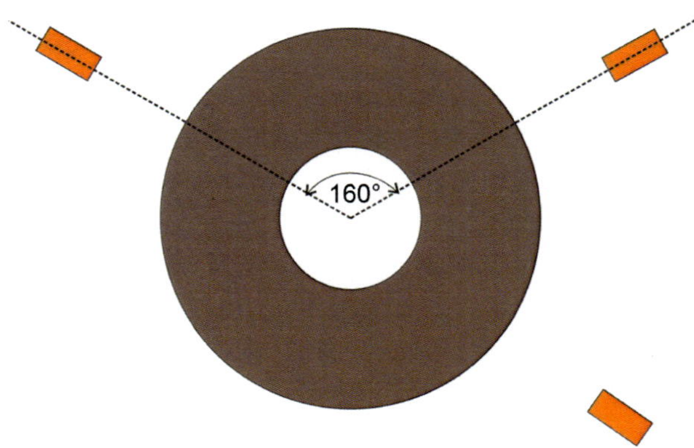

Fig. 9.2: Angle between the two superior scleral ports

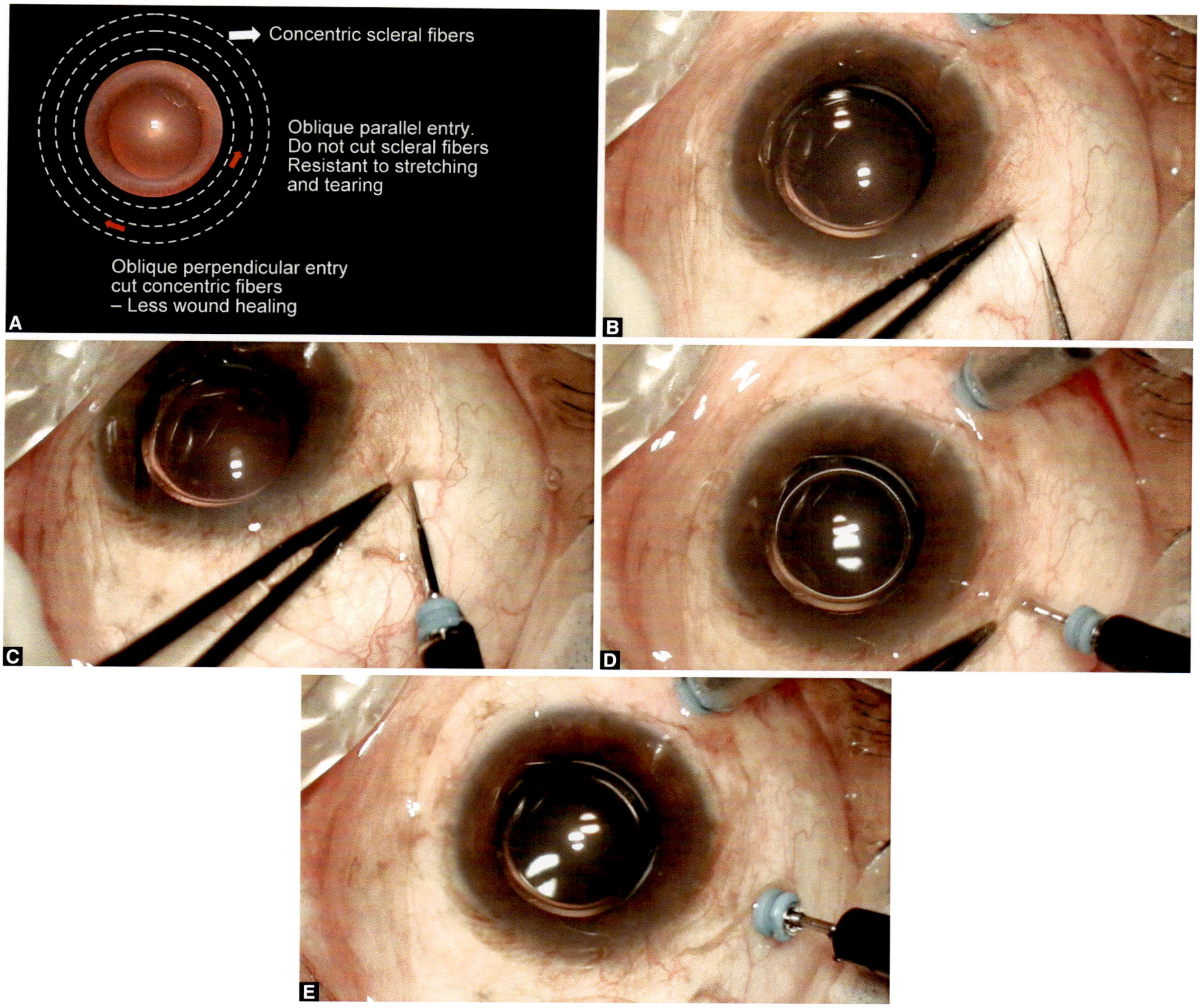

Figs 9.3A to E: Steps of making 25G ports with 25G trocar-cannula

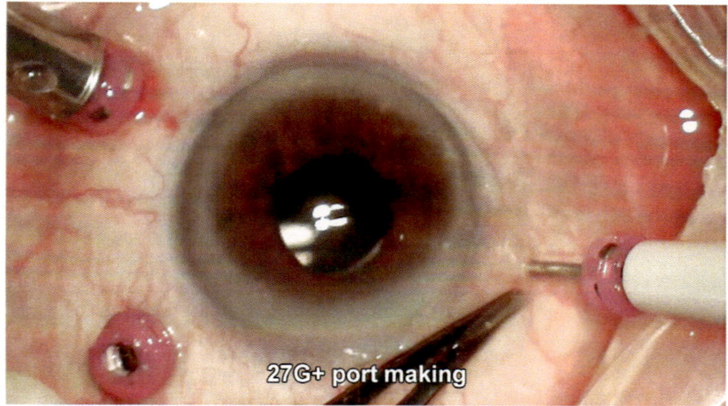

Fig. 9.4: Direct perpendicular one-step entry in 27G vitrectomy system

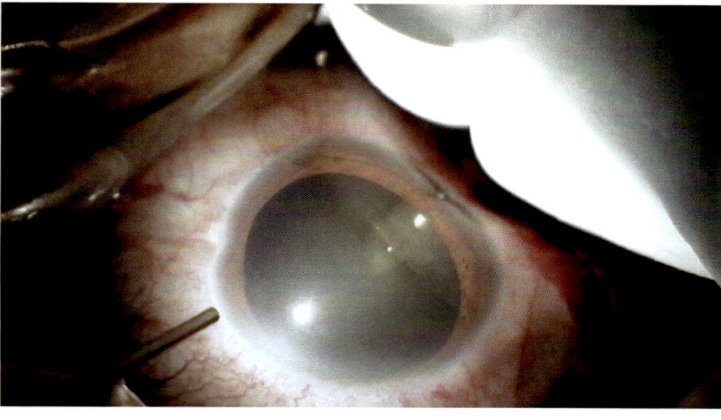

Fig. 9.5: Tip of infusion cannula is to be checked before turning infusion on

Wound Closure

- It is achieved by sideway wound apposition by edematous scleral fibers (Fig. 9.6)
- The aim is to collapse the open scleral tunnel. This can be achieved by externally exerting pressure over the outer lip, or internally by exerting pressure from inside by air or gas or silicone oil (Figs 9.7A to C).
- Gentle massage over the scleral ports with a blunt tip instrument for a few seconds are necessary for proper closure of ports (Fig. 9.8).
- If we consider the scleral tunnel architecture, short length scleral tunnel will produce relatively unstable valve action.
- When angle of entry is 45°, the length of scleral tunnel is 1.154 mm, considering scleral thickness 1 mm (Fig. 9.9A).
- But when the angle of entry is reduced to 30°, the length of scleral tunnel will be increased to 1.414 mm (Fig. 9.9B)
- This longer length scleral tunnel will exert relatively stable valve action. So by reducing angle of entry 15°, tunnel length is increased by 30%.

Cannulas should be blocked by plug before removal. As because, there is chance of vitreous incarceration inside the hollow cannula. And a plugged cannula will keep vitreous fibrils away (Fig. 9.10).

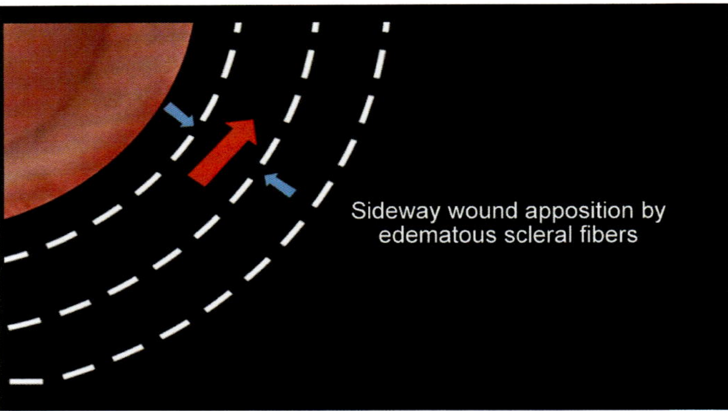

Fig. 9.6: Wound closure by side way apposition of edematous scleral fibers after removal of cannula

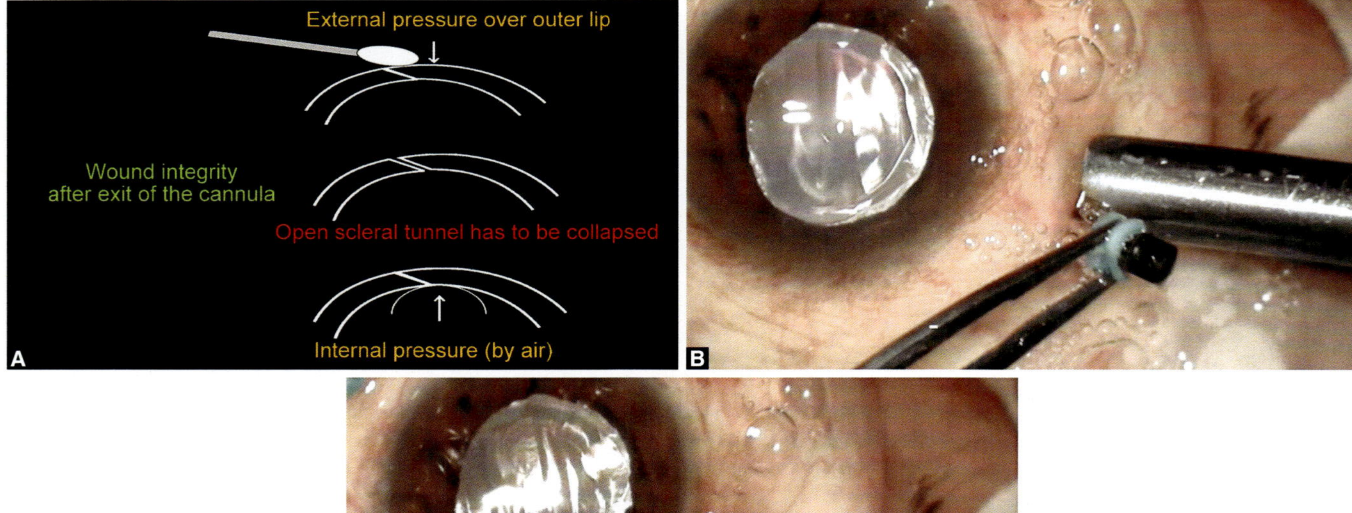

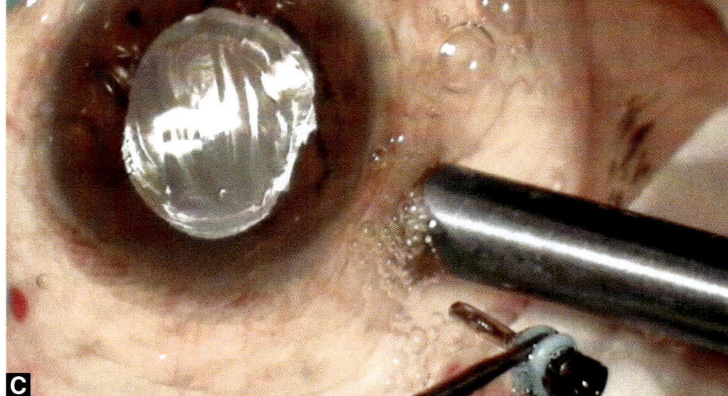

Figs 9.7A to C: Collapse of the open scleral tunnel by externally exerting pressure over the outer lip, or internally by exerting pressure from inside by air or gas or silicone oil

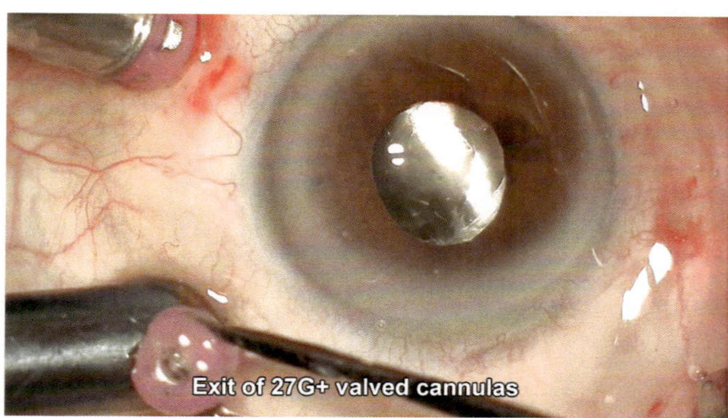

Fig. 9.8: Closure of ports by gentle massage over the scleral ports

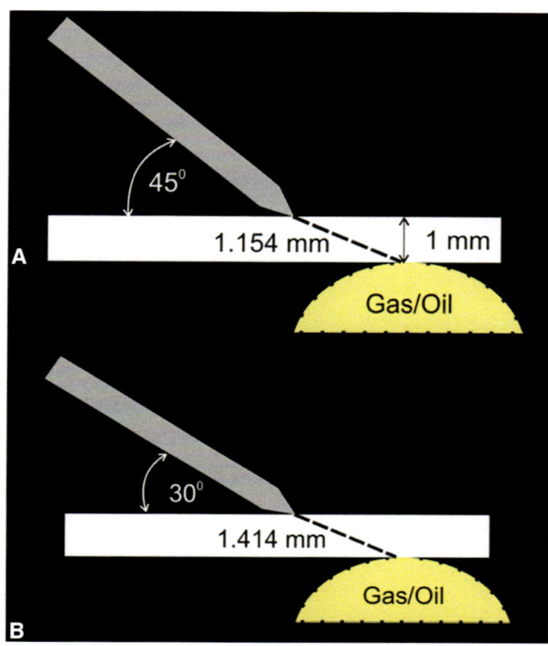

Figs 9.9A and B: Length of scleral tunnel is directly proportional to the stability of the wound

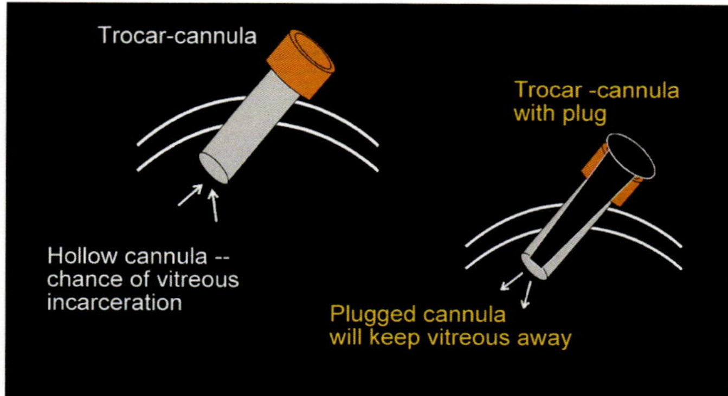

Fig. 9.10: Cannulas should be blocked by plug

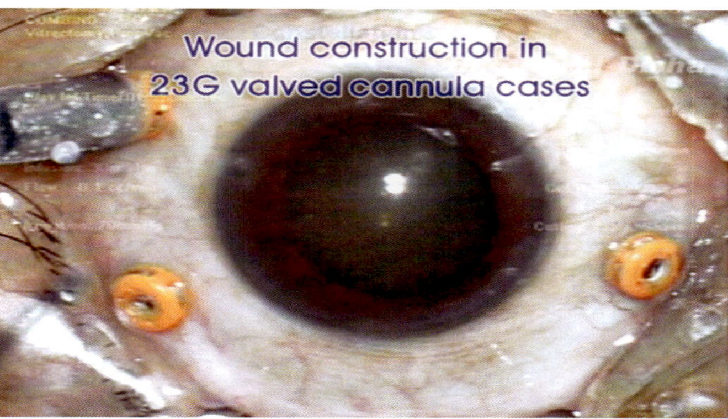

Fig. 9.11: Surgery with 23G valved cannulas

Ensure Wound Integrity

Ensure the wound integrity by checking any wound leak. Valved cannula will produce true closed eye environment at all the time during surgery without any undue fluid leakages through the ports at the time of surgery (Fig. 9.11).

Kindly scan the QR code below to access the online Video.

CHAPTER 10

Vitrectomy with Recent Developments

ANIMATION FOR VITRECTOMY *(VIDEO 1, CHAPTER 10)*

As the cutter is cutting the vitreous fibrils and aspirating it through the same cutter port, the whole vitreous cavity should be replaced by balanced salt solution plus (BSS plus, enriched with customized ingredients), coming through the infusion cannula. This whole procedure should be under direct visualization by the endoilluminator (Fig. 10.1A). This is basic of three port pars plana vitrectomy. One has to follow the shadow of cutter to avoid retina touch (Fig. 10.1B).

STEPS OF VITRECTOMY IN VITREOUS HEMORRHAGE *(VIDEO 2, CHAPTER 10)*

For standard three port vitrectomy, a 4 mm infusion cannula is placed through a sclerotomy located 3.5 mm behind the limbus.

It is important to visualize the tip of the cannula in the vitreous cavity before turning on the infusion.

1. *Anterior vitrectomy and core/mid vitrectomy:* Both anterior and core vitrectomy are to be completed with high suction (around 200–400 mm Hg) and low cutting rate (around 4000 cpm) for fast removal of vitreous (Fig. 10.1C). One should be careful with posterior lens capsule in phakic cases to avoid lens touch.
2. *Intravitreal applications of triamcinolone acetonide (TA) particles:* This is important to stain mostly invisible residual vitreous as well as posterior vitreous cortex.
3. *Posterior Vitrectomy with PVD induction:* The process of lifting up of posterior hyaloid from the retinal surface is called induction of posterior vitreous detachment. TA-stained posterior hyaloid face is to be removed to gain access to the retinal surface. It can be accomplished in following ways:
   - PVD induction with suction of cutter with accelerated suction (from 200 to maximum 600 mm Hg) from the optic disc margin or temporal to macula or nasal to the disc (Fig. 10.1D).
   - PVD induction with silicone-tipped backflush needle to lift up posterior hyaloid face passively from the retinal surface to release its macular attachments.
4. *Peripheral vitrectomy:* It should be always done keeping the low suction and maximum cutting rate (shave mode) (Fig. 10.1E).
5. Free flow of fluid indicate completion of vitrectomy (Fig. 10.1F).
6. *Vitreous base excision:* It should be done by external scleral depression by a blunt-tipped depressor or cotton-tip applicator (Fig. 10.1G).
7. Endolaser around the cauterized bleeders as well as full scatter (Fig. 10.1H).
8. Fluid air exchange (Fig. 10.1I) and intravitreal long-acting gas C_3F_8 injection.

VITRECTOMY IN SPECIAL SITUATIONS OF VITREOUS HEMORRHAGE

1. *Steps to manage retrolental or retro-IOL blood (Video 3, Chapter 10):* The retrolental or retro IOL blood layer of vitreous hemorrhage (Fig. 10.2A) has to be removed to allow further visualization. Although retro IOL blood removal can be done safely with the vitrectomy cutter, but retrolental blood is to be removed with caution with the help of suction (Fig. 10.2B) of cutter only from central to periphery to avoid lens damage.
2. *Core Vitrectomy:* To remove the central vitreous to clear vitreous hemorrhage if present (Fig. 10.2C).
3. *Steps to approach subhyaloid hemorrhage (Video 4, Chapter 10):* After core vitrectomy, there is posterior hyaloid (Fig. 10.3A). As there is incomplete posterior hyaloid separation, the vitreous cutter can easily incise the posterior hyaloid. After an opening has been created it can be easily enlarged to get access into subhyaloid space (Fig. 10.3B). Subhyaloid blood are not clotted and can be easily removed by either suction of cutter (Fig. 10.3C) or active or passive suction of soft-

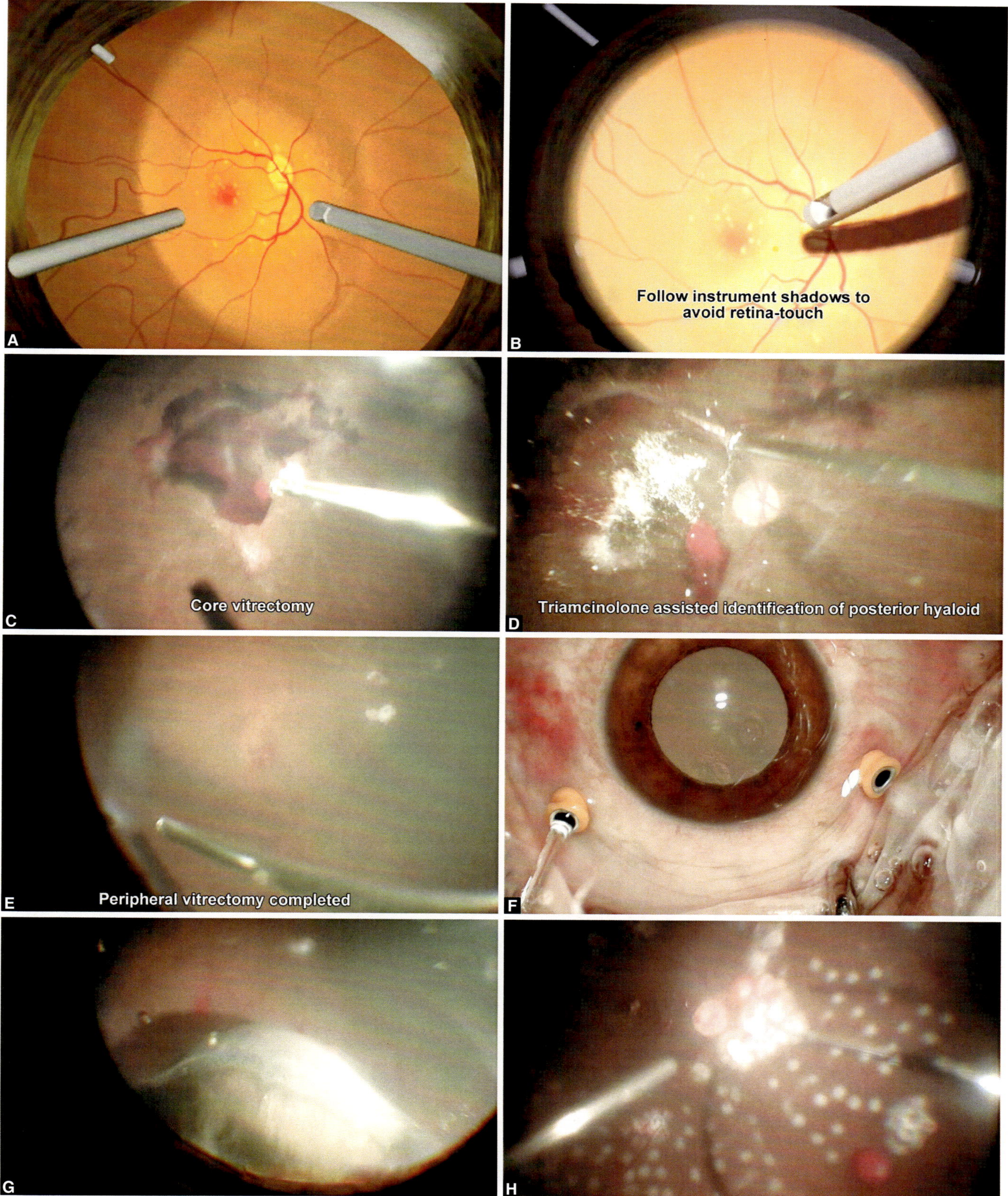

Figs 10.1A to H

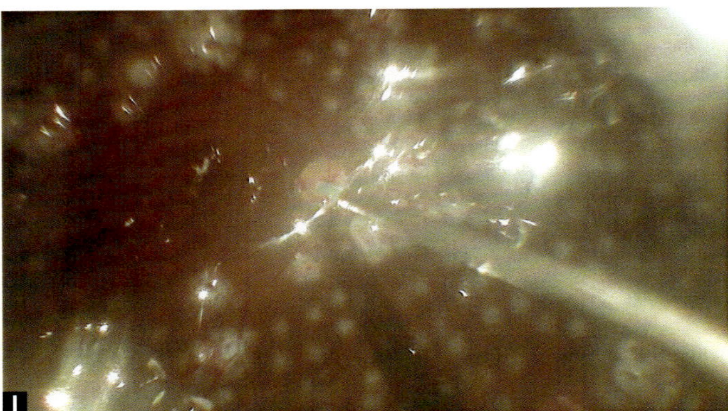

Figs 10.1A to I: (A) Three-port vitrectomy with infusion line, vitrectomy cutter and endoilluminator; (B) One has to follow the shadow of cutter to avoid retina touch; (C) Core vitrectomy with high suction (around 200– 400 mm Hg) and low cutting rate (around 4000 cpm); (D) PVD induction with suction of cutter; (E) Peripheral vitrectomy; (F) Free flow of fluid indicate completion of vitrectomy; (G) Vitreous base excision by external scleral depression; (H) Endolaser around the cauterized bleeders; (I) Fluid-air exchange

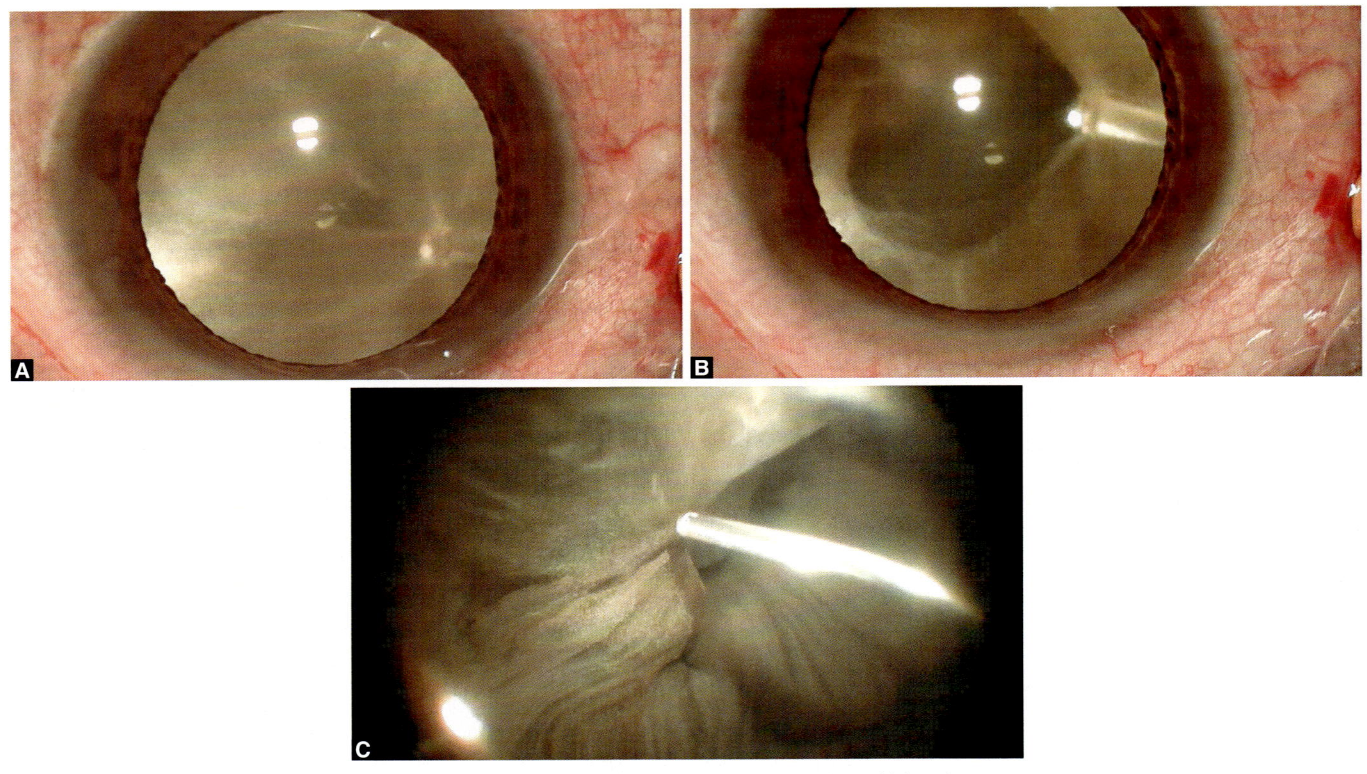

Figs 10.2A to C: Steps to manage retrolental blood

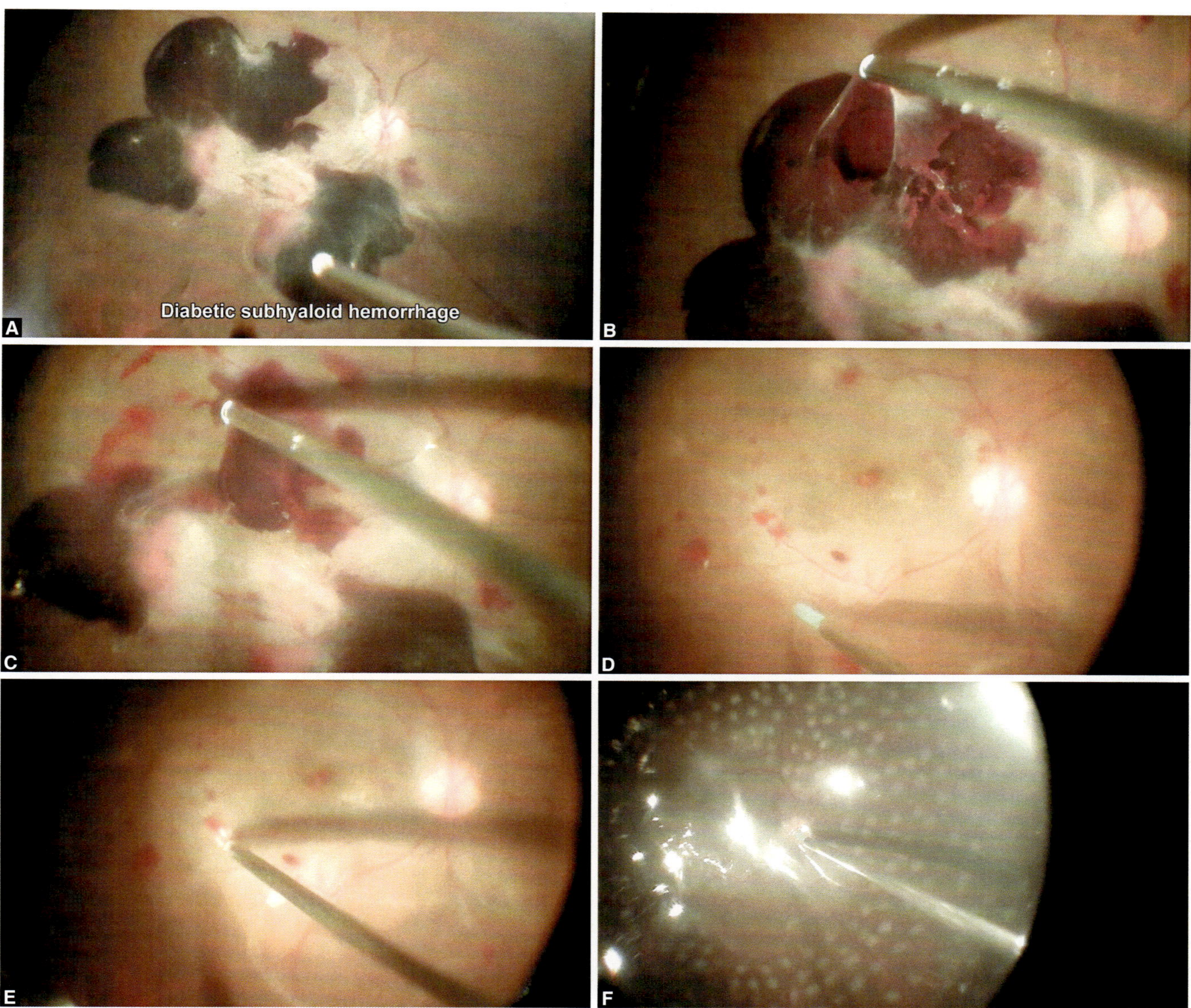

Figs 10.3A to F

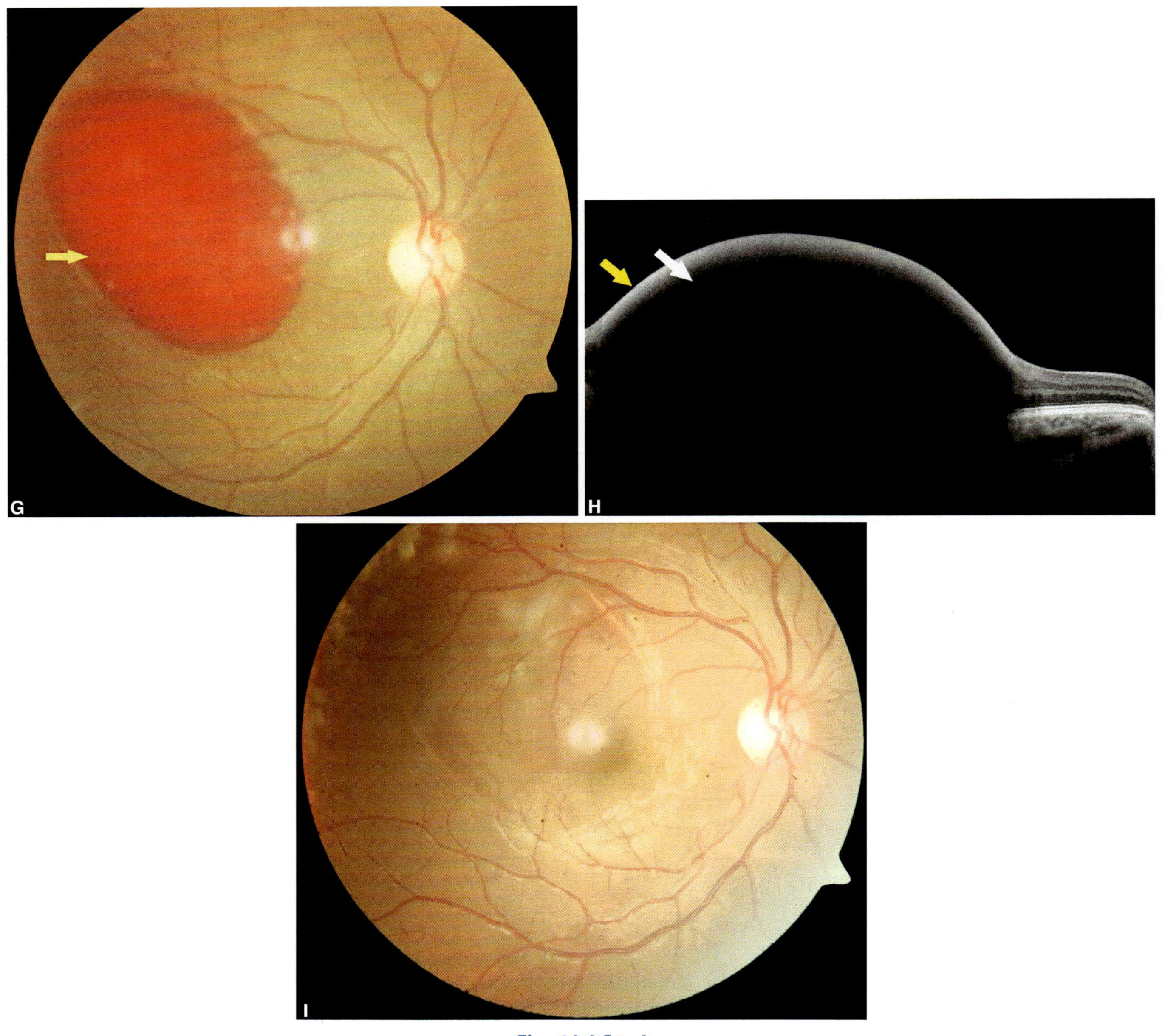

Figs 10.3G to I

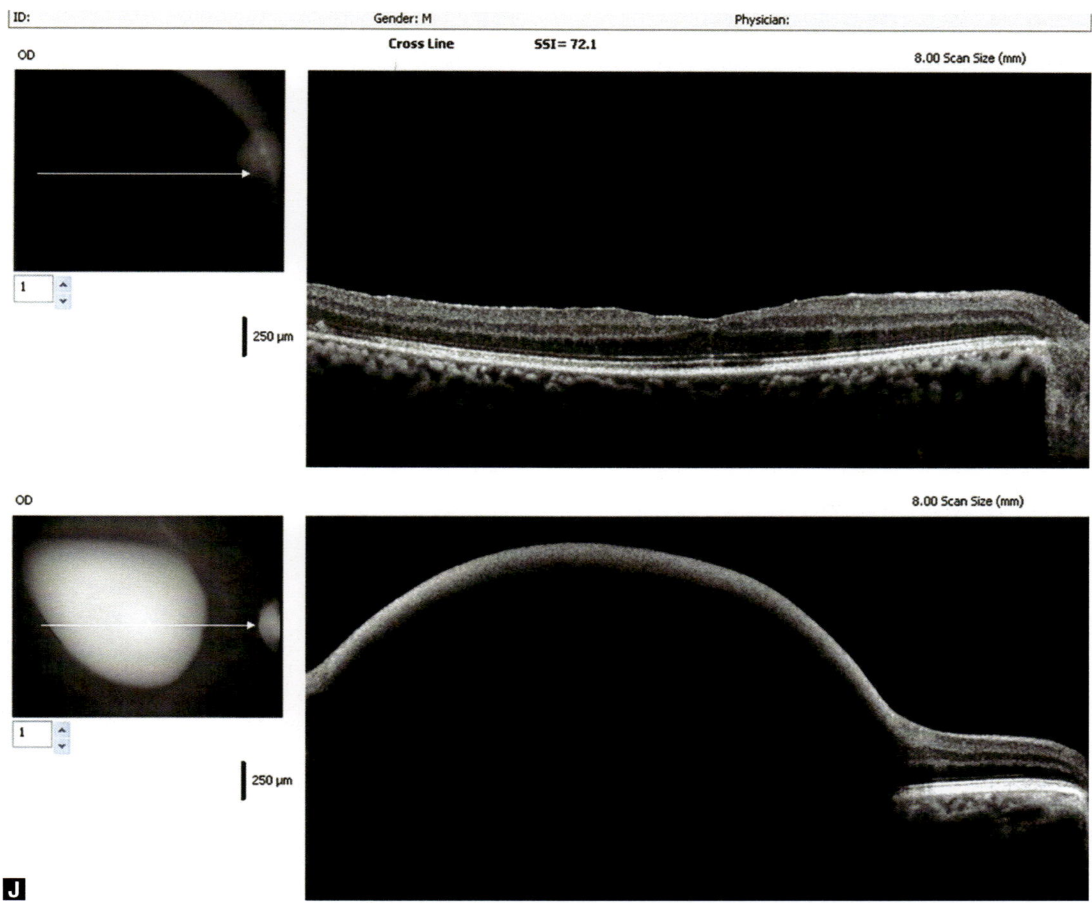

Figs 10.3A to J: (A to D) Steps to manage subhyaloid hemorrhage; (E) Steps to manage bleeder by cautery; (F) Fluid-air exchange; (G) Post-traumatic sub-ILM hemorrhage; (H) OCT of subinternal limiting membrane hemorrhage; (I) Postoperative fundus after vitrectomy and ILM peeling in case of sub-ILM hemorrhage; (J) Pre- and postoperative OCTs, after vitrectomy and ILM peeling in case of sub-ILM hemorrhage

tipped back-flush needle. Thus, this can improve the visualization of underlying retina (Fig. 10.3D).

4. *Cautery/diathermy and endolaser photocoagulation according to the etiology:* Diathermy of all bleeders should be done as soon as they appear (Fig. 10.3E). Sometimes surgeon has to increase the IOP to stop bleed. Even pure point laser photocoagulation has some diathermy-like effect to stop bleed.
5. Fluid-air exchange (Fig. 10.3F).

   Sub-ILM hemorrhage (Figs 10.3G to J): Sub-ILM hemorrhage may occur as a result of blunt trauma or Valsalva maneuver. After PVD induction, ILM has to be stained and ILM peeling has to be done overlying the hemorrhage. Sub-ILM blood usually comes out with the help of soft-tipped cannula.

HYPERVIT SYSTEM (FIG. 10.4)

- Very high-speed dual-pneumatic cutter (20000 cuts per minute)
- Dual-blade vitrectomy probe is driven by dual-pneumatic technology
- Continuously open port. So there is a near-continuous open port duty cycle.
- The cutter tip is beveled

Advantages:

- Increased vitreous flow with continuously open port, thus increasing efficiency for vitreous removal.
- Reduced fluidic turbulence, thus improving fluidic stability, which diminishes pulsatility during vitrectomy.
- Dual-cutting 20000 cpm probes result in less backflow and less retropulsion. A dead recirculatory flow zone is apparent inside the probe tip, contributing to backflow or retropulsion. The beveled-shaped tip reduces backflow by reducing the space of the dead flow zone.
- Reduced peak traction force on both on and off the retina
- Increased efficiency of the cutter.

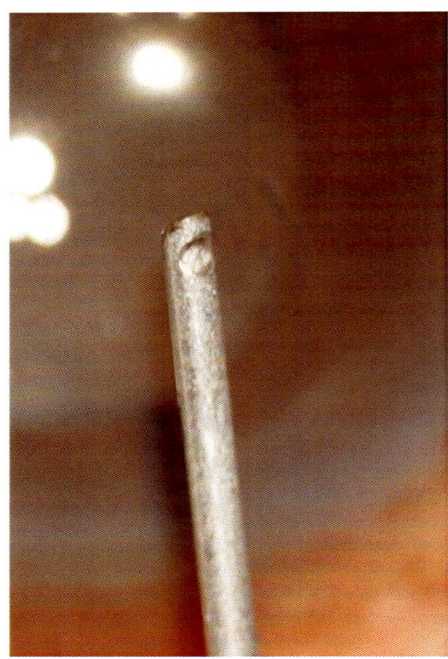

Fig. 10.4: Shows a Hypervit cutter with a beveled tip

Case discussion: Video 5, Chapter 10

- While using a hypervit dual-pneumatic cutter with 20000 cuts per minute, the port remains continuously open. Thus, there is increased vitreous flow.
- We can go very close to a mobile retina with a large tear with less suction of the cutter (Fig. 10.5A).
- With stable fluidics, there is reduced pulsatility of a mobile retina
- The peak traction force on the off retina is also less; thus, trimming vitreous, anterior to a retinal flap is also easier.
- After stabilizing the posterior pole, the vitreous base excision is also safe (Fig. 10.5B).

DIGITALLY-ASSISTED VITREOUS SURGERIES AND INTEGRATED INTRAOPERATIVE OCT

One of the latest innovations in vitreoretinal surgery is digitally-assisted vitreoretinal surgery (DAVS). It refers to real-time digital image guidance of vitreoretinal surgery, contemporarily utilizing an ultra-high-definition three-dimensional (3D) flat-panel display. DAVS provides a stereoscopic view of the surgical field on a large monitor that can be viewed by multiple individuals simultaneously, including the surgeon, assistants, and observers. This 3D heads-up system can be used for both vitreoretinal and cataract surgery, improving the quality of surgical visualization.

DAVS System (Fig. 10.6):

- A high-dynamic range (HDR) digital camera is mounted on the operating microscope, replacing the eyepiece of the microscope. This HDR camera is wired to a central processing unit (CPU)
- The camera projects a digital image onto an advanced 3D 4K OLED 55-inch surgical display
- Displayed images are viewed through a pair of passive, circular polarized glasses

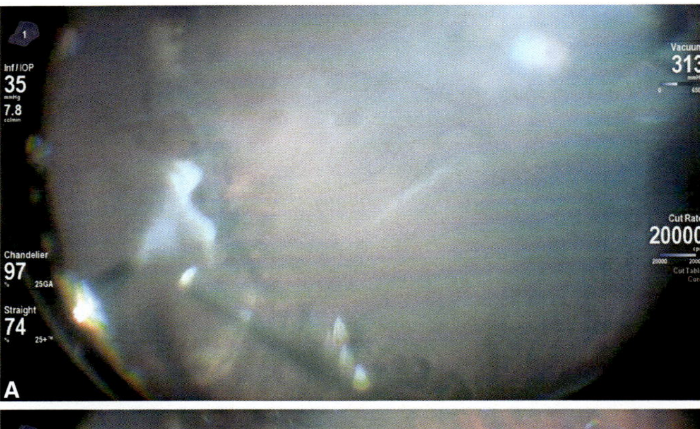

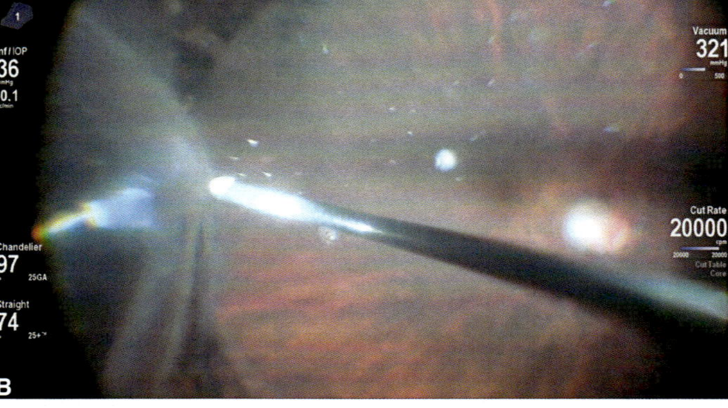

Figs 10.5A and B: (A) Shows a Hypervit cutter, trimming vitreous very close to a mobile detached retina with a large tear; (B) Shows a Hypervit cutter performing vitreous base excision with a relatively low vacuum (321 mm Hg)

Advantages over conventional microscopes:

- DAVS provides a better real-time view of the surgical field with better stereopsis, better depth of field, enhanced field of view and better resolution.
- DAVS allows the surgeon to make changes based on what they see on the screen
- DAVS need lower levels of illumination during surgery, increasing patient comfort. Thus, it improves safety as there is less phototoxicity
- It improves the ergonomics of the surgeons. There is a reduction in physical stress and neck pain among surgeons operating the DAVS in a "heads-up" position compared to the conventional operating microscope
- The learning curve is also steep
- DAVS is a better learning tool for trainees
- Options of digital filters to visualize vitreous fibrils, epiretinal membranes or ILM. Black-and-white (BW)

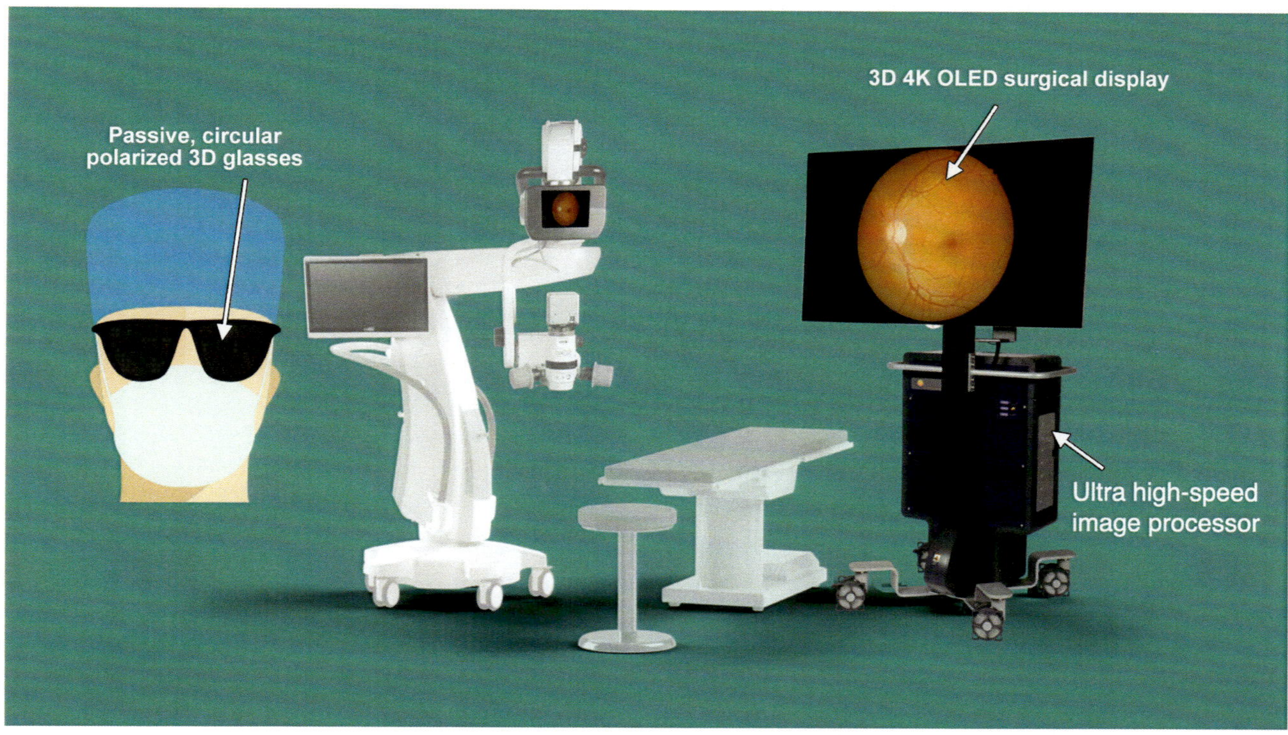

Fig. 10.6: The complete DAVS system.
Courtesy: Alcon

filters have classically been used to enhance medical image quality and tissue contrast. "Vitreous blue filter" can be used for better identification with enhanced contrast and clarity of the peripheral uncut vitreous. So, more complete removal of vitreous is possible using a blue filter. "Peeling blue filter" is required for ERM removal surgery. The filter's ability to enhance blue wavelengths enhances the dye's staining properties, making ERM more distinguishable against the retinal background, especially in high myopic eyes, where the natural contrast is already diminished. The "peeling blue filter" and "green filter" are important during ILM peeling surgery in the case of macular holes, as they enhance the tissue contrast. These additional filters also reduce the need for repeated staining.

Disadvantages: Sometimes there is difficulty in switching between DAVS and an analog microscope

Commercially available DAVS platforms: NGENUITY® 3D Visualization System (Alcon) and ARTEVO 800 (Carl Zeiss Meditec).

Case discussion (Video 6, Chapter 10):

- This is a proliferative diabetic retinopathy with extensive membrane formation, done using DAVS NGENUITY.
- It gives a digitally enhanced, expansive, immersive view of the surgical field
- The surgeon can delicately dissect all membranes and extract the posterior hyaloid face in an outside-in manner using passive polarized glass.
- Then, we can complete the PRP
- In the case of a macular hole, the surgeon can complete the PVD induction using triamcinolone particles and peel the BBG dye-stained ILM using a digital filter in an onion-peel manner.

Intraoperative Optical Coherence Tomography (Fig. 10.7)

Intraoperative optical coherence tomography (iOCT) is a relatively recent technology, offering real-time, high-resolution imaging of ocular structures during surgical procedures. It enables the detection of alterations in vitreoretinal structures during surgery, thereby promoting informed surgical decisions grounded on real-time input. One of the most promising applications of 3D visualization technology is its use in conjunction with intraoperative optical coherence tomography (OCT).

Currently commercially available iOCT options are the Leica Envisu handheld system, the Zeiss Rescan 700, and the Haag-Streit Surgical iOCT system.

Conventional viewing systems, like traditional microscopes, have visualization quality and ergonomics limitations. They need beam splitters and laser filters for

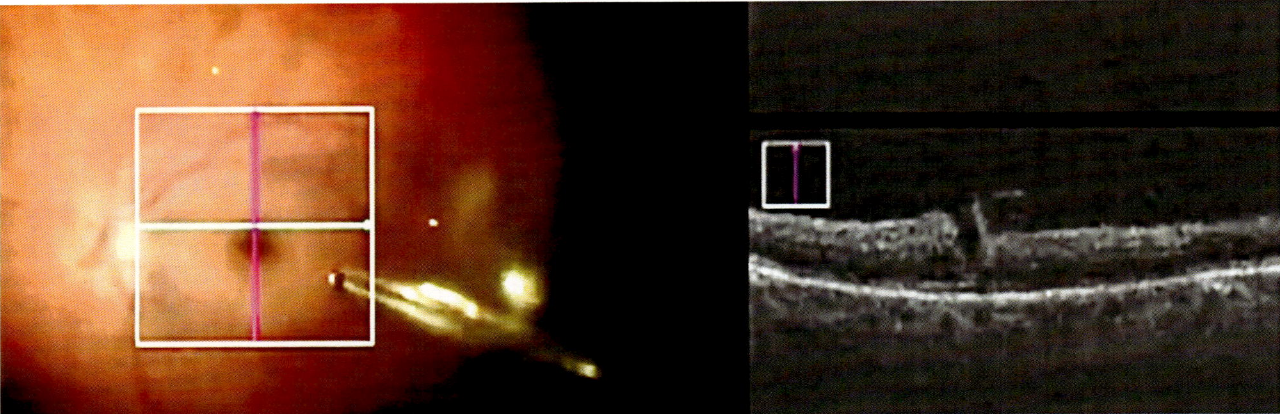

Fig. 10.7: Intraoperative OCT display during surgery.

secure and efficient functioning and fail to offer the same level of detail or adaptability as digital displays. In contrast, use of 3D visualization technology in conjunction with intraoperative optical coherence tomography (OCT) is more promising. By projecting the OCT on a high-resolution screen, surgeons could scrutinize the data without reverting to the microscope's external display system. Currently, commercially available 3D-DAVS with iOCT options are NGENUITY (Alcon) combined with Rescan 700 (Zeiss) and Artevo 800 (ZEISS) combined with Rescan 700.

The utility of iOCT in the OR is as follows:

1. Membrane dissection in diabetics and epiretinal membrane
   - To detect relief of vitreomacular traction on table
   - To confirm the complete removal of ERM
2. Macular hole surgery
   - To locate the macular hole, especially in high myope where the retina-choroidal contrast is very poor.
   - To confirm any iatrogenic retinal break formation due to tissue pull, especially when there is bleeding during ILM peeling.
   - Whether the ILM flap is in place covering the macular hole under air or not.
   - To confirm the closure of the macular hole on the table.
   - To confirm the complete plugging of the macular hole area by autologous retinal graft in case of re-surgery for failed open macular hole cases.
3. Retinal detachment
   - To detect the presence of subretinal fluid, when there is any doubt whether the retina is well-attached under PFCL or not.
   - To detect retinoschisis changes
   - To accurately detect retinal tear
4. *Myopic macular detachment:* To confirm the accurate position of the macular buckle over the detached the macula, in the case of myopic tractional maculopathy with macular RD due to a macular hole.
5. *Submacular surgery:*
   - To inject recombinant tissue plasminogen activator and anti-VEGF drug accurately between the photoreceptor layer and RPE layer in cases of submacular hemorrhages. Confirmation of tip of 38G or 40G subretinal cannulas in subretinal space, creation of bleb formation and overstretching of overlying neurosensory retina and even the accidental foveal-blowouts can be confirmed by iOCT.
   - To detect accurate delivery of drugs for subretinal gene therapy in certain hereditary retinal disorders like Leber's congenital amaurosis and retinitis pigmentosa.
   - To take the chorioretinal biopsy
   - To get real-time feedback for the correct position and orientation of Argus II retinal prosthesis over the macula in advanced RP.

Kindly scan the QR code below to access the online Video.

CHAPTER 11

Diabetic Vitreous Surgery

Changes in Retina and Vitreous in Diabetic Patients

A. Retinal vascular changes in diabetics:

1. *Microvascular damage:* Microaneurysms, retinal capillary nonperfusion, cotton wool spots, increased numbers of hemorrhages, venous abnormalities (e.g., dilation, beading, loops), and intraretinal microvascular abnormalities (IRMAs) (vascular changes).
2. *Increased vasopermeability:* Retinal thickening (edema) and/or exudates that may lead to a loss in central visual acuity (macular edema).
3. Gradual closure of arterioles and venules results in increasing signs of ischemia including venous abnormalities (e.g., dilation, beading, loops), IRMA, and more severe and extensive vascular leakage characterized by increasing retinal hemorrhages and exudation with the secondary proliferation of new vessels on the disk, retina, iris, and in the filtration angle (proliferative stage).

B. Vitreous changes in diabetics:

1. *Nonenzymatic glycation of proteins:* This nonenzymatic glycation of vitreous proteins can lead to degenerative changes in vitreous gel, which can lead to abnormal or anomalous posterior vitreous detachment (PVD) as this PVD is attached to multiple sites, especially areas of fibrovascular fronds.
2. There is also a progressive vitreous contraction in eyes with diabetic retinopathy and this progressive contraction of vitreous can continue even after successful regression of proliferative changes by pan retinal photocoagulation (PRP).
   Proliferative diabetic retinopathy further alters the vitreous by the inclusion of vasogenic cells and fibrous tissue. In the case of bleeding inside the vitreous cavity, there is further augmentation of the contractile property of the vitreous by the inclusion of vasogenic and fibrogenic elements. This can lead to the formation of fibrovascular tissue in the vitreous cavity and finally result in tractional retinal detachment (TRD), secondary rhegmatogenous retinal detachment, persistent macular edema, premacular hemorrhage and recurrent vitreous hemorrhage.

STEPS TO MANAGE VITREOMACULAR INTERFACE DISORDERS

- Diabetic macular edema is the significant source of visual deterioration in patients with diabetes mellitus. It occurs due to breakdown of both inner and outer blood retinal barriers resulting in leakage of intraretinal fluid from microaneurysms and abnormal retinal capillaries.
  - Its pathogenesis is multifactorial, involving vasopermeability factors [like vascular endothelial growth factors (VEGF), interleukin-6 and histamine], retinal anoxia/ischemia and vitreomacular attachments
  - Attached posterior hyaloid become taut, resulting in *anomalous posterior vitreous detachment* and cause tangential macular traction. Another factor is *progressive vitreous contraction* which is quite common in diabetics, can result in transvitreal vitreomacular traction and persistent macular edema, even responsible for progression of fibrovascular proliferation, tractional retinal detachment (TRD), then combined tractional-rhegmatogenous retinal detachment and recurrent vitreous hemorrhage
  - Spectral domain OCT, especially 3D view can reveal all kinds of vitreomacular attachments, starting from vitreomacular adhesion, symptomatic vitreomacular adhesion, epiretinal membrane (ERM), vitreofoveal traction (VFT), more severe form vitreomacular traction (VMT) and macular TRD.

Removal of Visible Tractions

Identification of Posterior Hyaloid Face (Video 1, Chapter 11)

Application of triamcinolone acenonide to stain posterior hyaloid (Fig. 11.1A), triamcinolone acetonide particles have to be injected after anterior and core vitrectomy.

Fluid-Air Exchange

- Removal of posterior hyaloid face by cutter *(Video 2, Chapter 11):* Modern small gauge high speed cutter technology, we can go very close to the retina to shave membranes with minimal traction on it, considering its attachment with underlying retina at multiple sites (Figs 11.1B and C).

Identification and Removal of Vitreoschisis (Video 3, Chapter 11)

Many times after posterior hyaloid removal, TA-stained vitreoschisis layer is well-revealed. Its removal with the suction of cutter (Fig. 11.1D) or end grasping forceps is important for complete removal of posterior hyaloid.

Symptomatic Vitreomacular Adhesion (VMA) (Video 4, Chapter 11)

Steps of surgery:

- In cases of symptomatic vitreomacular adhesions (Fig. 11.1E), where ocriplasmin injection has limited role, sometimes surgery helps
- Triamcinolone-stained adherent posterior hyaloid face can be lifted up by making an opening with a bent 24G needle (Fig. 11.1F)
- Needle is bent in such a way that tip is always visible to the surgeon and it is parallel to the retinal surface
- Suction of the cutter is used to complete PVD
- Postoperatively, smooth foveal contour can be achieved.

Vitreomacular Traction

i. Release of VMT by bent 24 G needle *(Video 5, Chapter 11)*-OCT PRE/POST
   - In case of diabetic taut posterior hyaloid with multifocal vitreomacular traction on 3D OCT (Fig. 11.1G), a bent 24G needle helps to tear the TA-stained posterior hyaloid face followed by its removal by end grasping forceps and then by cutter suction (Fig. 11.1H).

ii. Release of VMT by Visco dissection *(Video 6, Chapter 11)*
   - In case of diabetic taut posterior hyaloid face with broad-based VMT on both 2D and 3D OCT (Fig. 11.1I), an opening was made with a bent 24G needle to have an access to subhyaloid space
   - Now a bent 24G cannula is used to inject viscoelastic between taut hyaloid and retina to separate the elevated fovea from posterior hyaloid (Fig. 11.1J)
   - Then cutter can shave the separated loose hyaloid face safely.

Vitreomacular Traction with Tractional Retinal Detachment (Video 7, Chapter 11)

- In a case of diabetic thick posterior hyaloid with macular tractional detachment (Fig. 11.1K), after TA-stained PVD induction done, trypan blue dye injected to stain ERM
- After ERM removal (Fig. 11.1L), BBG dye injected to stain ILM. As ILM was already removed along with ERM, residual ILM was also removed. Postoperatively macula TRD settled.

Epiretinal Membrane (Video 8, Chapter 11)

- In case of ERM formation on 3D OCT (Fig. 11.1M) in a case of lasered PDR, TA-assisted vitrectomy done, followed by application of trypan blue dye under air to stain ERM
- Dye-stained ERM removed by ILM forceps (Fig. 11.1N)
- Again BBG dye applied to stain ILM. ILM was already removed along with adhered ERM. Residual ILM was also peeled. Postoperatively, OCT shows absence of ERM.

Removal of Invisible Tractions

Postvitrectomy Taut ILM

This is a newly diagnosed entity, where macular edema after diabetic vitrectomy, detected on OCT, is not relieved by intravitreal anti-VEGF injection; but ILM peeling is the only treatment of choice.

Refractory Diabetic Macular Edema (Video 9, Chapter 11)

They are diffuse diabetic macular oedema caused by excessive breakdown of both inner and outer blood retinal barriers and refractory to previous anti-VEGF and laser photocoagulation treatment. Its multifactorial origin and final role of surgery is to remove invisible tractions by both vitrectomy and ILM peeling to decrease macular thickness.

Steps of surgery:

- In case of recalcitrant diabetic macular edema, TA-assisted vitrectomy done followed by PVD induction and removal of macular vitreoschisis (Fig. 11.2A)
- Then application of BBG dye in saline and peeling of ILM (Fig. 11.2B) to ensure complete removal of any remnant of posterior hyaloid as well as removal of all tractions.
- Postoperatively, recalcitrant macular edema resolves (Fig. 11.2C) in most of the situations, but visual improvement may or may not occur.

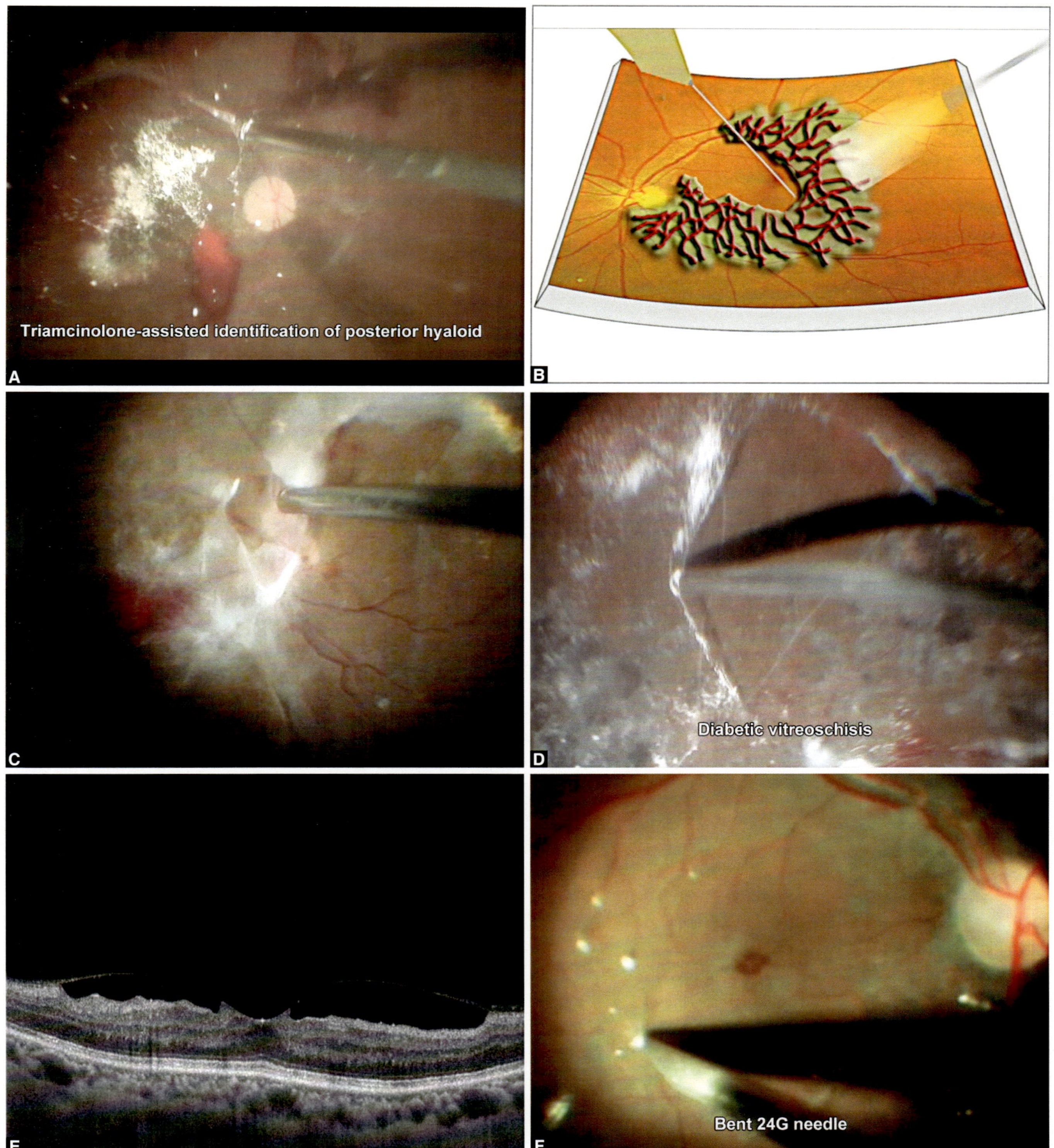

Figs 11.1A to F

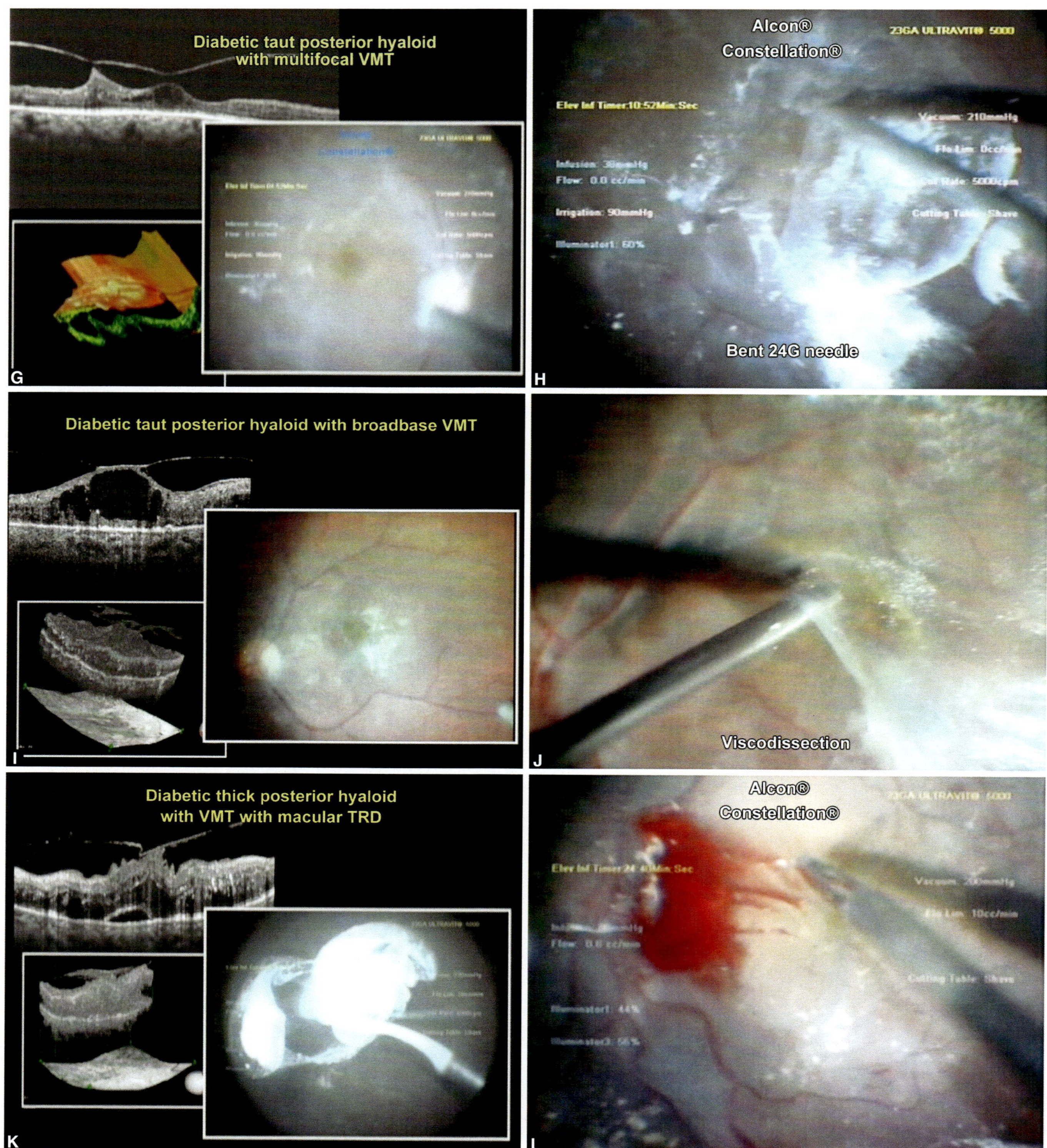

Figs 11.1G to L

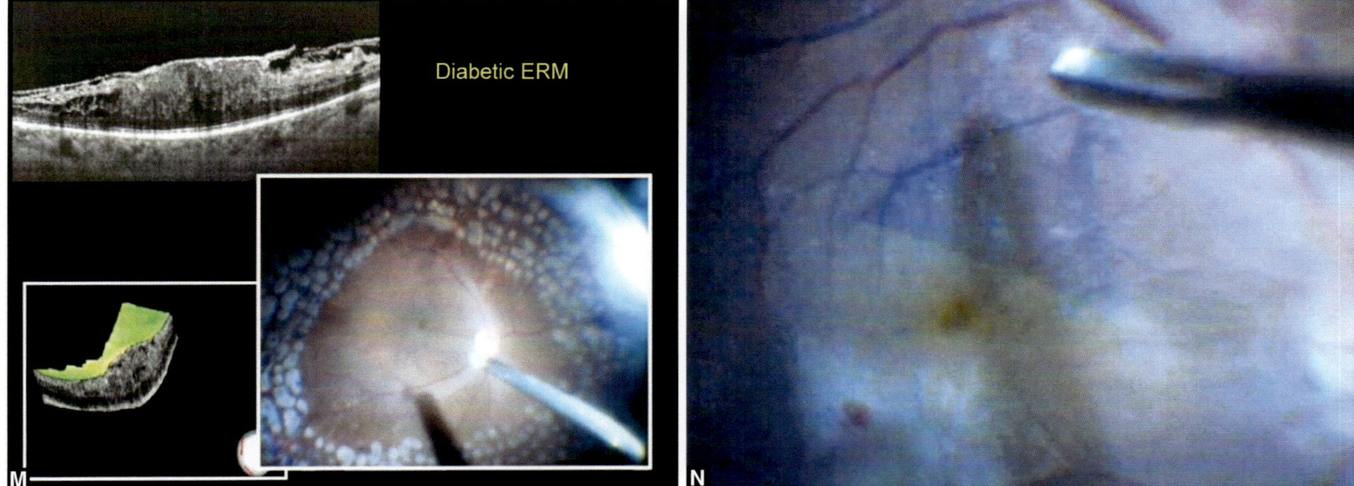

Figs 11.1A to N: (A) Triamcinolone acenonide particle to stain posterior hyaloid; (B and C) Removal of posterior hyaloid face by cutter; (D) Removal of triamcinolone-stained vitreoschisis membrane by the suction of a cutter; (E) OCT scan of macula of a 67-year-old patient having symptoms of metamorphopsia shows vitreomacular adhesion with foveal traction; (F) Intraoperative photograph shows making an opening in posterior hyaloid by a bent 24G needle in a case of symptomatic vitreomacular adhesion; (G) 3D OCT scan of macula shows diabetic taut posterior hyaloid with multifocal vitreomacular traction; (H) Intraoperative photograph shows tear in TA-stained posterior hyaloid face by a bent 24G needle in a case of multifocal vitreomacular traction; (I) Diabetic taut posterior hyaloid face with broad-based VMT on both 2D and 3D OCT; (J) Intraoperative photograph shows viscodissection by a bent 24G cannula, injecting viscoelastics between taut hyaloid and retina; (K) Both 2D and 3D OCT shows diabetic thick posterior hyaloid with macular tractional detachment; (L) Intraoperative photograph shows removal of trypan blue-stained ERM in a case of thick posterior hyaloid with macular tractional detachment; (M) Both 2D and 3D OCT shows diabetic epiretinal membrane formation in a case of lasered PDR; (N) Intraoperative photograph shows removal of trypan blue stained ERM in a case of diabetic epiretinal membrane formation in a case of lasered PDR

Abbreviations: VMT, vitreomacular traction; TRD, tractional retinal detachment

Diabetic Macular Hole (Video 10, Chapter 11)

- In chronic diabetic macular edema cases, macular hole formation can occur (Fig. 11.2D)
- Many times, associated ERM is present.

Steps of surgery:

- In case of diabetic macular hole, after completing vitrectomy TA-stained vitreoschisis was removed (Fig. 11.2E)
- Associated ERM stained with trypan blue also removed. (Fig. 11.2F)
- Then BBG dye applied in saline and dye-stained ILM peeled (Fig. 11.2G) followed by fluid-air exchange and
- Long-acting gas C_3F_8 injection done
- Pre- and postoperative OCT (Fig. 11.2H) shows closure of macular hole.

MEMBRANE DISSECTION

- In the stage of PDR, ischemic retina releases vascular growth factors (VEGF, insulin-like growth factors, b-Fibroblast growth factors) which can lead to formation of neovascular buds or vascular epicenter from retinal blood vessels
- Fibrovascular tissue proliferates in the potential space between the vitreous and retina
- Finally invasion of lamellae of cortical vitreous produce a very firm adhesion
- These adhesions can be of two basic types: i. Focal (point-like attachment, can be—single or multiple); and ii. broad
- Broad adhesions may or may not associate with folding of underlying retina, clinically appears gray with variable vascularization as a consequence of fibrotic posterior hyaloid between multiple focal adhesions that coalesce and contract.

Membrane peeling: The key step in diabetic VR surgery, needs to be done with high precision. We know, vitrectomy relieves centripetal traction and membrane peeling relieves tangential traction. Let us follow the principles of membrane peeling:

1. *Forceps peeling (Video 11, Chapter 11):* Forceps peeling means peeling a membrane from the underlying elevated retina with the help of forceps only (Fig. 11.3A). In this PDR case with TRD with fibrovascular membranes, membrane was tried to be separated from underlying TRD with the forceps gently, separating its

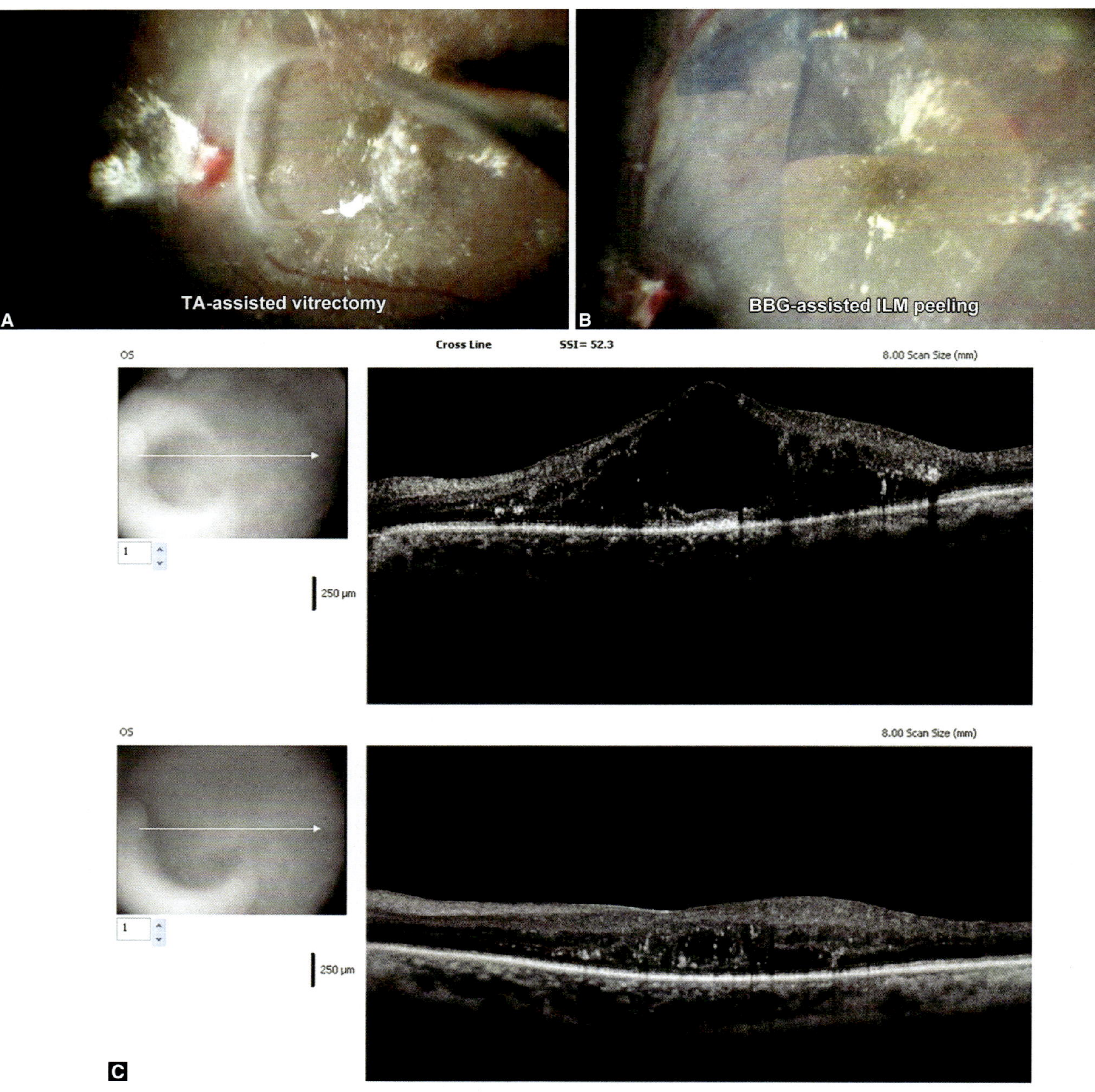

Figs 11.2A to C

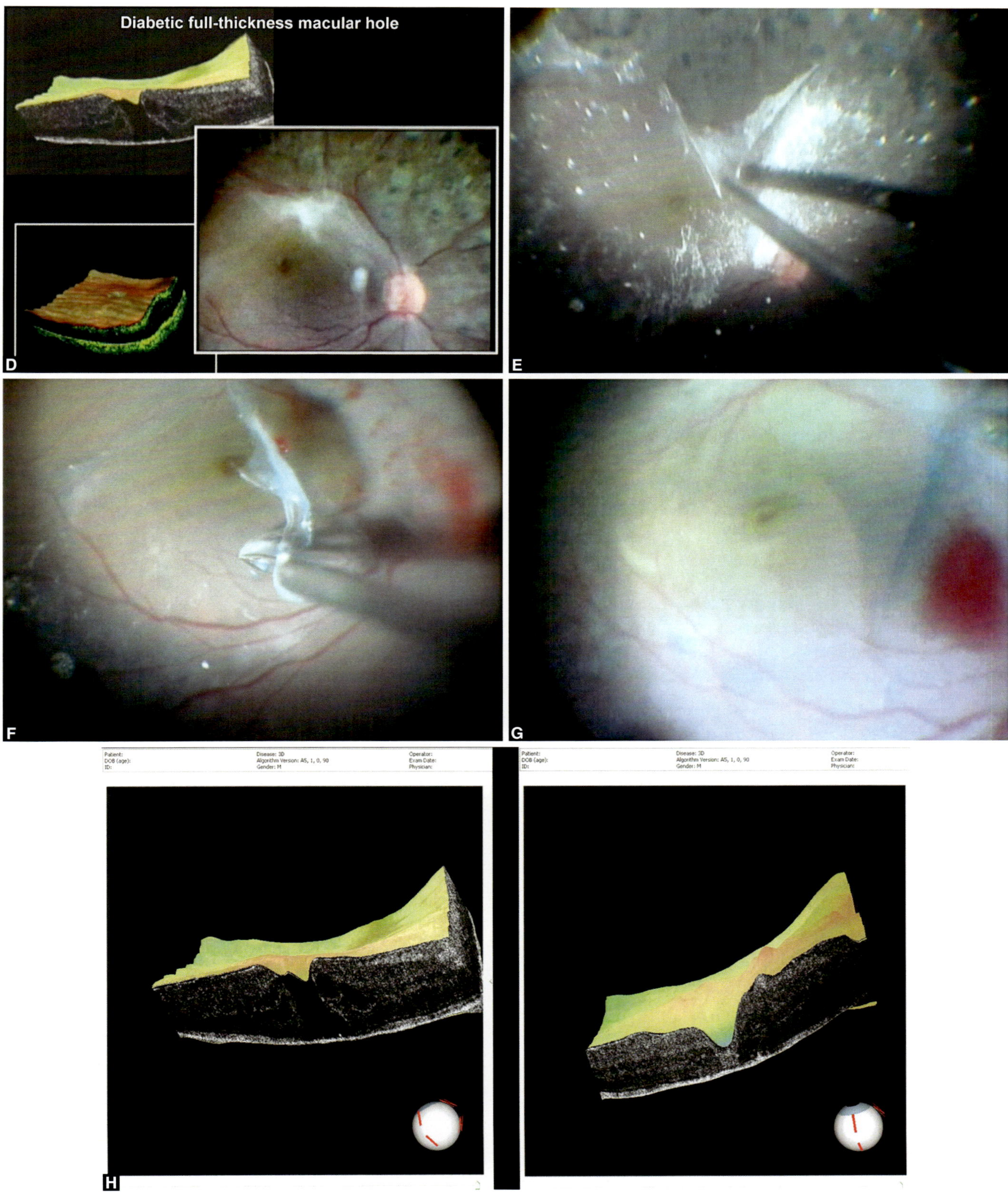

Figs 11.2A to H: (A and B) Intraoperative steps to manage recalcitrant diabetic macular edema; (C) Preoperative and postoperative comparative OCT in case of recalcitrant diabetic macular edema; (D) 3D OCT shows diabetic full thickness macular hole; (E to G) Shows intraoperative photographs of salient steps in diabetic macular hole surgery; (H) Pre- and postoperative comparative OCT in case of diabetic macular hole surgery

Abbreviations: TA, triamcinolone acetonide; ILM, internal limiting membrane extension from the surrounding retina and peeling it completely. If there is excessive traction during forceps peeling, one should use cutter to trim the membrane (Fig. 11.3B).

2. Chop-stick peeling, i.e holding the membrane with both light-pipe and cutter and then peeling it (Fig. 11.3C).

   Surgical steps (Video 12, Chapter 11):
   - In this case of PDR with a superior broad-based fibrovascular membrane, suction of the cutter was initially tried to separate the membrane and surrounding blood (Fig. 11.3D)
   - Then light pipe was introduced beneath the membrane and cutter was kept over the membrane and just like chop stick, the membrane was tried to be separated with both hands
   - And with the final attachment, cutter is used to trim it.
3. Suction peeling, i.e membrane peeling with suction of a cutter *(Video 13, Chapter 11)*. Focal vitreoretinal adhesions are easier to remove by cutter suction than broad-based adhesions, especially with those retinal folds (Fig. 11.3E).
4. *Segmentation of a membrane (Video 14, Chapter 11):* In case of bridging TRDs, segmentation of the bridging membrane between TRDs help. The segmentation can be performed by curved scissor or by the cutter (Fig. 11.3F). Segmented membranes should be trimmed with cutter leaving a small island on the top of TRDs (Fig. 11.3G).
5. *Delamination of that membrane (Video 15, Chapter 11)*: After segmentation, the segmented membranes can be:
   - Amputed by curved scissor or delaminated from the underlying elevated retina by cutter only or bimanually with forceps and cutter (Fig. 11.3H)
   - As a multifunctional tool, cutter delimitation can be of like 'lift and cut', where cutter is used to lift the membrane and then cut (Fig. 11.3I)
   - 'Fold back cutter delamination' for thinner flexible membrane, where placing the cutter on the anterior surface of ERM membrane just behind the leading edge result in fold back of membrane into the port (Fig. 11.3J)
   - 'Conformal delamination' for rigid thicker ERM membrane, where cutter is constantly rotating along the long axis to cause rotation of the port away from the retina, maintaining apposition of cutter port to ERM (Fig. 11.3K). The name 'fold back' and 'conformal delamination' coined by Dr Steve Charles. Delamination can be 'inside out', i.e managing diabetic ERM from inside outwards or 'outside in', i.e managing membranes from outside inwards. As central retina is thicker than the retina outside the macula, some prefers 'inside out' delamination as a safer technique.
6. *Hydrodissection (Video 16, Chapter 11):* It is the method of separating or dissecting the membrane from underlying retinal surface by BSS fluid. This hydrodissection can be performed by a tip-curved cannula or the 'proportional reflux' mode of cutter where fluid flow will come out from the cutter port (Fig. 11.3L) that can safely separate the membrane from the thin detached retina or very tightly adhered diabetic membranes (Fig. 11.3M).
7. *Viscodissection (Video 17, Chapter 11)*: The advanced thick broadly attached membrane (Fig. 11.3N OCT) sometimes difficult to separate from the detached thin retina. Use of viscoelastic (hydroxypropyl methyl cellulose) especially helpful in this broad-base VMT cases. A bent tipped 24G cannula (Fig. 11.3O) can be used to inject viscoelastic by viscous fluid control (VFC) syringe, made for silicone oil injection (Fig. 11.3P). In this case of PDR with broad-base VMT, visco dissection technique used to separate the posterior hyaloid from elevated fovea followed by routine use of cutter suction to induce PVD from other part of retina (Fig. 11.3Q).
   - So in clinical practice, all these principles should be used in combination.

STEPS TO MANAGE TRDS (BY CUTTER ONLY, AS A MULTIFUNCTIONAL TOOL)

Vitreous membranes caused by proliferative retinopathies or penetrating injuries can pull the sensory retina away from the pigment epithelium, causing TRD.

Characteristic configuration:

- Detached retina has a smooth surface and it is immobile.
- TRD is concave anteriorly and rarely extends to the ora serrata.

The commonest indication of diabetic vitrectomy is TRD involving macula or threatening macula. Studies showed that macular reattachment was achieved in 66–75% of eyes and a visual acuity of 5/200 or better was achieved in 59–67% of eyes.

In more complex advanced cases, there is little posterior vitreous separation, very fibrotic membrane and ERM surrounding the vitreo retinal adhesion.

Unimanual dissection—by the cutter itself using as a multifunctional tool:

1. By changing the parameter of cutting rate and suction, cutter can be used to deal various membranes. For thicker membranes, higher suction (250–400 mm Hg) and lower cut rate (3000–4000 cpm) can manage. To

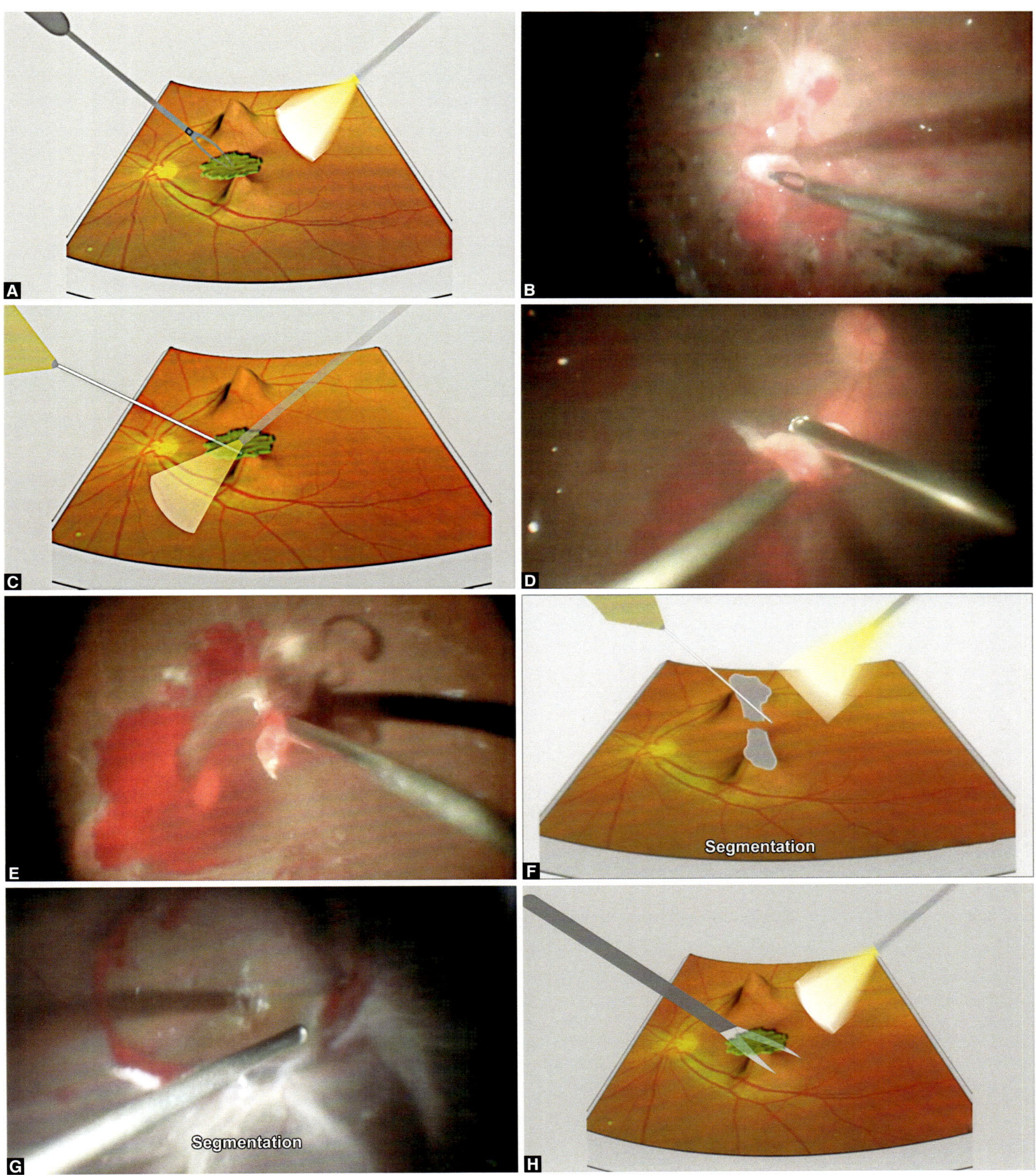

Figs 11.3A to H

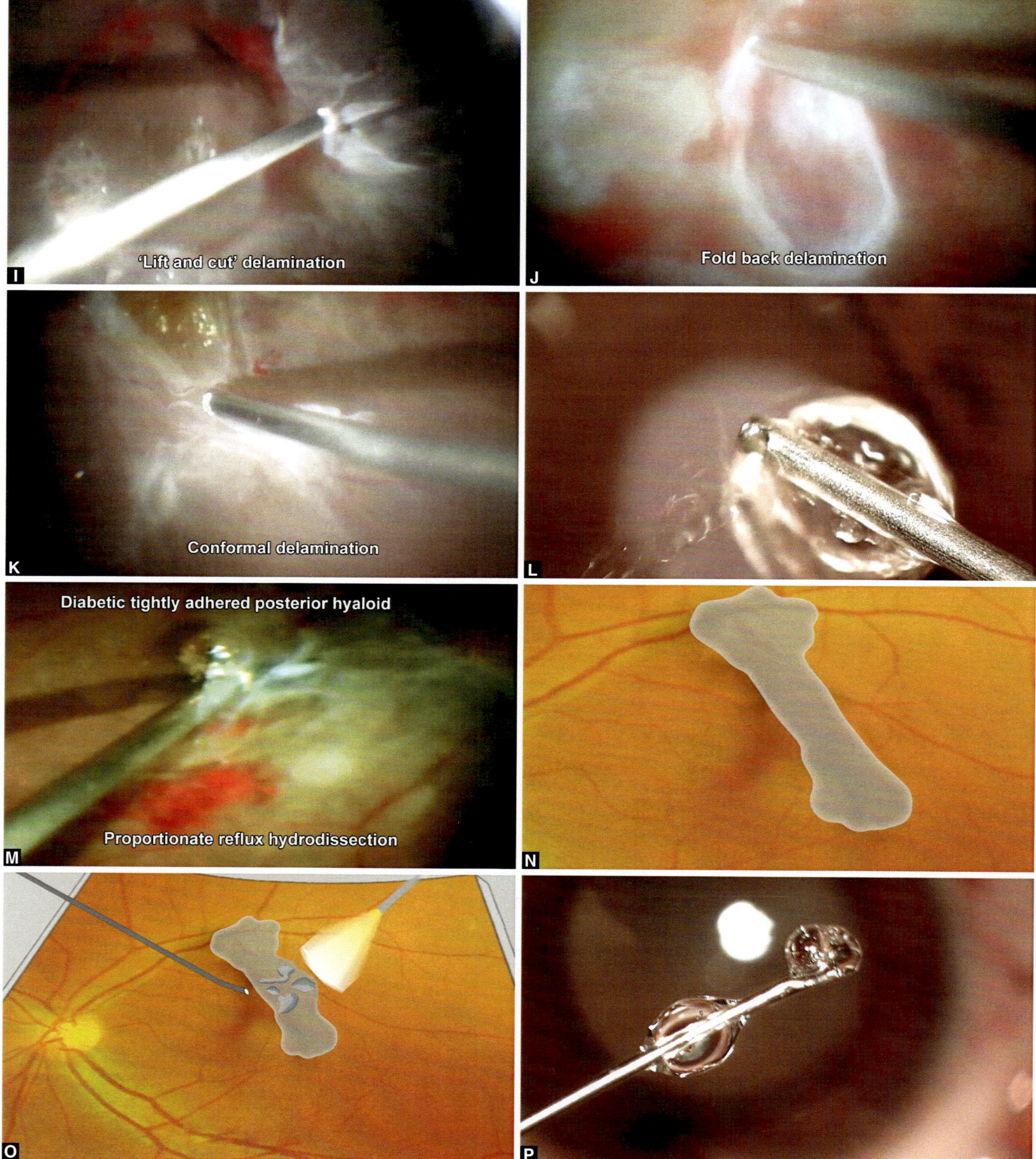

Figs 11.3I to P

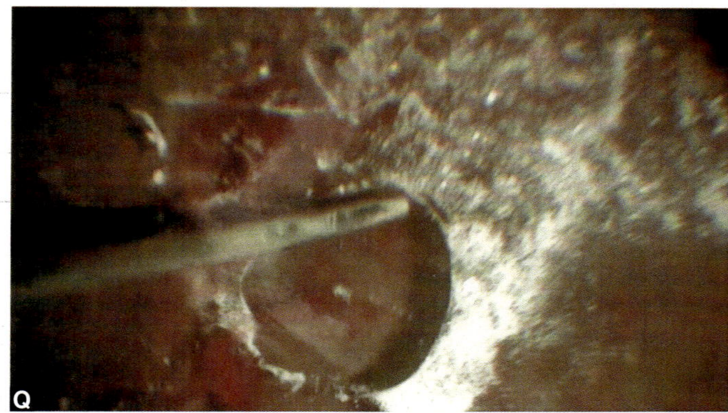

Figs 11.3A to Q: (A and B) Shows intraoperative photographs of forceps peeling; (C and D) Chop stick peeling; (E) Suction peeling; (F and G) Segmentation of diabetic fibrovascular membrane; (H) Delamination by curved scissor; (I) 'Lift and cut' delamination; (J) 'Foldback cutter delamination' for thinner flexible membrane; (K) 'Conformal delamination' for rigid thicker ERM membrane; (L and M) Proportional reflux hydrodissection; (N to Q) Steps of visco dissection in a case of advanced thick broadly-attached membrane

manage thin membranes maximum cut rate and lower suction is necessary.

2. Proportional reflux hydrodissection—To dissect adhered membrane by jet of BSS fluid through the cutter port. The fluid flow rate can be controlled by foot pedal. Fluid flow cause plane of cleavage between the membrane and thin retina and can separate safely the membrane from underlying thinned out retina. Risk of iatrogenic break formation is very low in this maneuver. This newly added property to the cutter improved the function of cutter to manage relatively complex cases unimanually.
Bimanual dissection: Situations where one have to use both hands are relatively more complex advanced diabetic cases with thick proliferative membranes.
One has to use chandelier's illumination as the fourth port make both hands free.

Management of Tractional Retinal Detachments

Managing Extramacular TRD (Video 18, Chapter 11)

Extramacular TRD is relatively safer situation. One has to remove surrounding vitreous along with removal of membrane attachment. Traction free elevated retina will be settled under endotamponade in due course of time (Fig. 11.4A).

Macula Threatening or Macula Involving Tractional Retinal Detachment Cases

These cases are to be intervened as early as possible.

Managing macula-threatening TRD:

- A case of advanced PDR with fibrous membrane formation with macula threatening TRD on OCT (Fig. 11.4B).

Case discussion (Video 19, Chapter 11):

- In case of macula threatening TRD, after TA-assisted vitrectomy, PFCL injected to stabilize macula (Fig. 11.4C)
- Surrounding fibrovascular membrane peeled with the suction of cutter (Fig. 11.4D)
- Iatrogenic break can be formed during membrane removal
- More PFCL then to be injected to make posterior pole more stable
- Overlying posterior hyaloid removed
- Bleeders are secured with cautery
- Fluid-air exchange started and PFCL removed
- Breaks are laser barraged and PRP done
- Silicone oil injected as tamponade
- Pre- and postoperative OCT (Fig. 11.4E) shows flattened macula five and half months after surgery with postoperative ERM formation.

Managing Macula Involving Advanced TRDs

Case discussion (Video 20, Chapter 11):

- A case of advanced proliferative diabetic retinopathy with elevated macular tractional detachment (Fig. 11.4F)
- TA-assisted vitrectomy done
- Posterior hyaloid was tightly adhered at the posterior pole and PVD seen at periphery
- An opening in posterior hyaloid made at periphery and cutter introduced in subhyaloid space (Fig. 11.4G)
- Posterior hyaloid separation started from 'outside-in' manner (Fig. 11.4H)
- Segmentation of the membranes done
- Thick fibrous membrane delamination done by 'lift and cut' technique (Fig. 11.4I)

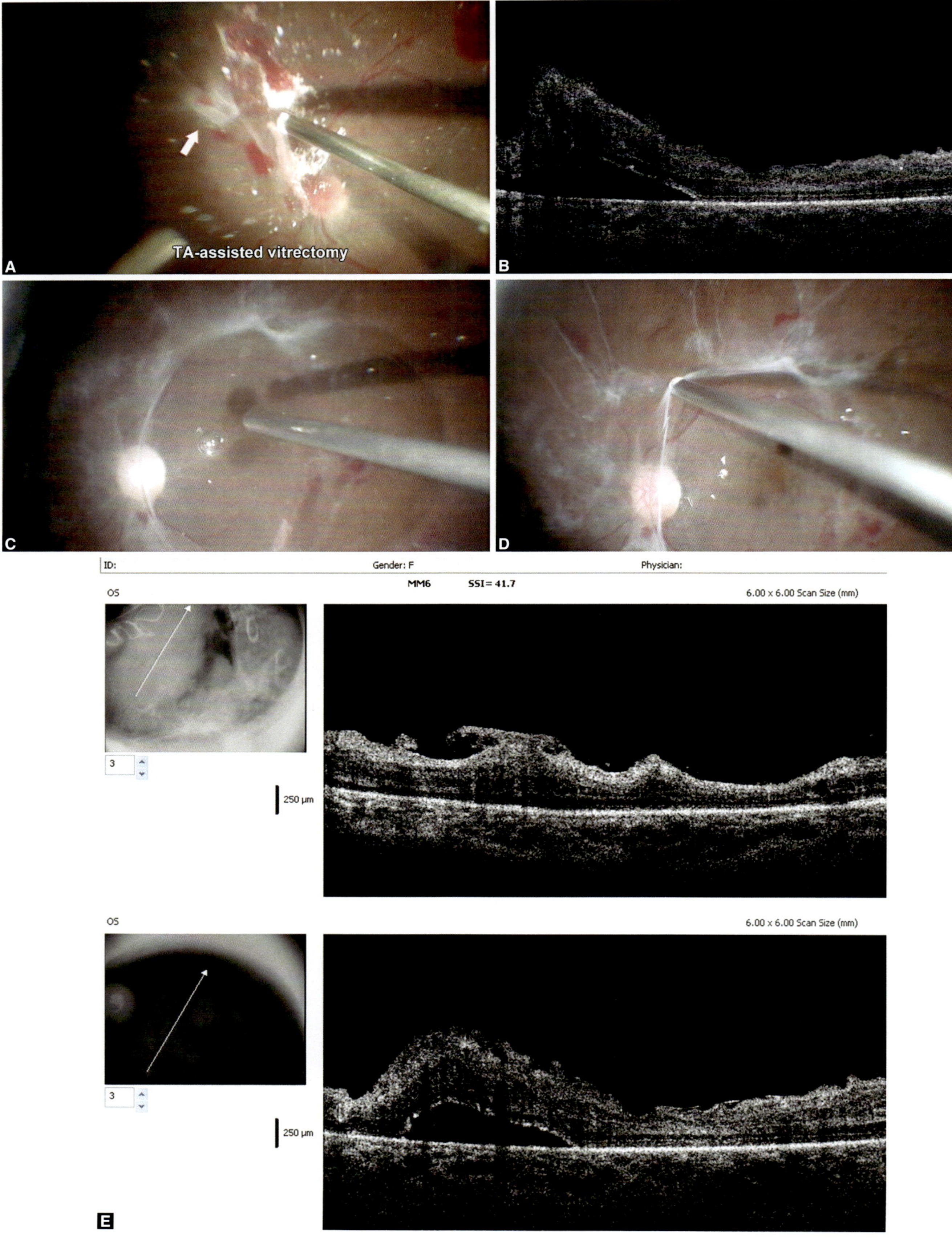

Figs 11.4A to E

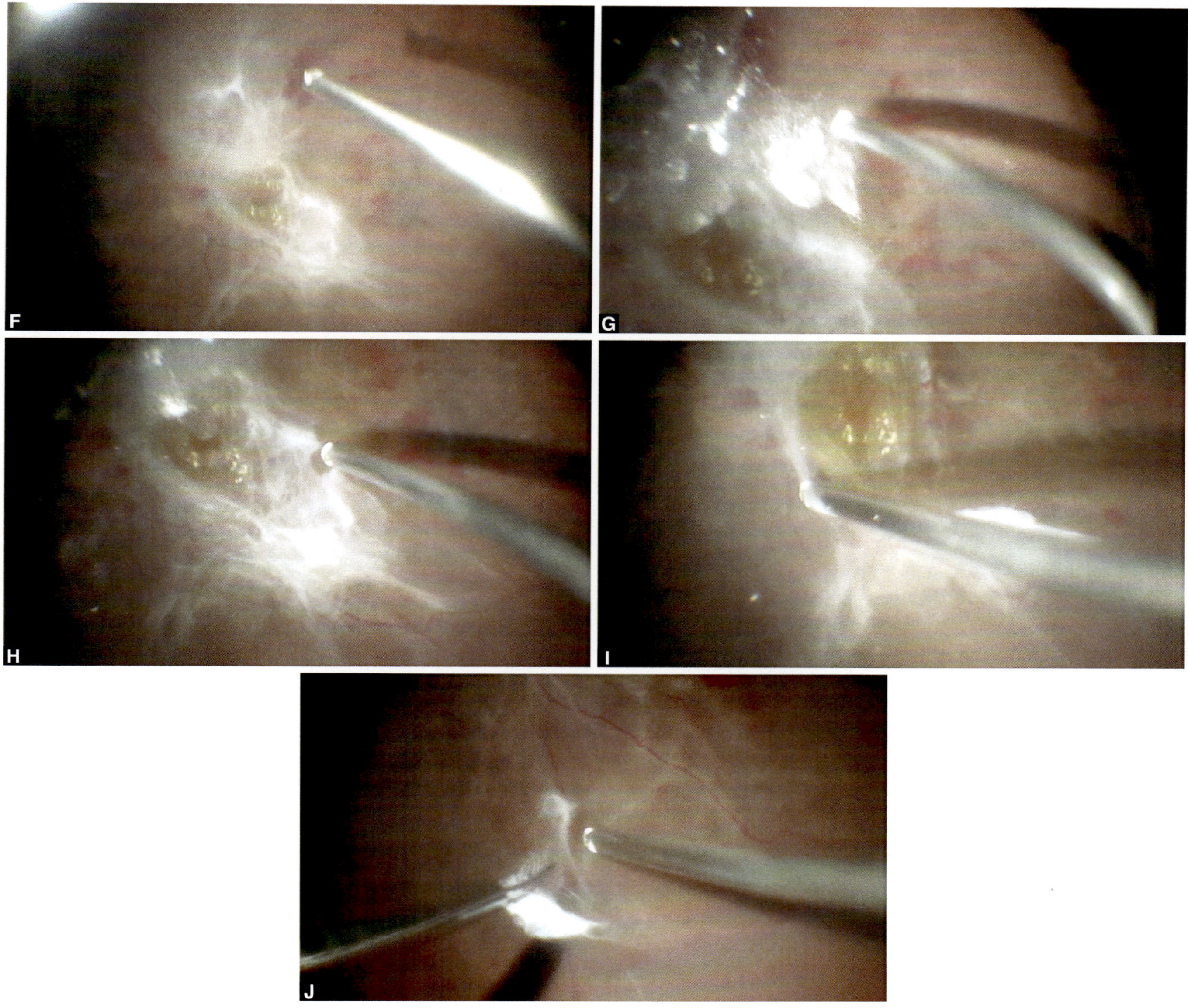

Figs 11.4F to J

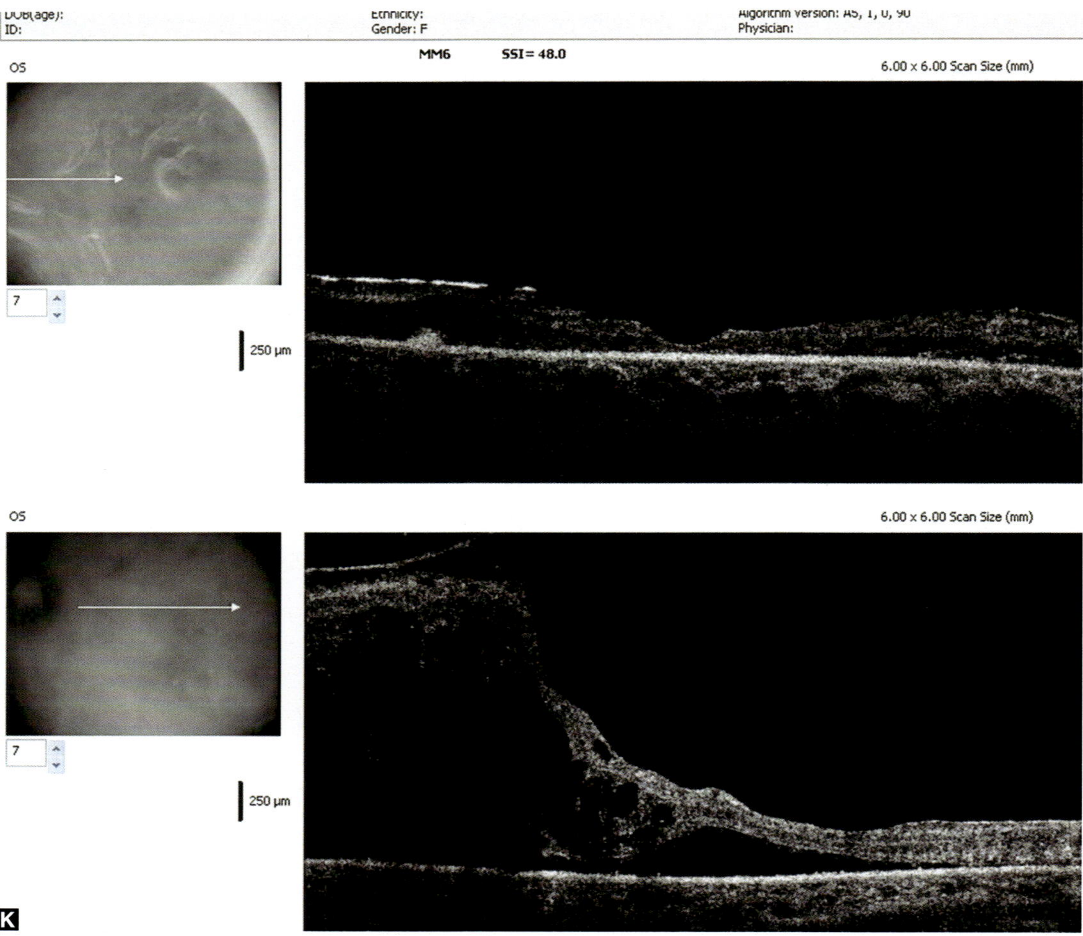

Figs 11.4A to K: (A) Extramacular nasal tractional retinal detachment (white arrow); (B) OCT shows macula threatening tractional retinal detachment; (C and D) Shows intraoperative steps of managing macula threatening tractional retinal detachment; (E) Pre- and postoperative OCT in a case of macula-threatening tractional retinal detachment— shows flattened macula five and half months after surgery with postoperative ERM formation; (F to J) Shows intraoperative steps of managing macula involving tractional retinal detachment; (K) Pre- and postoperative OCT in a case of macula involving tractional retinal detachment—shows flattened macula one month after surgery with silicone oil reflection

- Finally bimanual membrane separation, segmentation and delamination completed (Fig. 11.4J)
- PFCL injected
- Fluid-air exchange started to settle retina through the break
- Laser completed
- Silicone oil injected
- Pre- and postoperative OCT (Fig. 11.4K) shows flattened macula 1 month after surgery with silicone oil reflection.

Steps to Manage Combined Tractional - Rhegmatogenous Retinal Detachments

Progressive vitreous contraction and contraction of fibrovascular membranes lead to worsening of TRD and sometimes create retinal break formation, producing a combined tractional-rhegmatogenous detachment with different configuration convex, bullous shaped (not concave like TRDs).

Breaks (holes) are often found next to the areas of traction, hidden underneath areas of vitreo retinal adhesions or neovascular frond. Surgical repair has led a 48–53% improvement in visual acuity.

However, approximately 10–20% of diabetic vitrectomies (for TRD and combined RD) resulted in vision of no light perception.

Advanced cases of PDR has very thick fibrotic membrane and associated combined TRD-rhegmatogenous retinal detachments are usually chronic with atrophic thinned retina. Bullous configuration of this kind of RD is due to contracted posterior hyaloid and anterior-posterior traction. Excising posterior hyaloid and delamination of fibrotic membrane can result in settling of detached retina. However, residual fibrovascular tissue may exert traction with associated posterior break. In these cases, retina surrounding the area of traction may have to be excised to reapproximate the retina. If there is minimal separation of posterior hyaloid, an MVR blade or membrane pic or bent 24G needle can be used to separate the hyaloid face.

Simple localized combined RD (Video 21, Chapter 11):

- A macula-off diabetic combined retinal detachment with thick posterior hyaloid with subhyaloid hemorrhage
- Posterior hyaloid face cut and subhyaloid hemorrhage removed
- Posterior hyaloid removed around the elevated detached retina (Fig. 11.5A)
- Underlying breaks detected (Fig. 11.5B, white arrow shows underlying break)
- Preretinal blood removed by soft-tip cannula
- Triamcinolone particles injected to check residual blood and peripheral vitrectomy completed (Fig. 11.5C)
- PRP completed (Fig. 11.5D)
- Combined retinal detachment was localized involving macula (Fig. 11.5E)
- Fluid-air exchange started and localized subretinal fluid drained through the break (Fig. 11.5F)
- Laser done around the break
- Silicone oil injected for tamponade (Fig. 11.5G).

Complex combined RD (Video 22, Chapter 11)

Preoperative OCT shows macula-off combined rhegmatogenous-TRD (Fig. 11.5H).

- A case of macula-off combined retinal detachment in advanced diabetic retinopathy with extensive posterior pole fibrovascular proliferation (Fig. 11.5I)
- Triamcinolone-assisted vitrectomy done
- An opening made in posterior hyaloid (Fig. 11.5J)
- Posterior hyaloid with fibrovascular membrane was tried to separate from the underlying detached retina with proportionate reflux hydrodissection mode of the cutter (Fig. 11.5K)
- Then a bent tip 24G cannula used for viscodissection (Fig. 11.5L), attaching with the VFC syringe, filled with viscoelastic hydroxypropyl methyl cellulose
- Then the bent tip cannula introduced in between the vascular membrane and detached retina and viscoelastic materials injected using VFC in viscous fluid injection mode (Fig. 11.5M)
- Bimanually the membrane everted with an ILM forceps and viscoelastic injected again to separate the membrane from the detached retina (Fig. 11.5N)
- Multiple underlying attachments bluntly cut
- Underlying break detected (Fig. 11.5O)
- Membrane trimmed (Fig. 11.5P)
- Preretinal blood removed
- Cautery done for all bleeders
- Laser done around the cauterized bleeders
- Fluid-air exchange done
- Laser done around the break
- PRP completed (Fig. 11.5Q)
- Disc hemorrhage secured with triamcinolone particles
- Silicone oil injected
- Pre- and postoperative OCT (Fig. 11.5R) shows flattened macula 2 weeks after surgery.

Bimanual Surgery for Complex Diabetic Retinal Detachments

Bimanual dissection can be followed in the following manners:

1. *End-grasping forceps and curved scissor:* For segmenting as well as delaminating a membrane. Membrane can be cut between TRDs introducing an arm of a scissor between membrane edge and retina. After segmentation end-grasping forceps has to hold one edge of the segmented membrane and then delaminate it from the underlying elevated retina.
2. *End-grasping forceps and cutter:* Cutter is more frequently used instead of scissor to segment a membrane and to delaminate it from the underlying elevated retina (Fig. 11.6A -animation).
3. *End-grasping forceps and proportionate reflux hydrodissection mode of cutter:* After elevating an edge of a membrane cutter can be introduced.

Case discussions (Video 23, Chapter 11):

Case-I

- Case of advanced PDR with macula-involving TRD
- Vitrectomy was done
- Bridging vitreous between and around the TRDs with proliferations were cut (Fig. 11.6B)
- Triamcinolone acetonide particles were injected and residual vitrectomy was done
- Fibrovascular polyp from the optic disc was removed
- Triamcinolone-stained ERM from macula was removed
- Fibrovascular membrane was cut bimanually by end-gripping forceps and curved scissors using BIOM noncontact lens (Fig. 11.6C)
- Preretinal blood was removed
- All bleeders were cauterized
- Vitreous base excision was done by external scleral depression
- PRP was done avoiding areas of TRDs
- Fluid-air exchange was done
- Laser was done around the break
- Silicone oil was used for tamponade.

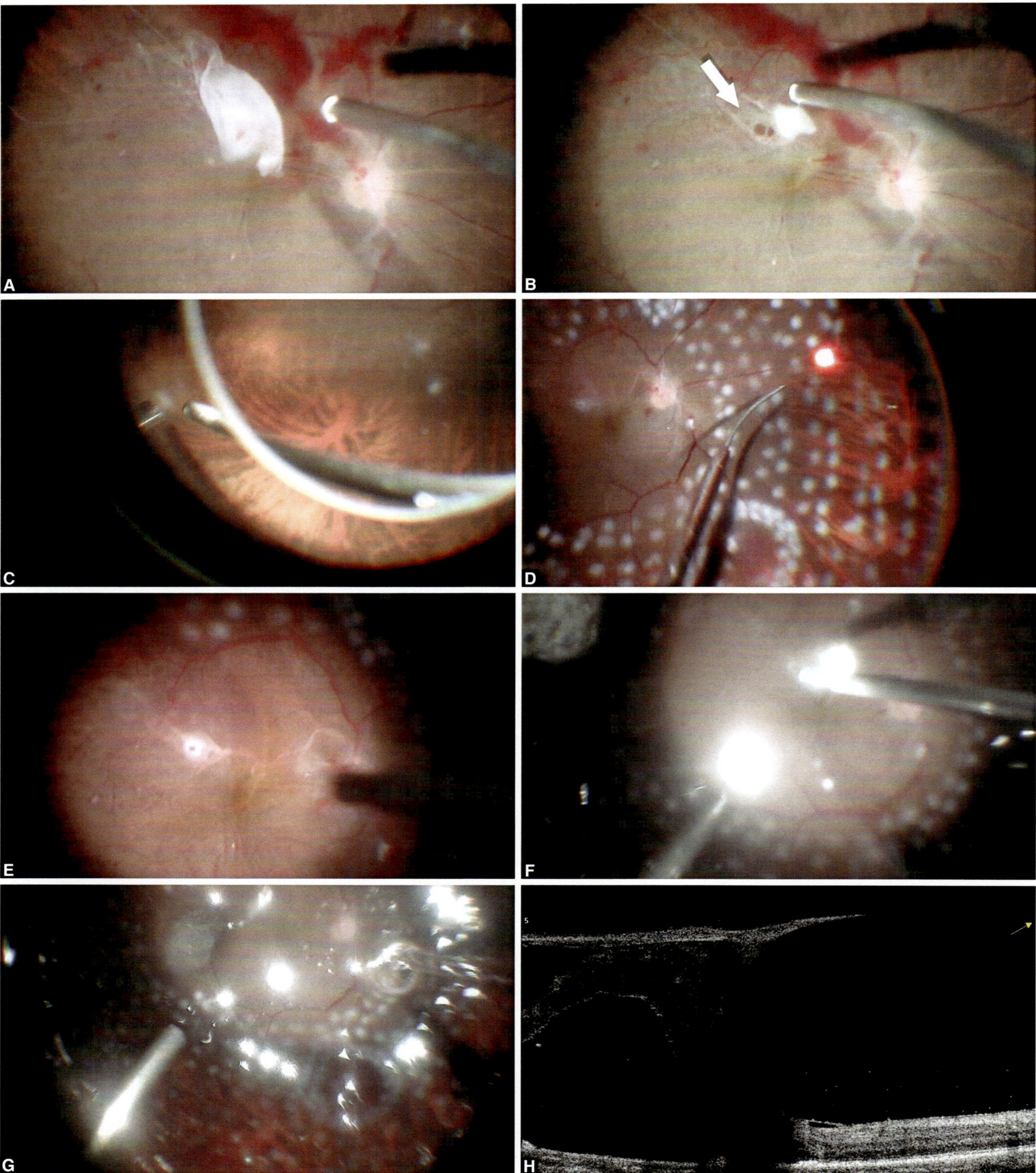

Figs 11.5A to H

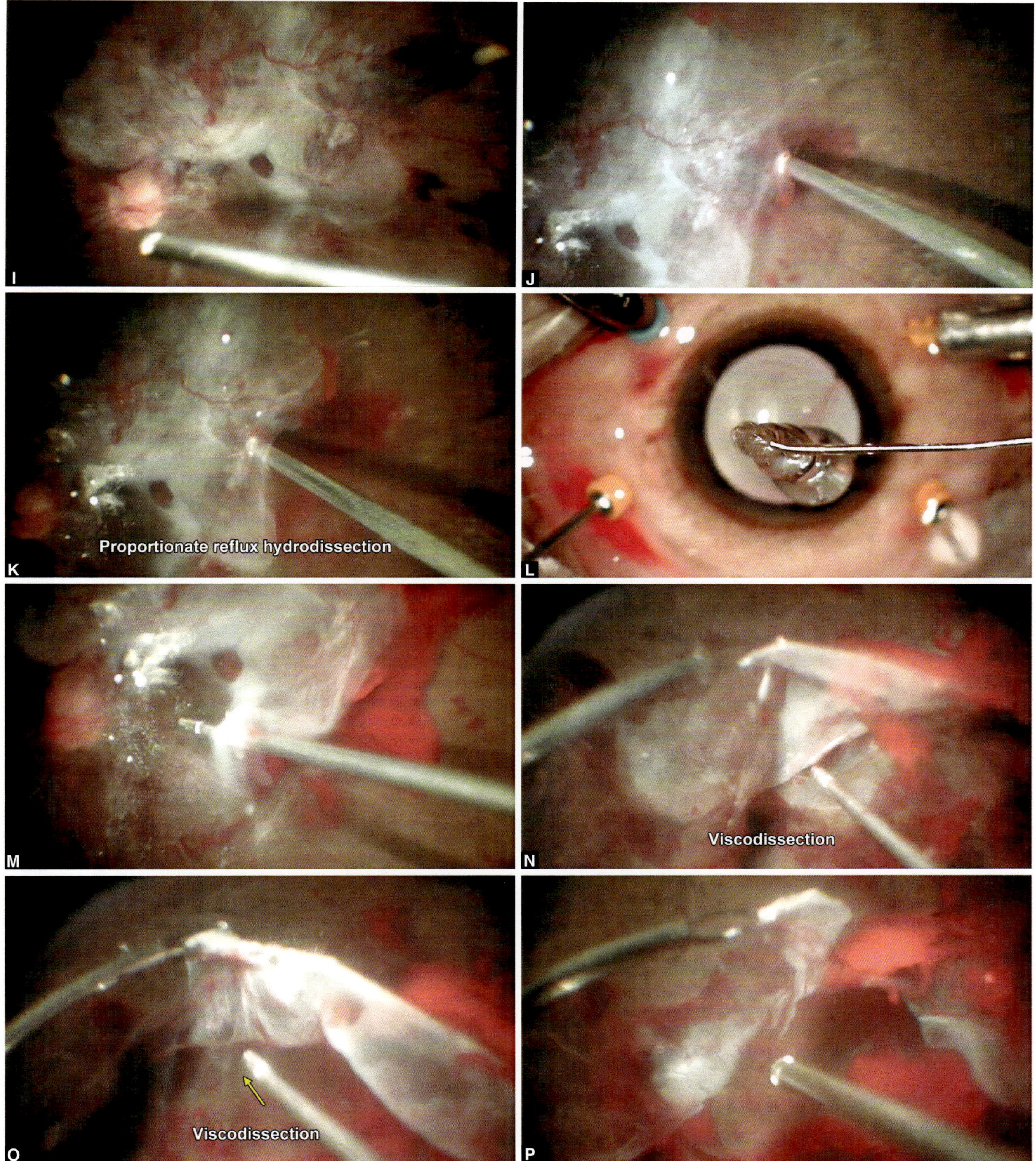

Figs 11.5I to P

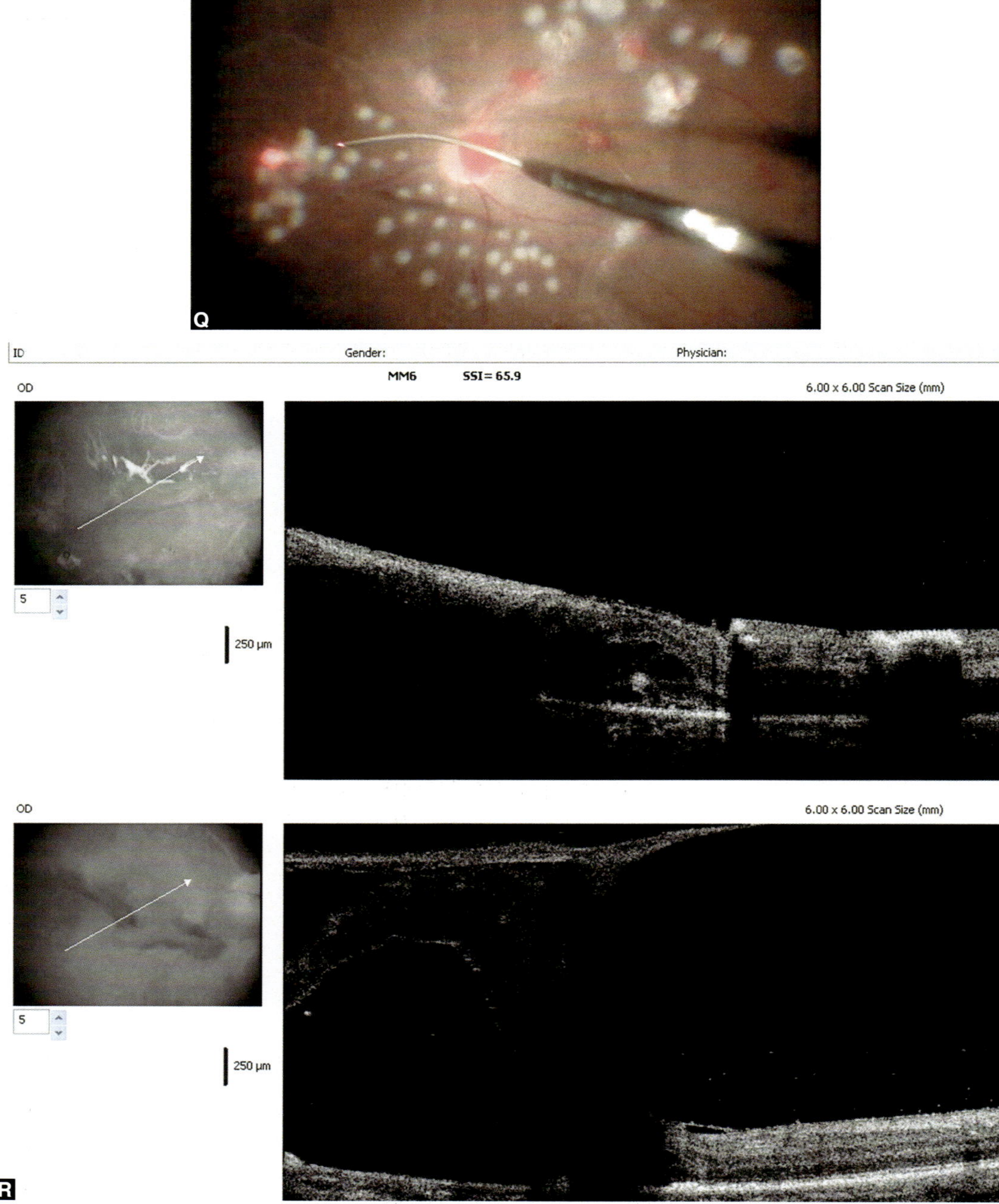

Figs 11.5A to R: (A to G) Shows intraoperative steps of managing simple combined retinal detachment; (H to Q) Shows intraoperative steps of managing macula-off combined rhegmatogenous- tractional retinal detachment; (R) Pre- and postoperative OCT in a case of macula-off complex combined rhegmatogenous- tractional retinal detachment—shows flattened macula two weeks after surgery

Case-II:

- Advanced PDR with posterior pole TRDs
- Preoperatively intravitreal injection Bevacizumab (0.05 mL) was given 3 days back
- Here proportionate reflux was used to separate the thick membrane from underlying detached retina (Fig. 11.6D)
- Bimanual dissection is always helpful in these advanced cases
- Careful segmentation and delamination is required (Fig. 11.6E)
- Again proportionate reflux was used to separate the membrane up to periphery
- PRP was done after fluid-air exchange.

Case-III:

- A four port 25G+ bimanual approach in advanced PDR with subhyaloid hemorrhage

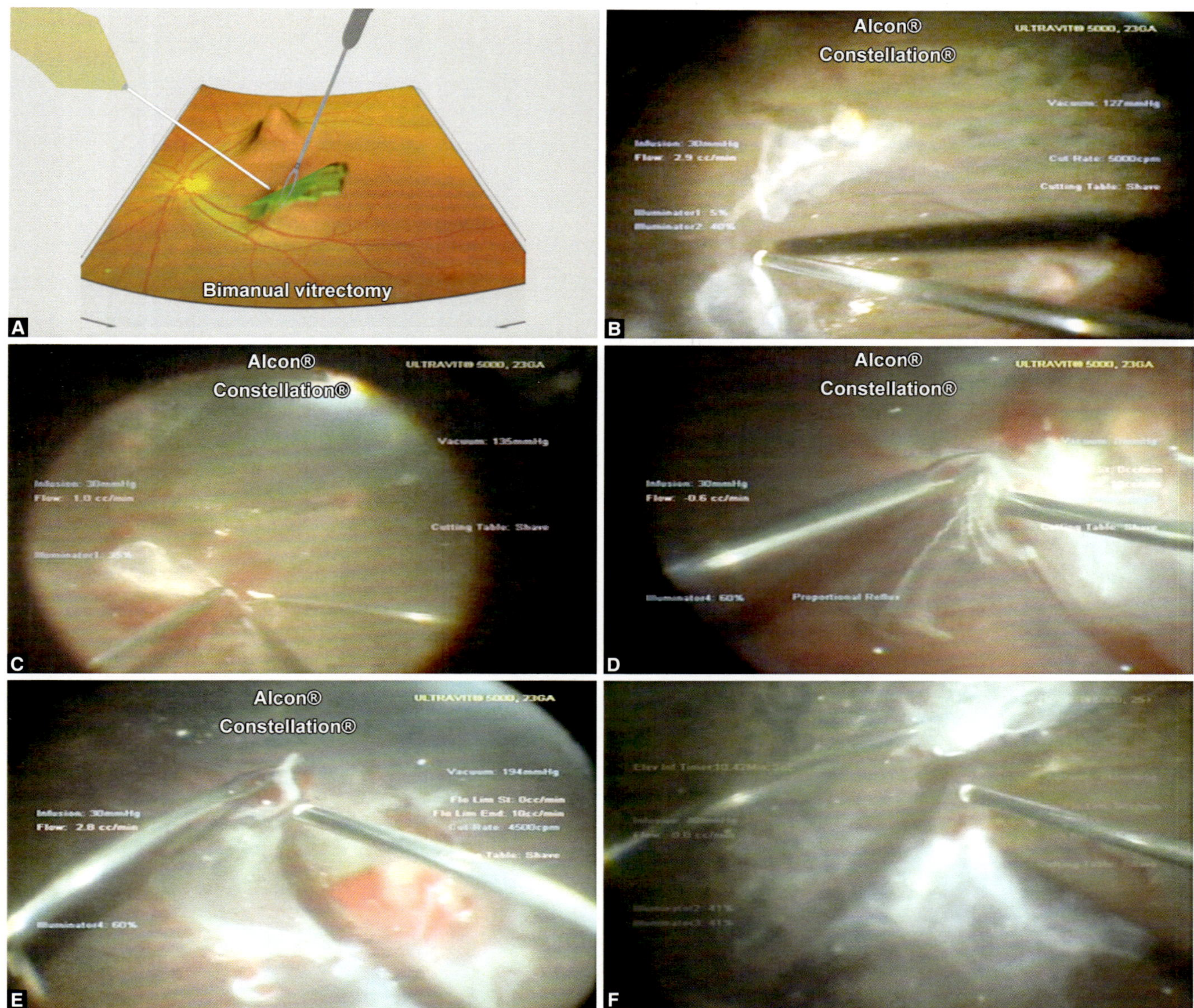

Figs 11.6A to F: (A) Shows bimanual dissection by end-grasping forceps and cutter in a case of advanced PDR with TRD; (B) Shows dissection of bridging vitreous by cutter in a case of advanced PDR with macula involving TRD; (C) Shows bimanual dissection in a case of advanced PDR with macula involving TRD by end-grasping forceps and curved scissor; (D) Shows bimanual dissection in a case of advanced PDR with posterior pole TRD by end-grasping forceps and cutter using proportionate reflux; (E) Shows bimanual membrane dissection in a case of advanced PDR with posterior pole TRD by end-grasping forceps and cutter; (F) Shows bimanual membrane dissection in a case of advanced PDR with posterior pole TRD by ILM forceps and cutter.

- Tip of infusion cannula was checked before turning it on
- Vitrectomy was done
- Thick posterior hyaloids face was trimmed out all around
- It was previously lasered
- Triamcinolone acetonide particles were injected
- Thick fibrous band was cut bimanually (Fig. 11.6F)
- And the membrane was trimmed out
- Cautery should be done for bleeders without delay
- The other end of the membrane was again segmented and trimmed out accordingly bimanually
- All membrane dissections were completed

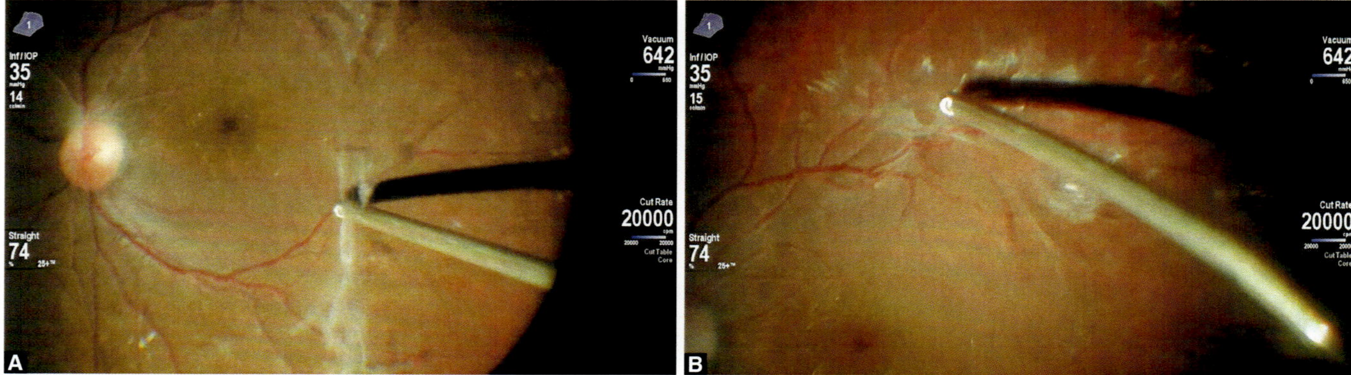

Figs 11.7A and B: Intraoperative steps of managing advanced PDR with multiple tractional retinal detachments with high-speed cutter.

- Cautery was done for all bleeders and breaks
- Fluid-air exchange was done
- PRP was completed and laser was done also around the breaks
- Silicone oil injected as an endotamponade
- 25G cannulas were plugged and removed
- *Managing advanced PDR with multiple tractional retinal detachments with high-speed cutter:* With a high-speed dual-pneumatic beveled tip cutter having 20000 cuts per minute, one can truly shave the posterior hyaloid face and remove all the fibrovascular membranous attachment, reaching very close to the retinal surface. Moreover, fluidic stability is achieved because of reduced fluidic turbulence.

Case discussion (Video 24, Chapter 11):

- A case of PDR with a taut posterior hyaloid face with multiple tractional retinal detachment
- We used a 25 G Hypervit cutter in this case
- After core vitrectomy, the cutter was used to cut the membranous attachments in between bridging TRDs (Fig. 11.7A)
- The beveled-tip cutter was very useful for reaching near the retinal surface and trimming the fibrous proliferative membranes (Fig. 11.7B)
- This is almost the ideal mode of shaving the taut hyaloid face
- Now Triamcinolone-stained vitreoschisis membranes can be detached safely from the retinal surface

Kindly scan the QR code below to access the online Video.

CHAPTER 12

Subretinal Hematoma, Subretinal Recombinant Tissue Plasminogen Activator and Current Management Algorithm

Causes

1. Age-related macular degeneration (ARMD)
2. Polypoidal choroidal vasculopathy
3. Macroaneurysm
4. Trauma.

Prognosis of Submacular Hemorrhage

Unfortunately, submacular hemorrhages usually have a poor visual prognosis if left untreated. This is the result of the following factors:

- A barrier effect that prevents metabolic exchange between the retina and choriocapillaris
- Toxicity of iron released by the hemoglobin
- Fibrin infiltration between the inner and outer segments of photoreceptors can result in destructive shearing of the cells
- Shearing of the outer segments of the photoreceptors from contraction of the hemorrhage.
- The prognosis of submacular hemorrhage is further worsened if the hemorrhage is thick and is associated with age-related macular degeneration.

Prerequisite for subretinal hematoma drainage are:

- Good photoreceptor
- Recent drop or still good visual acuity
- OCT
- Duration of loss of reading capacity
- Central visual field defect

Intraoperative risk factors:

- Hypertension
- Patient is on anticoagulant therapy.

But it all depends on the strategy.

All submacular hemorrhages can be divided into three categories:

1. *If small:* Intravitreal anti-VEGF or pneumatic displacement and follow up.
2. *If medium-sized:* Intravitreal tPA (tissue plasminogen activator) injection + SF_6 gas injection + anti-VEGF injection. If it fails to displace the submacular blood, then one should go for vitrectomy + subretinal tPA injection.
3. *If large and elevated:* Then vitrectomy along with subretinal blood removal with or without full thickness RPE-choroid transplant can be performed.

Surgical Steps

Submacular Hematoma-subretinal Membrane Removal (Video 1, Chapter 12)

- Status post-AMD submacular hematoma
- There was subneurosensory retinal hematoma on OCT
- Heavy PFCL (Decaline) was injected to displace submacular hematoma after vitrectomy (Fig. 12.1A)
- An extramacular retinotomy was made at PFCL bubble margin over hematoma (Fig. 12.1B)
- PFCL bubble was rolled over hematoma to displace submacular blood
- An area of localized retinal detachment was created to remove submacular blood
- Submacular blood was removed bimanually using suction
- Subretinal neovascular membrane was removed using forceps (Figs 12.1C and D)
- Fluid-air exchange was performed to settle induced detachment
- Laser was done around the retinotomy (Fig. 12.1E) and silicone oil was injected.

Submacular Blood Removal with Full Thickness RPE-Choroid Transplantation (Video 2, Chapter 12)

- Initial vitrectomy done for vitreous hemorrhage with PVD induction (Fig. 12.2A)
- A temporal 180 degree retinectomy done (Fig. 12.2B) and retinal detachment induced

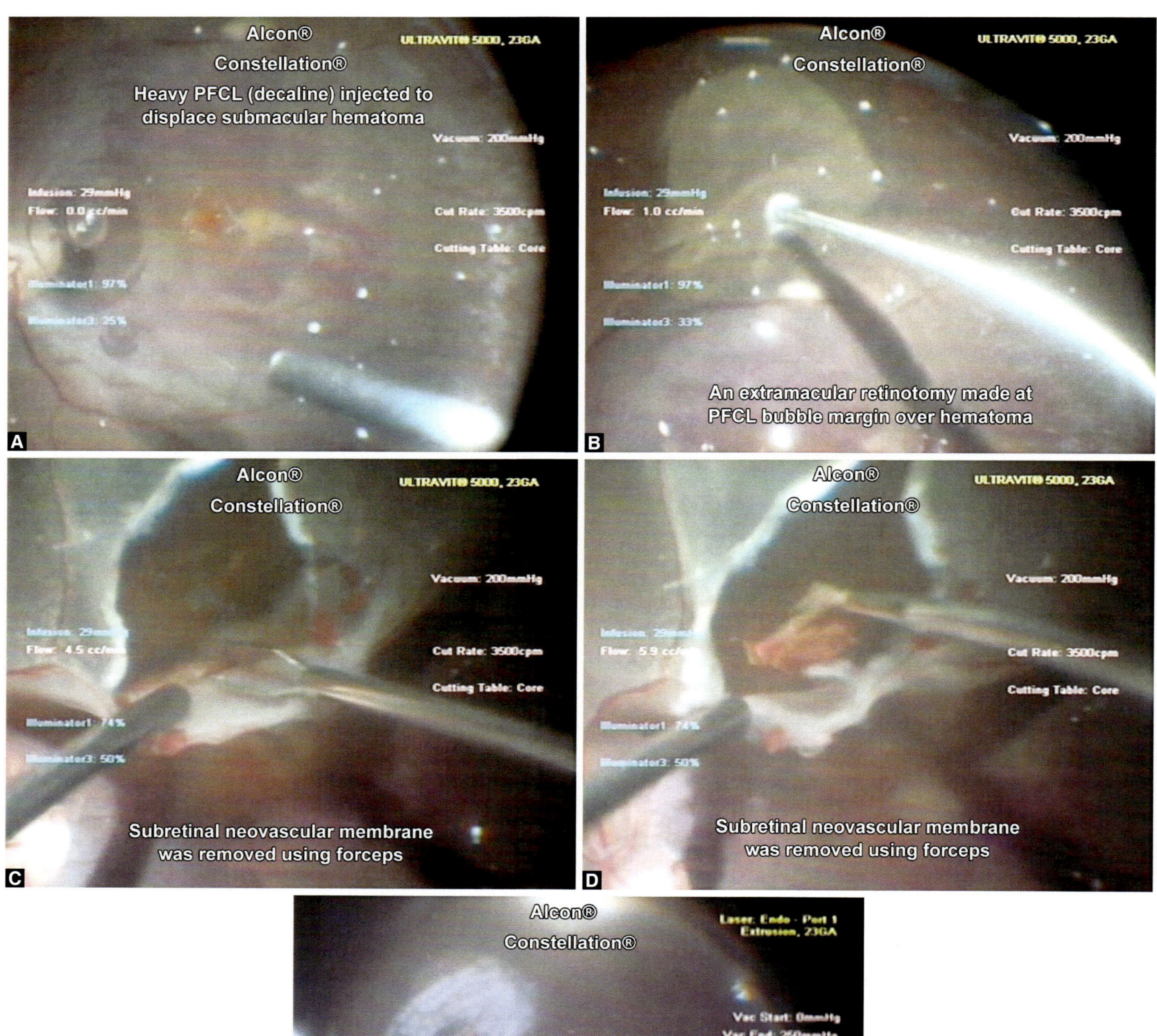

Figs 12.1A to E: Intraoperative steps of removal of submacular neovascular membrane

- Subretinal blood including submacular extensions removed bimanually with cutter and silicone tipped backflush needle in a similar manner (Figs 12.2C and D)
- A full thickness RPE-choroidal graft taken from the superotemporal quadrant and placed subfoveally (Figs 12.2E to G)
- Reapposition of retinal flap after injecting PFCL (Figs 12.2H and I)
- Fluid-air exchange done through the retinectomy margin
- Laser done (Fig. 12.2J)
- Direct silicone oil—PFCL exchange done (Figs 12.2K and L)
- Postoperative wide-field fundus photograph (Fig. 12.2M), two weeks after submacular blood removal with full thickness RPE-choroid transplantation, shows subfoveal RPE-Choroidal graft and OCT macular scan (Fig. 12.2N), after three months, shows subneurosensory retinal RPE-choroidal graft.

Plasminogen Activator (rt-PA)

- It is a protein involved in the breakdown of blood clots.
- A serine protease is found in endothelial cells that line the blood vessels. As an enzyme, it catalyzes the conversion of plasminogen to plasmin, the major enzyme responsible for clot breakdown.
- tPA cleaves the zymogen plasminogen at its Arg561-Val562 peptide bond.
- The molecular weight of human tPA is ~70 kDa in the single-chain form.
- Normally it is present in ocular tissues like aqueous humor (30 times more than plasma), trabecular meshwork, lens, vitreous, conjunctiva, and cornea protein, but not in retina or choroid.

Subretinal vs Intravitreal rt-PA Injection

a. Intravitreal rt-PA injection:
   - *Advantages:* It is easier to perform, less invasive, and takes less time
   - *Disadvantages:* Responses are variable

b. Subretinal rt-PA injection:
   - *Advantage:* Response is definitive
   - *Disadvantages:* It is more invasive and takes more time

Adverse effects of rtPA:

a. *Ocular side effects:*
   i. Photoreceptor cell loss
   ii. RPE pigmentary changes
   iii. Exudative retinal detachment
   iv. Iatrogenic large retinal break
   v. Foveal blow-out (secondary macular hole formation)

b. *Extraocular side effects:* If too high dose (>100 µg/0.05 mL), theoretical risk of
   i. Bleeding (intracranial/gastric)
   ii. Angioedema (airway obstruction)

Current Management of Submacular Hemorrhage

It all depends on the size of the submacular hemorrhage and the duration and distribution of SMH. A rational treatment algorithm is as follows (Flowchart 12.1):

A. Small SMH (less than 4 disk diameter in size) with less than 2 weeks duration

i. If post-nAMD or PCV—only anti-VEGF or intravitreal rt-PA injection
ii. If post-traumatic—pneumatic displacement, i.e., intravitreal C3F8/SF6 gas injection with or without intravitreal rt-PA injection

B. Significant SMH (more than 4 disk diameter in size)

I. SMH is less than 4 weeks duration, confined to the macula with or without inferior extension: A nondrainage technique, i.e., vitrectomy, subretinal cocktail injection of recombinant tissue plasminogen activator [rt-PA (Actilyse, Boehringer Ingelheim, Germany) 50 µg dosage in 0.05 mL of balanced salt solution], anti-VEGF (Ranibizumab 0.5 mg in 0.05 mL) and filtered air (0.03 mL) injection with a 38 gauge flexible/41-gauge metallic needle followed by 20% sulfur hexafluoride (SF6) gas (iso expansile concentration) tamponade is required.

This nondrainage technique by vitrectomy with a cocktail of subretinal rtPA, anti-VEGF, and filtered sterile air injection is enough in cases of SMH up to 4 weeks duration and mainly confined to the macula, as considerable visual improvement is possible without blood drainage because of displacement of submacular blood, either partially or completely.

Subretinal anti-VEGF injection: It is required to deliver the drug near the choroidal neovascular membrane and prevent its early washout from the vitreous cavity.

Subretinal filtered sterile air: It helps to lower the buoyancy of red blood cells, allowing higher gravitational force relative to buoyancy force to facilitate downward displacement of the lysed SMH.

Case discussion (Video 3, Chapter 12): When submacular hemorrhage is less than 4 weeks in duration and confined to the macula with or without inferior extension, it is better to plan for nondrainage technique.

- Triamcinolone-assisted vitrectomy performed (Fig. 12.3A)

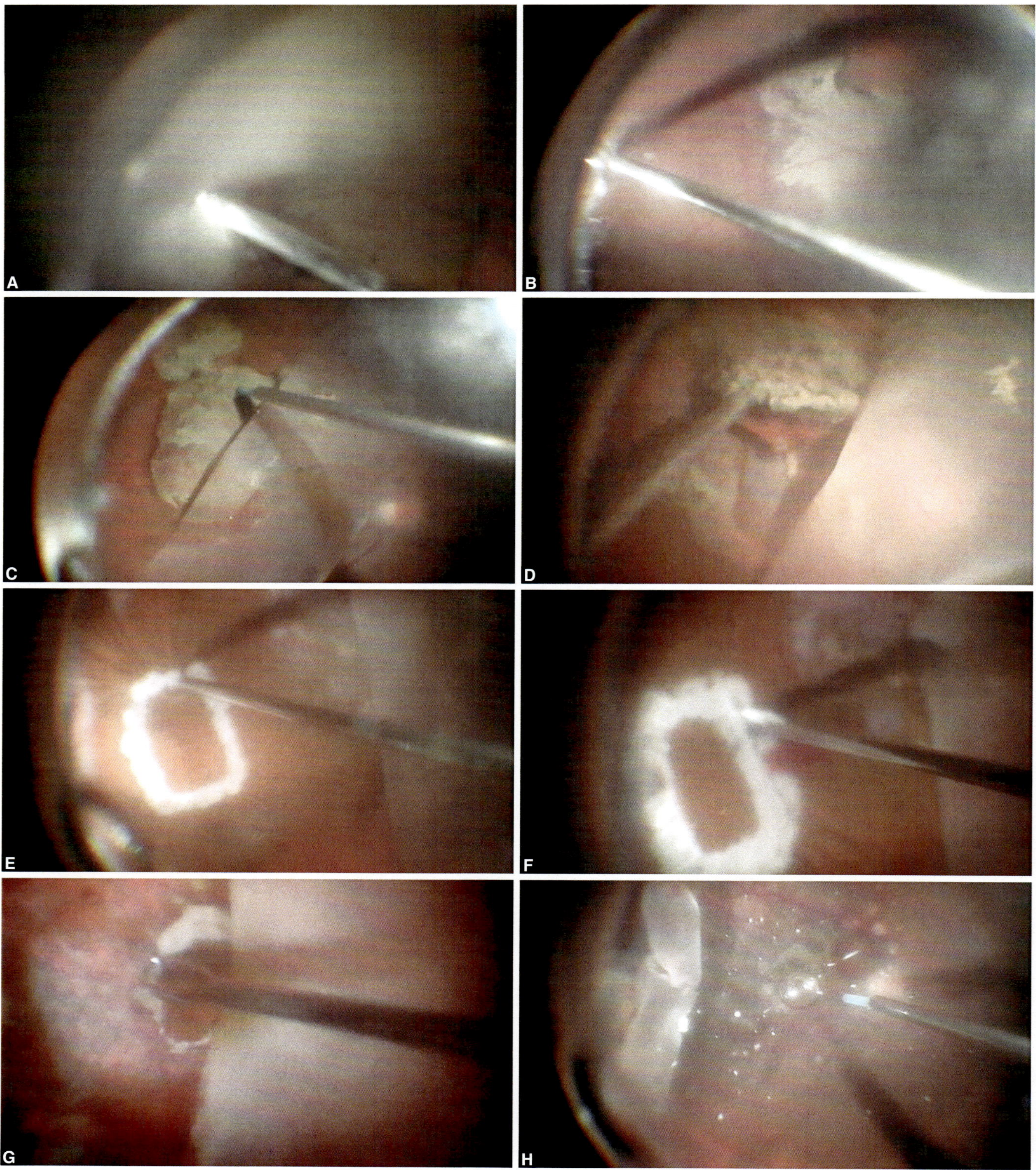

Figs 12.2A to H

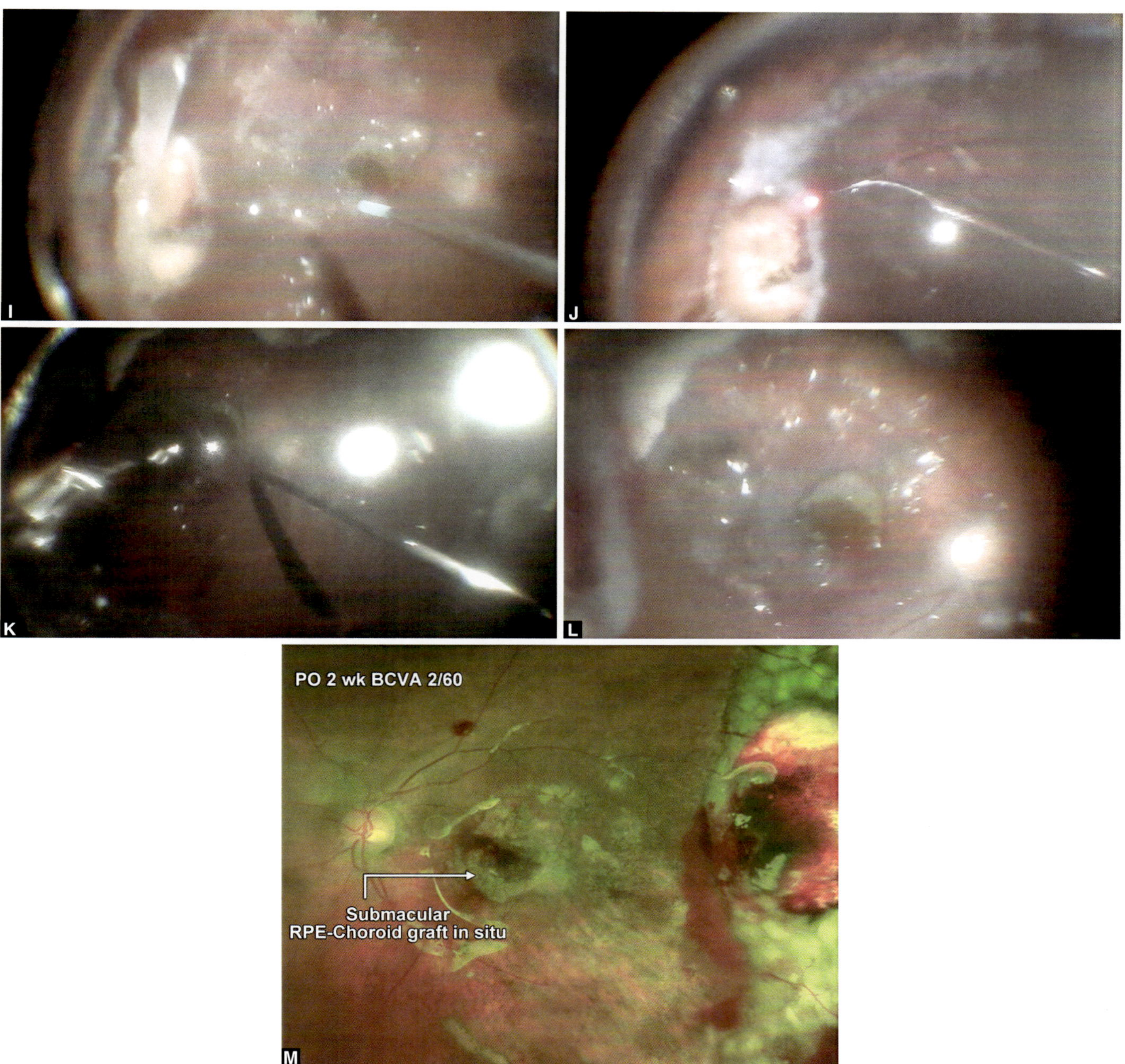

Figs 12.2I to M

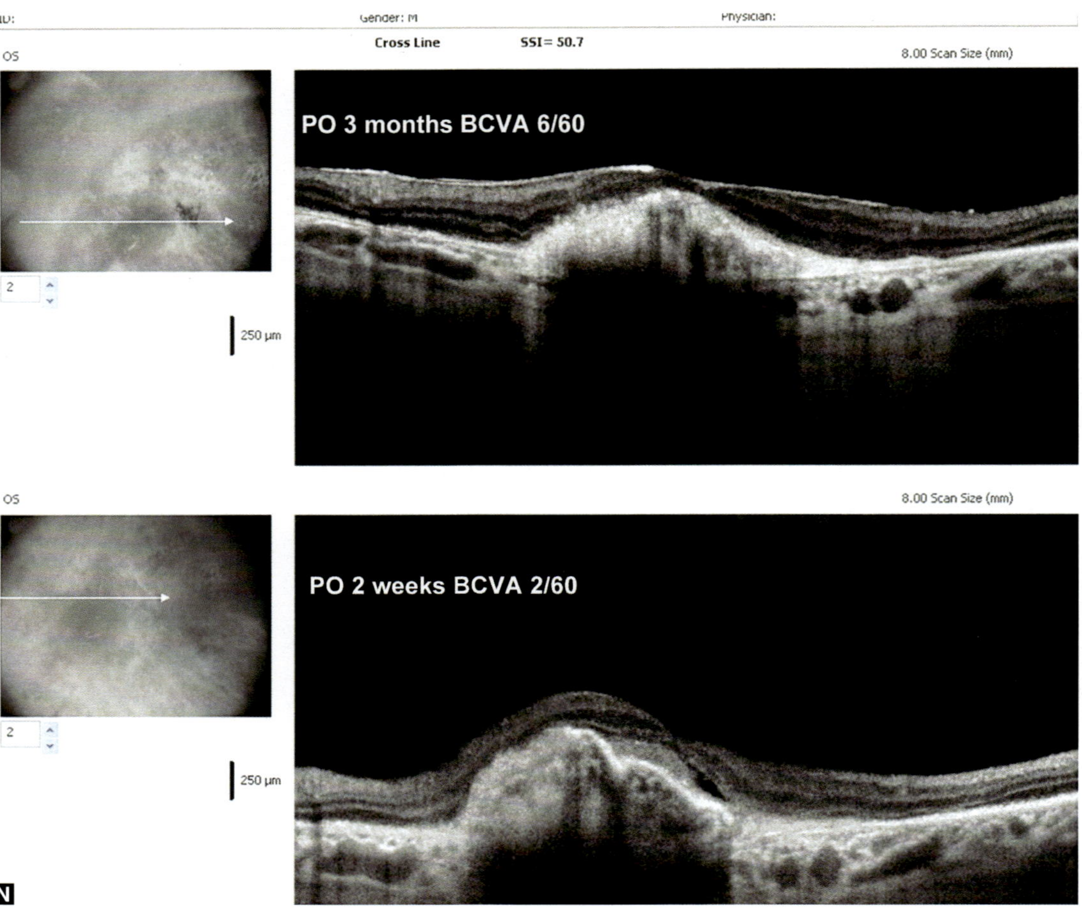

Figs 12.2A to N: (A to L) Intraoperative steps of submacular blood removal with full thickness RPE-choroid graft transplantation; (M) Postoperative subfoveal RPE-Choroidal graft, two weeks after submacular blood removal with full thickness RPE-choroid transplantation; (N) OCT macular scan shows postoperative subneurosensory retinal RPE-choroidal graft, two weeks and three months after submacular blood removal with full thickness RPE-choroid transplantation

Flowchart 12.1: Rational treatment algorithm in cases of submacular hemorrhage

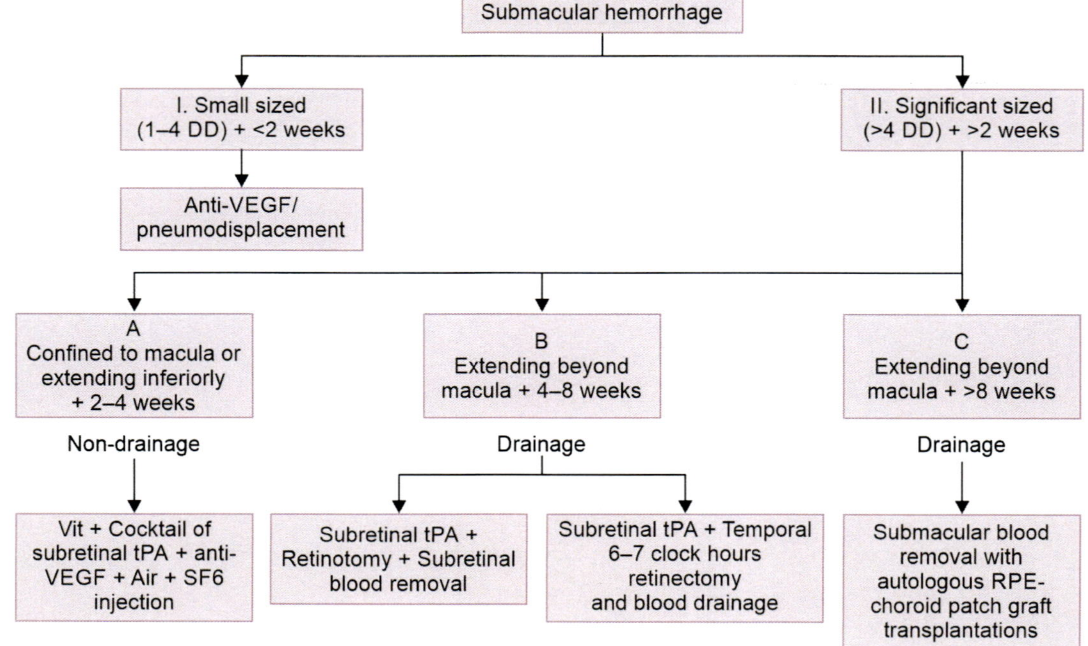

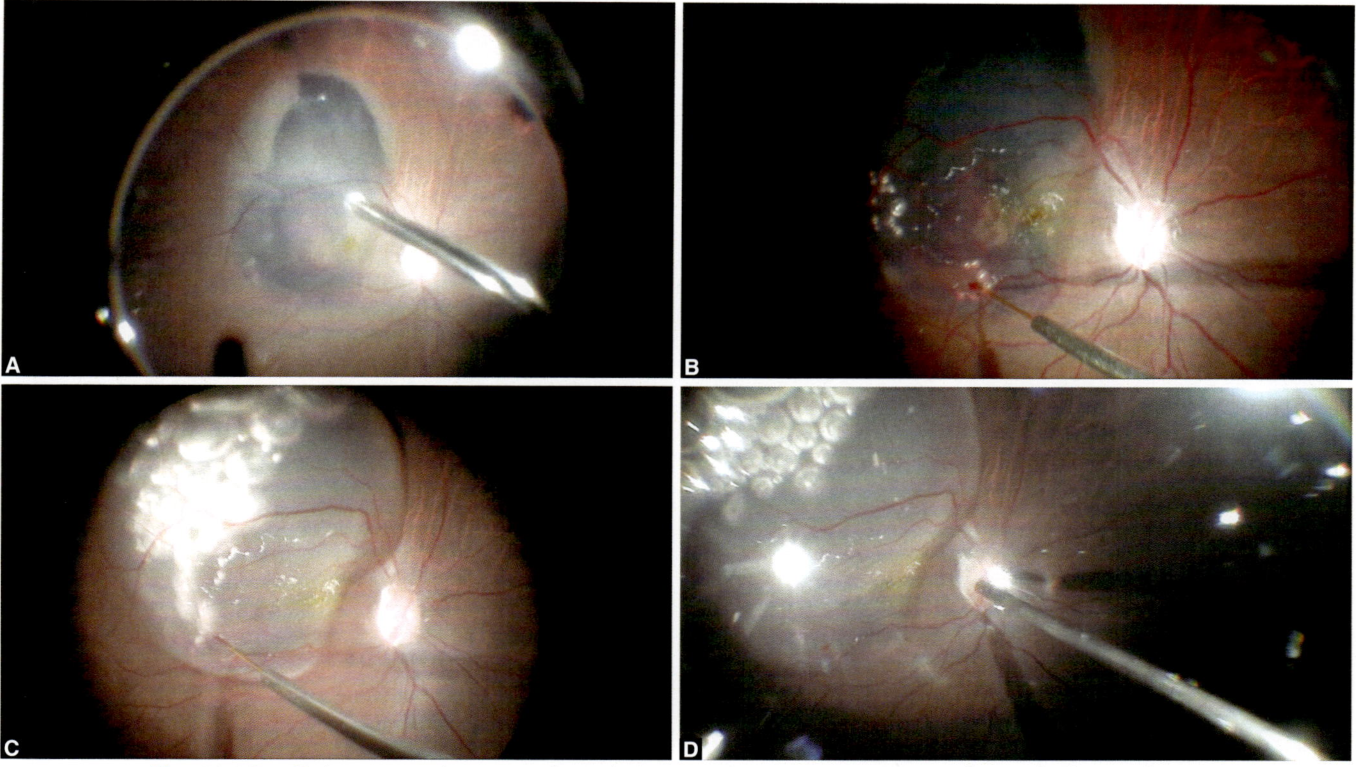

Figs 12.3A to D: Intraoperative steps of nondrainage technique in managing submacular hemorrhage.

- Then 0.05 mL recombinant tissue plasminogen activator was injected subretinally with a 38 gauge flexible nonmetallic needle (Fig. 12.3B)
- Then, a combination of 0.05 mL anti-VEGF drug and 0.03 mL filtered air was injected subretinally at a different site away from the macula with the same 38 gauge flexible nonmetallic needle (Fig. 12.3C) followed by fluid air exchange (Fig. 12.3D)
- The case was ended with 20% sulfur hexafluoride (SF6) gas injection in iso expansile concentration.

II. SMH is 4–8 weeks in duration, extending both superior and inferior to the macula: Drainage of SMH is necessary. Vitrectomy followed by injection of subretinal rt-PA (50 µg in 0.05 mL of balanced salt solution) is necessary. Then, 15–30 minutes of waiting time will be provided for adequate clot lysis. Subretinal blood is then drained either by paramacular retinotomies, which were a maximum of two in number in opposite quadrants, or by temporal 6–7 clock-hours (180° or more) retinectomy, followed by reposition of the retina, laser retinopexy and silicone oil (SO) tamponade. Submacular neovascular tissue is also to be removed along with SMH in the retinectomy cases. PFCL is used to settle the retinal flap in these cases.

- Complete drainage of SMH is possible in these cases after clot lysis by subretinal rt-PA injection, to minimize further damage of photoreceptors as well as RPE cell activities.

Case discussion:

- *Submacular Hemorrhage Drainage by Retinotomy (Video 4, Chapter 12)*
  - This is a case of a cataract with dense vitreous hemorrhage with hemorrhagic retinal detachment.
  - We first did phacoemulsification followed by intraocular lens implantation (Fig. 12.4A)
  - Then, vitrectomy started to clear the vitreous hemorrhage
  - Hemorrhagic retinal detachment was detected underneath (Fig. 12.4B).
  - Then 0.05ml recombinant tissue plasminogen activator was injected subretinally with a 40 gauge metallic needle at two sites (Fig. 12.4C) and waited 10 minutes for adequate clot lysis.
  - Then a retinotomy was made using endocautery at inferonasal quadrant.
  - The vitrectomy cutter was used to aspirate out the lysed blood (Fig. 12.4D)
  - Another retinotomy was made at the superotemporal quadrant and again the vitrectomy cutter was used to aspirate out the residual lysed blood
  - Subretinal blood drainage from diagonally opposite retinotomy sites ensures more complete drainage of subretinal blood (Fig. 12.4E)
  - The fluid air exchange was performed to settle the retina

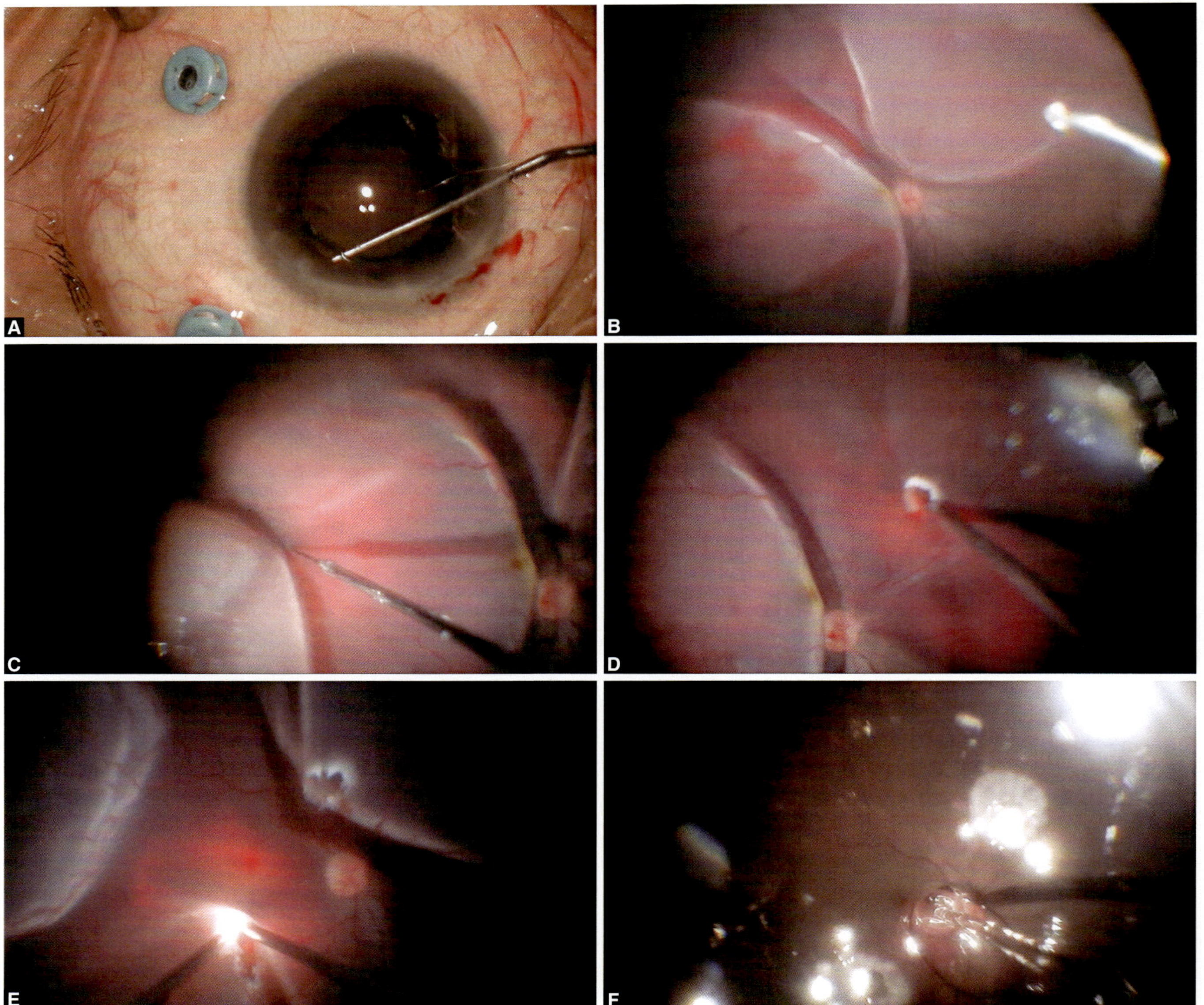

Figs 12.4A to F: Intraoperative steps of drainage technique by retinotomy in managing submacular hemorrhage.

- Endolaser are done around the sites of retinotomy.
- Silicone oil was used as a tamponade in this case (Fig. 12.4F)

- *Submacular Hemorrhage Drainage by Retinectomy (Video 5, Chapter 12)*
  - A case of post-PCV dense old vitreous hemorrhage with total hemorrhagic retinal detachment.
  - 3 port 25 gauge pars plana vitrectomy was planned
  - Vitrectomy started to clear old vitreous hemorrhage
  - An elevated old hemorrhagic retinal detachment was detected underneath (Fig. 12.5A)
  - PVD induction was performed carefully
  - 0.05 mL recombinant tissue plasminogen activator was injected subretinally with a 38 gauge nonmetallic needle at two sites (Fig. 12.5B) and waited 15 minutes for adequate clot lysis.
  - Then retinectomy was performed at the temporal periphery (Fig. 12.5C)
  - Subretinal lysed old blood was aspirated out by a cutter (Fig. 12.5D)
  - Then, the temporal retinal flap was repositioned again by putting PFCL at the posterior pole (Fig. 12.5E).
  - Fluid air exchange was permed and temporal retinal edges were settled.
  - Laser retinopexy was done around the retinal edges as well as all around (Fig. 12.5F).
  - Then, a direct silicone oil—PFCL exchange was performed by injecting silicone oil with the left hand and aspirating the PFCL bubble with the right hand under Chandelier's illumination (Fig. 12.5G).

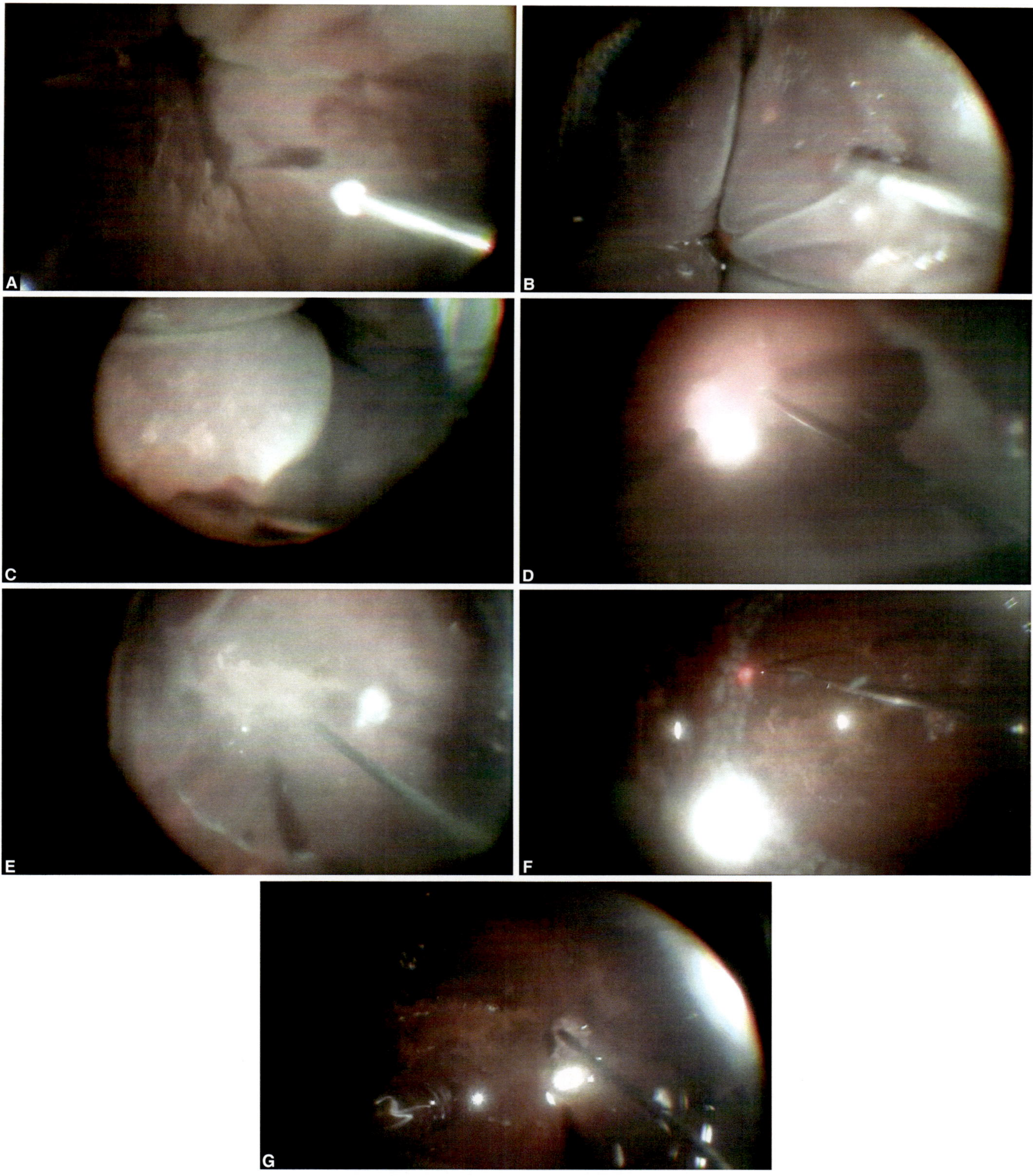

Figs 12.5A to G: Intraoperative steps of drainage technique by retinectomy in managing submacular hemorrhage.

III. *More than 8 weeks duration, extending both superior and inferior to the macula:* Drainage of SMH along with transplantation of an autologous RPE-choroid patch graft is warranted. Vitrectomy, followed by inducing retinal detachment by injecting balanced salt solution (BSS) using 38 G/ 41 G subretinal cannula, followed by submacular blood removal by creating temporal 6–7 clock-hours (180°) retinectomy, followed by harvesting autologous RPE-choroid patch graft from either superotemporal or inferotemporal quadrant from a relatively healthy-looking area and transferring the graft under the PFCL bimanually to the foveal area. Then the retinal flap is repositioned using PFCL, followed by laser retinopexy at the margin of retinectomy and 360°, then fluid-air exchange (FAE) and silicone oil tamponade.

Full-thickness RPE-choroid graft transplantation is necessary to provide relatively healthy autologous RPE cells when SMH persists for more than 8 weeks and extends both superior and inferior to the macula as there was already extensive damage of photoreceptor and RPE cells.

- *Case discussion (Video 6, Chapter 12)*
  - Vitrectomy, followed by induction of retinal detachment by injecting BSS subretinally by 38 G subretinal cannula at multiple sites (Fig. 12.6A)
  - Then gentle endocautery was performed at the temporal periphery to perform retinectomy
  - 180° retinectomy was performed at the temporal periphery to create a 6–7 clock-hour giant retinal tear (Fig. 12.6B)
  - Then submacular blood was removed (Fig. 12.6C)
  - Submacular scarred neovascular tissue should be separated carefully from the overlying retinal flap and be chewed up by a cutter with high suction (500–600 mm Hg) and very low (around 100 to 200) cuts per minute (Fig. 12.6D)
  - PFCL was injected subretinally from the posterior pole up to beyond mid-periphery to keep the retinal flap away from the working zone (Fig. 12.6E).
  - A superotemporal quadrant was chosen with a relatively healthy-looking area of RPE to harvest the full-thickness autologous RPE-choroid patch graft and marked with gentle endocautery (Fig. 12.6F).
  - Then, under Chandelier's illumination, the harvested RPE-choroid patch graft sheet was transferred under the PFCL bimanually by two forceps up to the foveal area (Fig. 12.6G).
  - The graft alignment was completed (Fig. 12.6H).
  - PFCL was removed from the subretinal space (Fig. 12.6I) and the retinal flap is repositioned again by injecting PFCL over the retina starting from the disk (Fig. 12.6J), followed by laser retinopexy at the margin of retinectomy, fluid-air exchange (FAE) and silicone oil tamponade.
  - Postoperatively, vision improved to 20/200 with graft in situ on wide-field fundus photo (Fig. 12.6K), FAF and OCT (Fig. 12.6L)

Postoperative Position

- After the nondrainage procedure, a 12-hour initial propped-up position is followed by a prone position for 14–16 hours a day for the next 3 weeks.
- After the drainage procedure, a strict prone position was advised for 16 hours a day for the next 3 weeks.

Postoperative complications specific to the different management modalities in managing SMH:

A. Complications in cases of nondrainage technique (Vitrectomy + Subretinal cocktail injection of rt-PA + anti-VEGF + filtered air + gas tamponade):
   1. Recurrent vitreous hemorrhage
   2. Recurrent submacular hemorrhage
   3. Macular hole formation due to foveal blow-out due to submacular volume overload during subretinal injections, close to the fovea.
   4. Retinal detachment (from inadvertent retinal tear during subretinal injection or from vitrectomy-induced peripheral break)

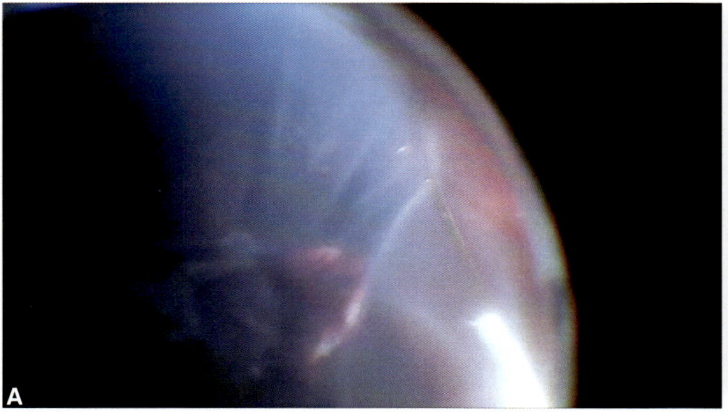

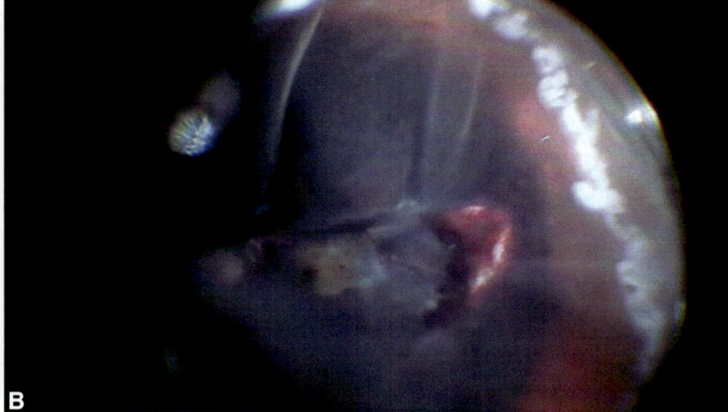

Figs 12.6A and B

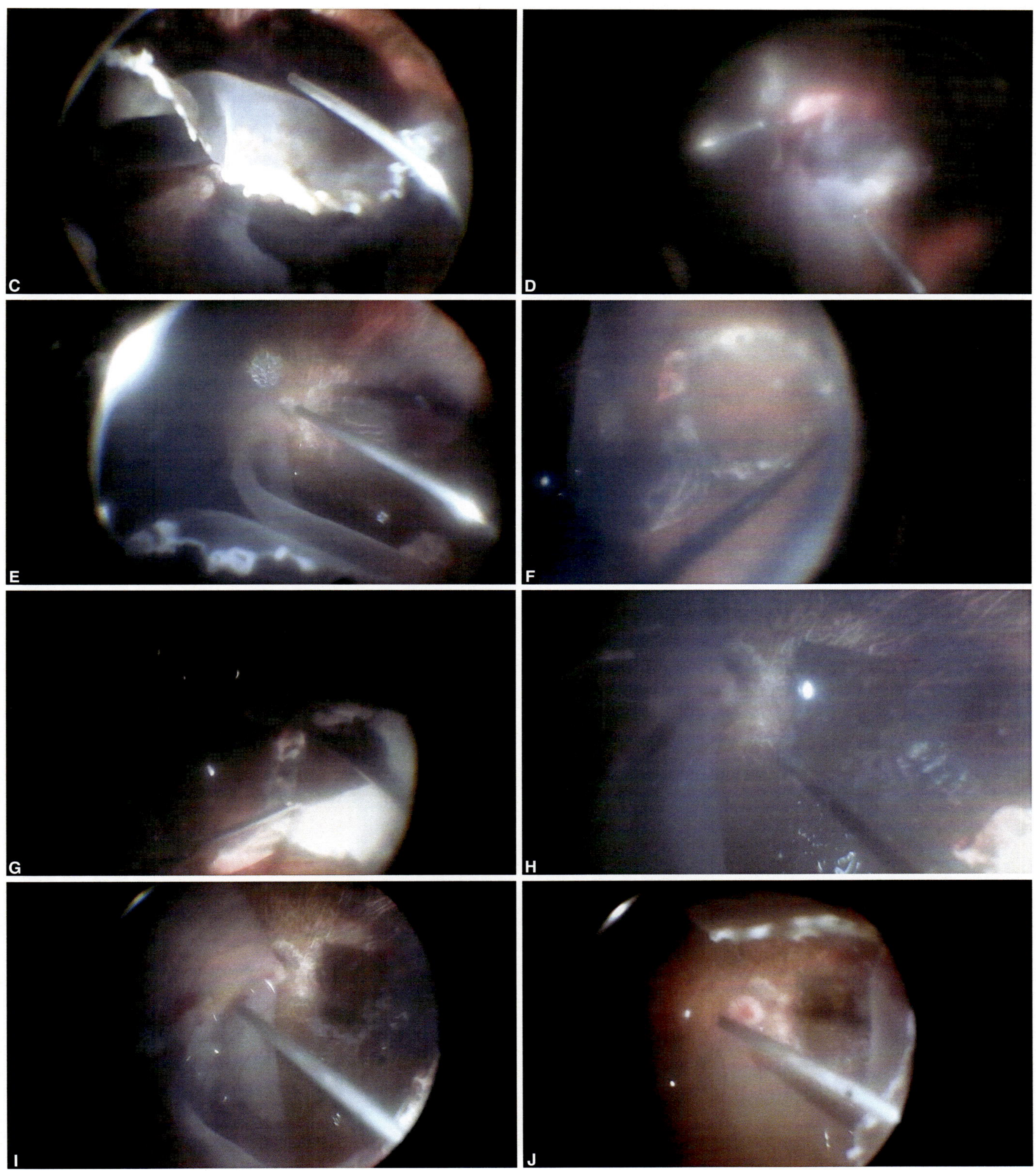

Figs 12.6C to J

Figs 12.6A to J: Intraoperative steps of drainage technique by submacular blood removal along with transplantation of an autologous RPE-choroid patch graft in managing submacular hemorrhage.

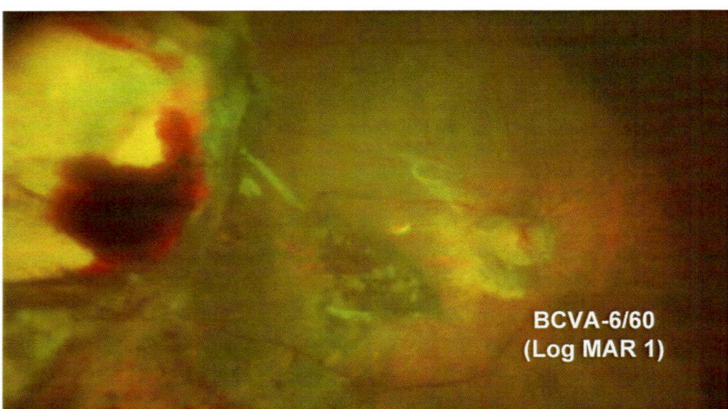

Fig. 12.6K: Postoperative wide-field fundus photo (Optos200) with graft in situ

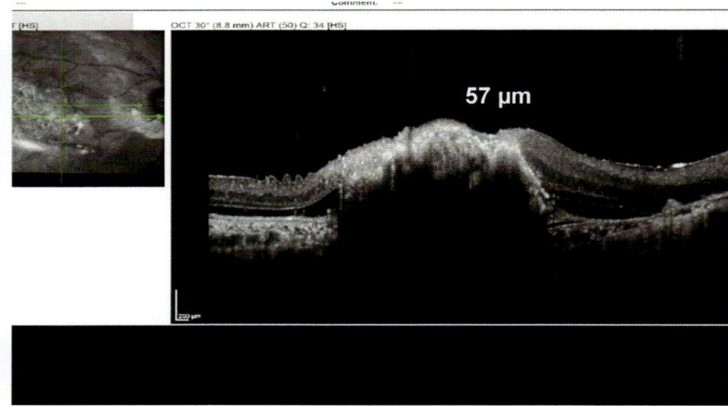

Fig. 12.6L: Postoperative OCT macular scan with submacular RPE-choroid graft in place.

B. Complications in cases of submacular hemorrhage drainage by retinotomy
   1. Recurrent submacular hemorrhage
   2. Hyphema and corneal blood staining if follow-up is not done early.
   3. Epiretinal membrane (ERM) formation
   4. Retinal detachment (from inadvertent retinal tear during subretinal injection or from vitrectomy-induced peripheral break)
C. Complications in cases of submacular hemorrhage drainage by retinectomy
   1. Recurrent submacular hemorrhage
   2. Hyphema and corneal blood staining
   3. ERM formation
   4. Retinal detachment
   5. Hypotony
D. Complications in cases of submacular hemorrhage drainage with an autologous RPE-choroid patch graft transplantation
   1. Recurrent submacular hemorrhage
   2. Recurrent choroidal neovascular membrane
   3. Choroidal hemorrhage
   4. Extensive subretinal scar formation
   5. Retinal detachment
   6. Hypotony
   7. Phthisis bulbi

Kindly scan the QR code below to access the online Video.

CHAPTER 13

Management of Retinal Detachment

The most common mechanism causing retinal detachments is the formation of rhegmas or full-thickness tears in the retina. Rhegmatogenous detachments account for 90% of detachments, resulting from the traction exerted on the retina by the posterior vitreous. As the rhegma forms, liquefied vitreous is allowed access to a pathway into the subretinal space. It subsequently acts as a wedge to separate the retina from the retinal pigment epithelial.

SCLERAL BUCKLING

In this era of MIVS, scleral buckling surgery still continues to be a principal approach in many clinical scenarios. Detachments that emanate from breaks anterior to the equator (the anterior-posterior circumferential midpoint of the globe) are more amenable to placement of buckles.

Basics of scleral buckling: Scleral buckling is based on the anatomic correction of the space created between the detached sensory retina and the underlying retinal pigment epithelium. This is done by the inward indentation of the sclera from the exterior, creating a ridge (or buckle) that reduces the retinal tear to allow for the reapposition of separated layers, thus reestablishing their physiologic connection.

The sclera itself is most commonly indented by placement of a permanent explant beneath the retinal tear.

Importance of cryoretinopexy: It is important that the retinal tears are sealed by the formation of chorioretinal adhesions. This is performed by inducing a thermal injury via the use of cryotherapy, diathermy, or laser energy. In conjunction with the generation of such adhesions, the physical closure of the break by the explant enables the attachment of the retina. The dynamic forces that generated the detachment (vitreoretinal traction and inflow of liquefied vitreous) are countered by these maneuvers.

Auxiliary procedures along with scleral buckling are:

1. External drainage of subretinal fluid
   - Incremental deepening of a 2–4 mm long scleral incision permits choroidal exposure and visualization
   - After scleral cutdown,the choroid can be coagulated by cautery or diathermy before mechanical puncture
   - Followed by drainage of SRF by choroidotomy with a sharp tipped blade.

   There is a risk of inadvertent choroidal puncture, retinal incarceration and potential reopening of the sclerotomy at reoperation.

   Needle drainage: The much smaller sclerochoroidal opening after hypodermic needle or suture needle drainage virtually eliminates the risk of incarceration while inviting choroidal hemorrhage with subretinal or suprachoroidal spread unless the intraocular pressure is maintained high enough and long enough for hemostasis to become established.
2. Injection of intravitreal gas C_3F_8.

Surgical Steps

Let's revisit the surgical steps of scleral buckling before discussing the role of MIVS in retinal detachment cases:

Scleral Buckling without Drainage of Subretinal Fluid (Video 1, Chapter 13)

- 360° conjunctival peritomy was done (Fig. 13.1A)
- Tenotomy was performed between the insertion of recti muscles
- Muscle hooks were passed underneath the recti muscles (Fig. 13.1B)
- 1'0 silk bridle sutures were passed (Fig. 13.1C)
- Localization of breaks and adequate cryotherapy for the breaks
- 6'o ethibond suture with tip spatula needles were passed through sclera over the areas of breaks (Care should be taken not to puncture the globe) (Figs 13.1D and E)
- Now, 276 Buckle was passed under the knots and recti muscles (Fig. 13.1F)
- Buckle sutures were tied (Fig. 13.1G)

- Now 240 encirclage was passed around the globe to support the vitreous base as well as to have permanent buckle effect
- Encirclage was tied over the buckle (Fig. 13.1H)
- Paracentesis was done to normalize the IOP
- Peritomy was closed (Fig. 13.1I)
- Central artery pulsation should be noted at the end of surge.

Scleral Buckling (Chandelier Illumination Assisted) with Drainage of Subretinal Fluid

Advantages of using Chandelier endoillumination during scleral buckling procedure:

- The surgical procedure can be sequentially performed through the surgical microscopes without the burden of repeated wearing and removal of indirect ophthalmoscope, usually needed for scleral buckling

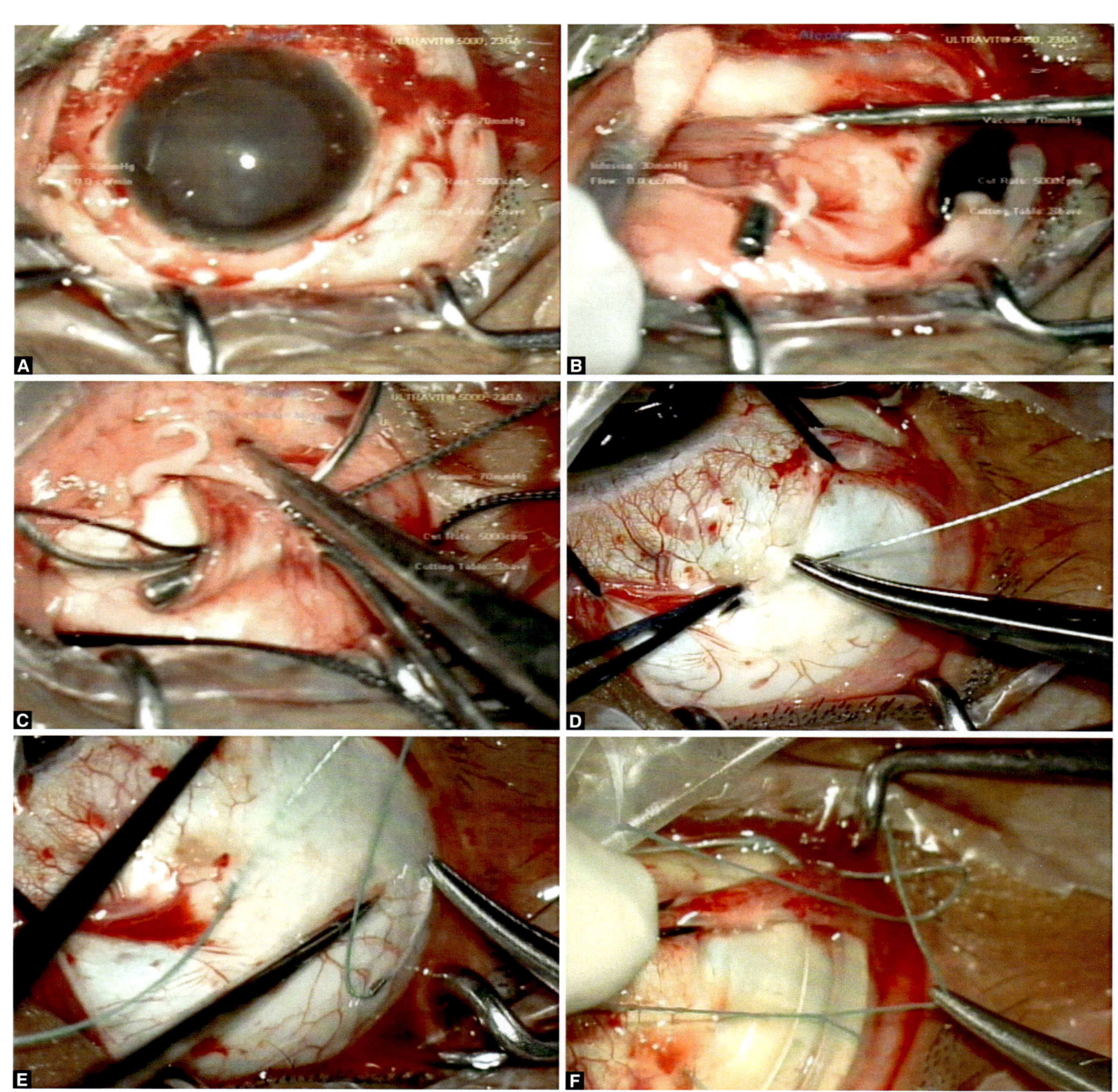

Figs 13.1A to F

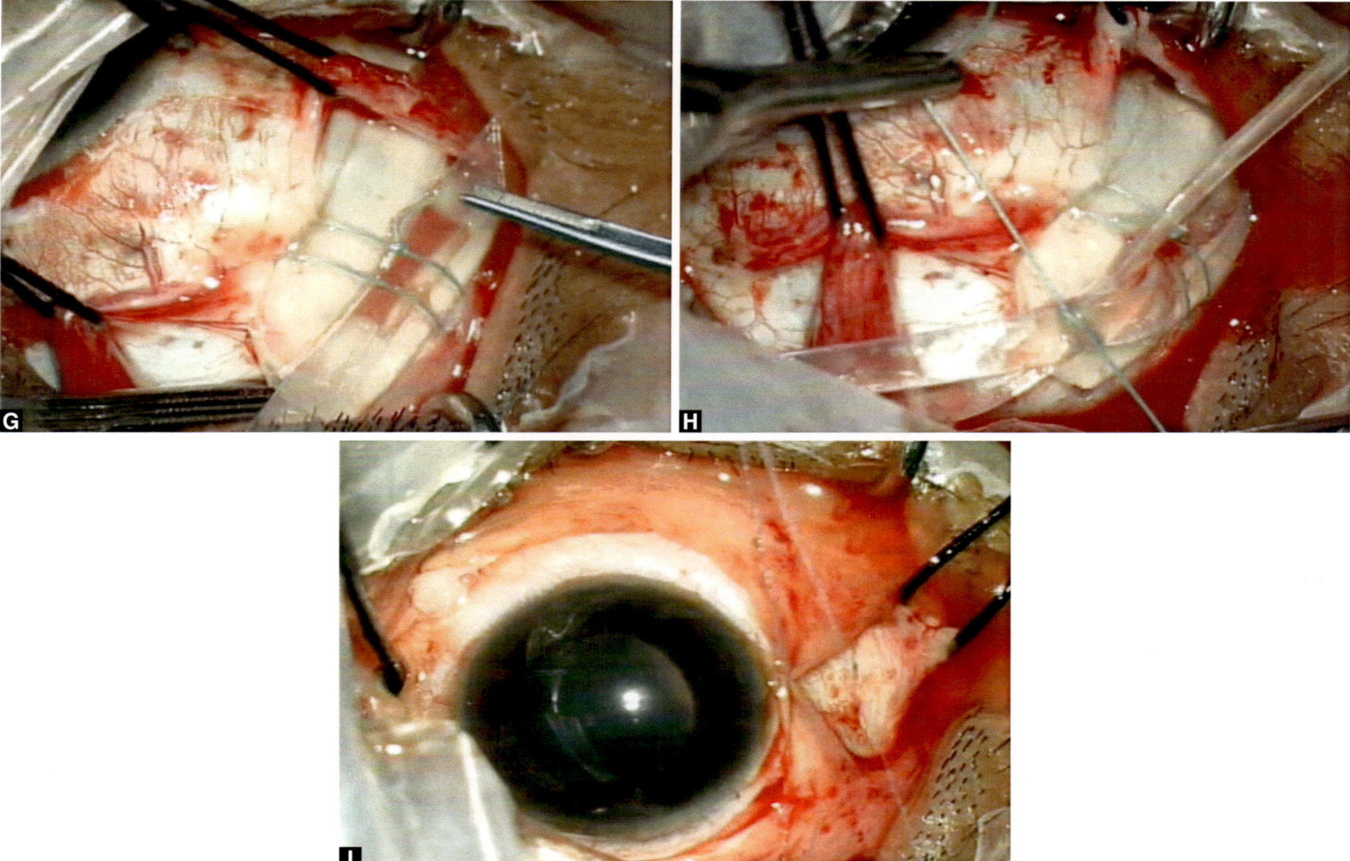

Figs 13.1A to I: Intraoperative steps of scleral buckling (without drainage of subretinal fluid)

- During cryoretinopexy, backache is a problem for the surgeon due to repeated bending to treat the retinal breaks. But chandelier endoillumination assisted scleral buckling resolves the issue
- One can adjust viewing focus and magnification under the microscope, which may be more helpful to identify preoperatively unrecognized tears.

Surgical steps (Video 2, Chapter 13)

- 360° conjunctival peritomy done
- Tenotomy was performed between the insertion of recti muscles
- Muscle hooks were passed underneath the recti muscles
- 1'0 silk bridle sutures were passed (Fig. 13.2A)
- 25G Chandelier's light introduced 4 mm away from the limbus (Fig. 13.2B)
- Localization of temporal breaks & adequate cryotherapy done for the breaks (Fig. 13.2C)
- A scleral incision made to drain sub retinal fluid (Fig. 13.2D)
- Underlying choroid exposed and cauterized (Fig. 13.2E)
- A horizontally bent 26G needle used to drain subretinal fluid (Fig. 13.2F)
- Fundus examination done again to exclude retinal incarceration or choroidal hemorrhage (Fig. 13.2G)
- Drainage area sutured
- 6'0 ethibond suture with tip spatula needles were passed through sclera over the areas of breaks (Care should be taken not to puncture the globe)
- Now 276 Buckle was passed under the knots and recti muscles
- Buckle sutures tied
- Now 240 encirclage passed around the globe to support the vitreous base as well as to have permanent buckle effect (Fig. 13.2H)
- Encirclage tied over the buckle (Fig. 13.2I)
- Paracentesis done to normalize the IOP
- Central artery pulsation should be noted at the end of surgery
- Peritomy was closed (Fig. 13.2J).

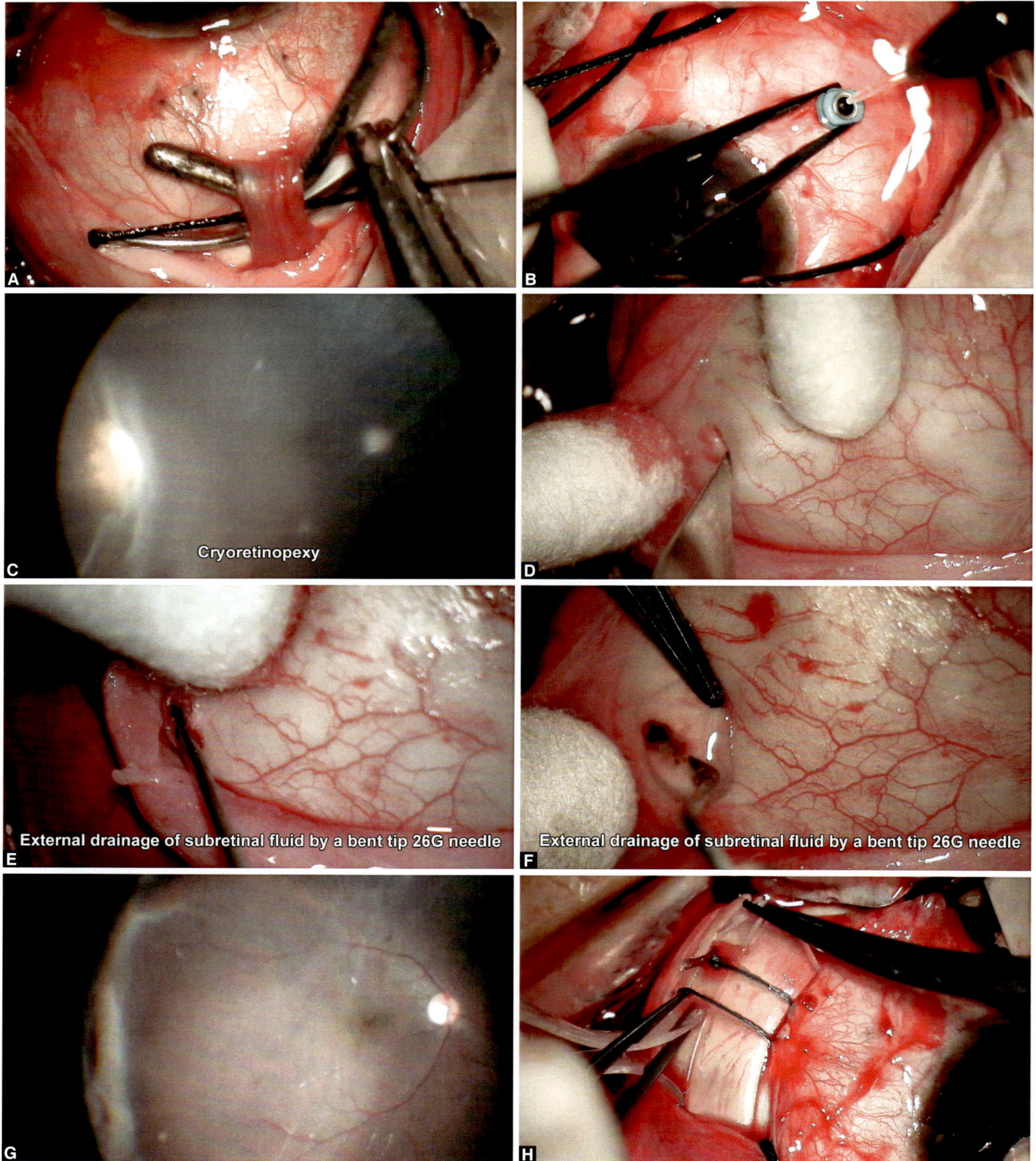

Figs 13.2A to H

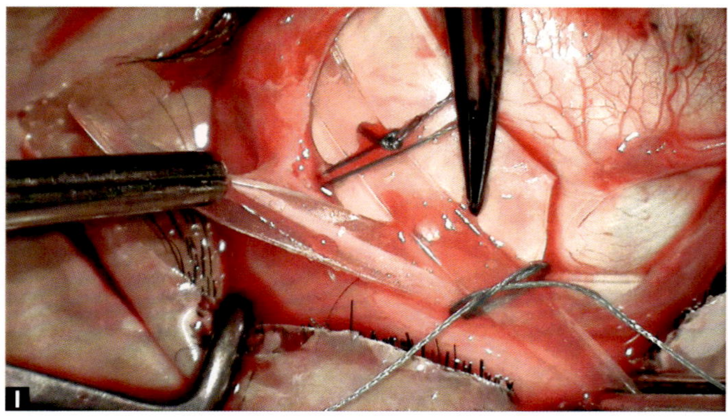

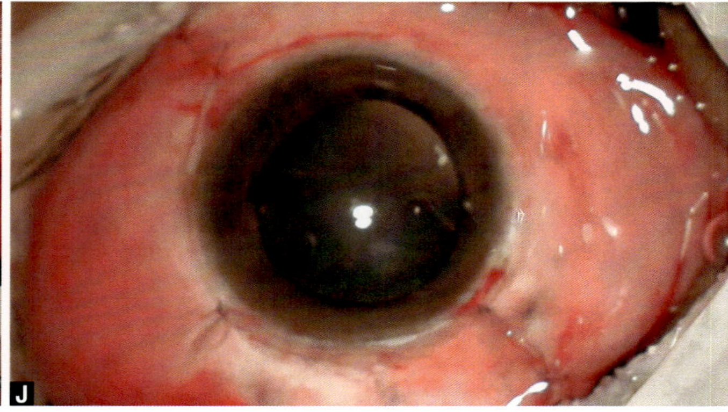

Figs 13.2A to J: Intraoperative steps of chandelier assisted scleral buckling with drainage of subretinal fluid

Contraindications of scleral buckling procedure:

1. Breaks significantly posterior to the equator are anatomically more difficult to approach due to hindrances from the bony orbit. Thus, these may be difficult technically.
2. In presence of opaque media like vitreous hemorrhage from associated PVD may preclude visualization of retinal tears, and thus proper accounting of the breaks.
3. In patients with significant vitreoretinal traction, such as with proliferative vitreoretinopathy and diabetic neovascularization, using a scleral buckle exclusively is usually insufficient to reattach the retina. However, buckling can be part of the surgical approach, in addition to vitrectomy.
4. In patients with vaso-occlusive disease, like sickle cell anemia, many surgeons prefer to avoid possible anterior ischemia caused by buckling.

VITREORETINAL APPROACHES

General Steps to Manage a Retinal Detachment *(Video 3, Chapter 13)*

- Initial vitrectomy (anterior and core vitrectomy) (Figs 13.3A and B)
- Identification of posterior hyaloid by adding TA particles (Fig. 13.3C)
- PVD induction
- Injecting heavy fluid-like PFCL to stabilize posterior pole (Fig. 13.3D)
- Vitreous base excision by external scleral depression and then removal of all peripheral vitreous as much as possible (Figs 13.3E and F)
- PVR management like release of fixed folds, removal of subretinal bands and retinectomy or relaxing retinotomy
- Diathermy at the margins of all breaks for better identification and to stop oozing of blood from the break margins
- Internal drainage of SRF by either creating a posterior retinotomy or draining SRF through the peripheral breaks by injecting heavy liquid PFCL over the posterior pole up to the posterior margin of breaks
- Fluid-air exchange (FAX) to drain residual SRF and making the smooth retinal reattachment to the underlying RPE-choroid complex (Fig. 13.3G)
- Laser retinopexy around all retinal breaks (Fig. 13.3H) as well as in 360 degree peripheral retina to create an artificial ora serrata (Fig. 13.3I)
- Use of proper endotamponade like C_3F_8 gas or silicone oil (Fig. 13.3J).

Vitrectomy (Core and Peripheral Vitrectomy)

- After initial anterior vitrectomy, core vitrectomy is to be performed, keeping the cutting rate a little on the lower side (3500–4000 cpm) with higher suction (300–400 mm Hg) for fast removal of vitreous (Fig. 13.4A). For peripheral vitrectomy, shave mode of the machine is preferable, keeping highest cut rate (5000 or 7500 cpm) and lower suction (<200 mm Hg) (Fig. 13.4B), as these parameters exert less traction on peripheral retina. *(Video 4, Chapter 13).*

PVD Induction

1. *Without PFCL (Video 5, Chapter 13)*
   - After core and peripheral vitrectomy, triamcinolone acetonide particles have to be injected to stain posterior vitreous face. Now one can use suction of the cutter to separate the posterior vitreous face from the detached retina. This posterior vitreous

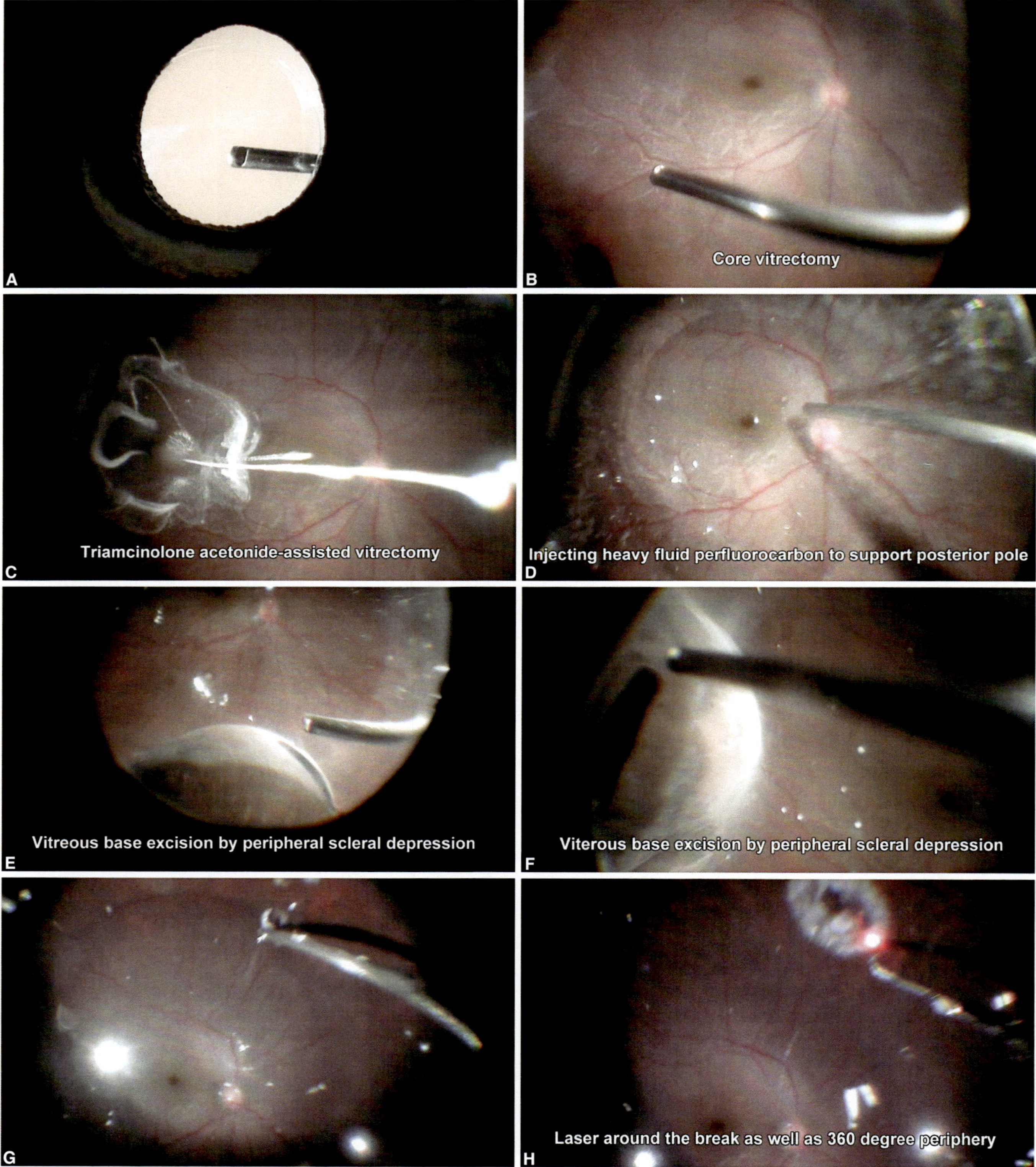

Figs 13.3A to H

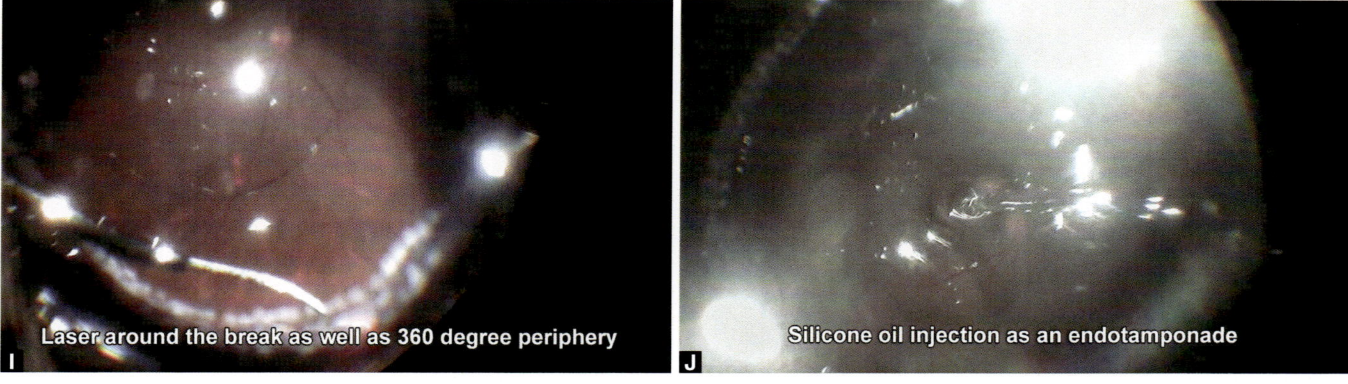

Figs 13.3A to J: Intraoperative steps of vitreoretinal approach to manage retinal detachment

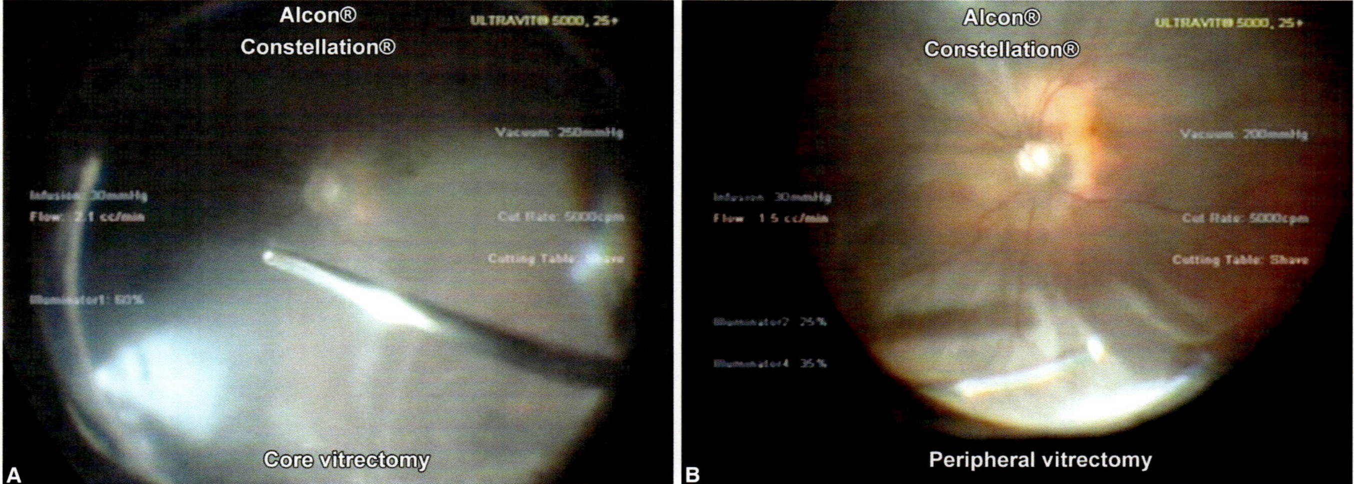

Figs 13.4A and B: Core vitrectomy (A), and peripheral vitrectomy (B)

detachment should start from the posterior pole then towards periphery (Fig. 13.5A). This process should be continued till the periphery.

ii. With PFCL *(Video 6, Chapter 13)*
   - During PVD induction, one can stabilize mobile posterior pole by PFCL and continue detaching posterior vitreous face from the peripheral detached retina as much as possible (Fig. 13.5B).

iii. By forceps *(Video 7, Chapter 13)*
   - Many times, complete PVD induction can be done separating the posterior hyaloid from the detached retina and around the optic nerve head using a forceps (Fig. 13.5C).

PVR Management

PVR complicates approximately 5–10% of rhegmatogenous retinal detachment and typically occurs 6–8 weeks postoperatively.

It may occur with long standing RD or it may occur following scleral buckling, pneumatic retinopexy or vitrectomy.

The major clinical finding in PVR is retinal starfold (Fig. 13.6A), which has been classified into Type 1–5 like focal, diffuse, subretinal, circumferential and anterior displacement.

Focal: Starfold posterior to vitreous base.

Diffuse: Confluent starfold posterior to vitreous base. Optic disc may not be visible.

Subretinal: Proliferation under retina, either 'Napkin ring' around the disc or 'clothes-line' or Motheaten-appearing sheets.

Circumferential: Contraction along posterior vitreous base with central displacement of retina.

Anterior displacement: Vitreous base pulled anteriorly by proliferative tissue with peripheral retinal trough. Ciliary process may be stretched or covered by membrane.

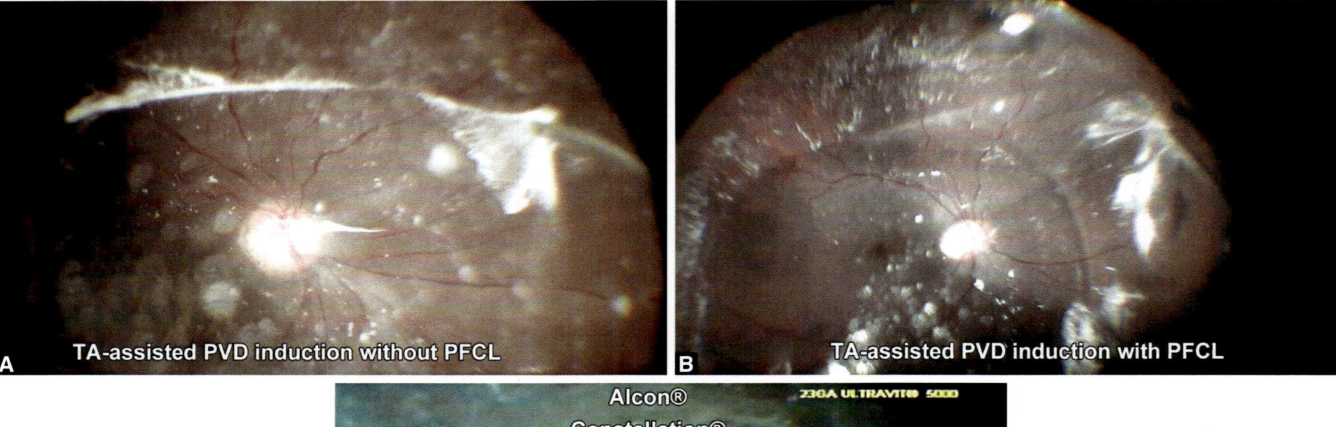

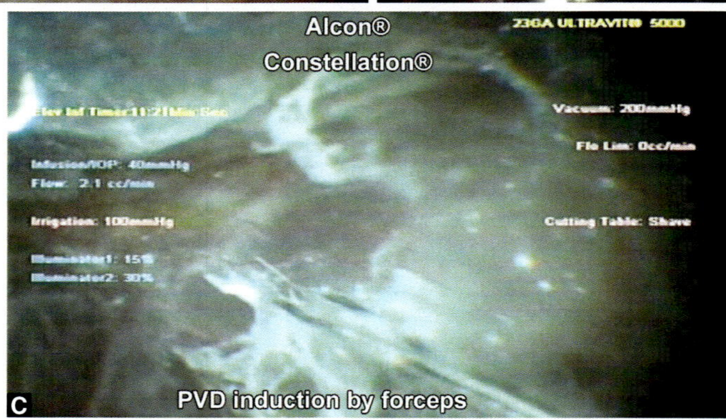

Figs 13.5A to C: (A) PVD induction without PFCL; (B) PVD induction with the support of PFCL; (C) PVD induction using a forceps
Abbreviations: PVR—proliferative vitreoretinopathy; PVD—posterior vitreous detachment; TA—triamcinolone acetonide; PFCL—perfluorocarbon liquid

The Retina Society Classification (published in 1983) described PVR according to the severity (Table 13.1).

A revised classification by Retina Society was published in 1991. The new system retains original grade A and B. Grade C has been modified to CP1–CP12 (posterior to anterior) and CA1–CA12 (anterior to posterior) retinal folds (focal, diffuse, subretinal, circumferential and anterior displacement).

Grade D has been eliminated in the revised classification.

PVR management can be done in these following ways:

1. *Release of fixed folds/Membrane peeling (Video 8, Chapter 13):* It should be carried out from posterior to anterior retina. Signs of presence of membranes include obscuration of retinal vessels or a soft gray appearance of the retina. Again fixed folds can be released in these following ways:
   i. *By forceps:* Starfold membranes are engaged by stripping towards the center of radiating fold. There is redundant retina obscured within the fold of retina, beneath the membrane (Fig. 13.6B).
   ii. *Sub PFCL membrane peeling:* After PVD induction, all fixed folds have to be released by peeling membranes at the fixed folds with forceps. Residual fixed folds have to be released after injecting heavy fluid PFCL and doing membrane peeling under PFCL to make retina tractionless (Fig. 13.6C).

TABLE 13.1: Retina society classification of retinal detachment with PVR

Grade	*Name*	*Clinical signs*
A	Minimal	• Vitreous haze • Vitreous clumps
B	Moderate	• Wrinkling of inner retinal surface • Rolled edges of retinal breaks • Retinal stiffness • Vessel tortuosity
C C1 C2 C3	Marked	Full-thickness, fixed retinal folds: • One quadrant • Two quadrants • Three quadrants
D D1 D2 D3	Massive	Fixed retinal folds in four quadrants: • Wide funnel shape • Narrow funnel shape • Closed funnel shape (optic nerve head not visible)

(The classification of retinal detachment with proliferative vitreoretinopathy. Ophthalmology 1989;90:121-5)

Sometimes in chronic retinal detachment, excessive star folds, thin retina and thick membranes, heavy fluid PFCL has to be injected to perform sub PFCL membrane peeling as thin retina needs counter support by PFCL fluid. Care should be taken not to inject PFCL directly over the break (PFCL may go subretinally).

iii. *Bimanual membrane peeling (Video 9, Chapter 13):* It can be done by two forceps (Figs 13.6D and E) or a forceps and an illuminated pic. The forceps will pull the hyaloid centrally and another forceps or illuminated pic is used to separate the vitreous from the retina. The blunt part of the second instrument should be used to create the plane of cleavage. After the traction has been released, the retina becomes very mobile and more bullous. Now PFCL is to be injected to stabilize the posterior pole to carry the vitreous base excision.

2. *Removal of subretinal bands (SRBs) (Video 10, Chapter 13):* It is possible by creating an extra retinotomy overlying a relatively thicker part of subretinal band. A forceps should be introduced through the retinotomy opening with closed fashion and then the forceps should be opened beneath the retina to catch the band and then remove it through the opening. Often bimanual approach by using two forceps help to remove the bands in toto (Fig. 13.6F). Another approach to remove subretinal bands is going beneath the retina by everting the flap of existing peripheral large tear. This approach is especially helpful to remove long posterior (especially macular region) SRBs bimanually with end gripping forceps and ILM peeling forceps (Fig. 13.6G).
3. *Relaxing retinotomy:* The concept of relaxing retinotomy was initially described by Machemer. Relaxing retinomies or retinectomies are most commonly indicated when PVR contractile changes cannot be relieved adequately by membrane dissection. This may vary from a small area of retinal defect to drain SRF to a 360 degree excision of peripheral retina. It is commonly performed circumferentially.

   Indications of RR—Relaxing retinectomy is indicated in:
   i. Proliferative vitreoretinopathies (focal star folds, diffuse contraction, circumferential contraction, intrinsic retinal contraction, anterior retinal displacement, GRT).
   ii. Proliferative vascular retinopathy with long standing fibrovascular proliferation in PDR.
   iii. Retinal incarceration (postpenetrating trauma, sclerotomy site).

   Following important facts are to be remembered during RR:
   - This is very important to extend the retinotomy past all areas of retinal traction
   - Posterior pole should always be stabilized by PFCL
   - Commonly inferior posterior RR is performed
   - It is always essential to maintain hemostasis at the margin of RR
   - After adequate RR, fluid air exchange has to performed, retina is to be inspected to notice any traction
   - If required, further RR has to be done after making the infusion on.

   Case Discussion: Relaxing retinotomy for intrinsic retinal contraction *(Video 11, Chapter 13)*
   - In a case of old retinal detachment, intrinsic retinal contraction was realized while doing fluid air exchange through the mid peripheral retinotomies, as detached retina was not settling and surrounding retina was taut under air
   - Infusion was made 'on' again
   - Liberal relaxing retinotomy done at the midperiphery after diathermizing the taut area (Fig. 13.6H)
   - Fluid-air exchange started again noticing the smooth settlement of retinal detachment.

   Complications of RR:
   1. Functional loss of visual field.
   2. Hemorrhage.
   3. Hypotony.
   4. Recurrent proliferation and recurrent PVR and recurrent retinal detachment.
4. *Anterior PVR management:* Membrane dissection is to be done meticulously as posterior hyaloid detachment is frequently not possible till ora serrata, especially if there are:
   - Fixed folds
   - Circumferential retinal contraction—Circumferential retinal contraction is more complicated, as it creates tight retinal folds that radiate posteriorly by the pull of hyaloid. Even after excision of hyaloid and sectioning circumferential membranes, the retina may remain in contracted state. Use of PFCL over posterior pole and peripheral hyaloid removal with membrane dissection with meticulous vitreous base shaving by scleral depression is to be done initially
   - Often large areas of relaxing retinectomy has to be performed. But peripheral retina is end-arterial system with minimal collateral circulation. Thus, in case of large anterior retinectomy, the remaining anterior retina is essentially non-viable. So the remaining anterior retina should be treated by either laser photocoagulation or cryoablation or extending retinectomy up to the ora serrata
   - Sometimes radial RR has to be done if anterior margin of a large tear is not settling with advanced contractile PVR.

Rarely, a broad encircling scleral band is required.

Case discussion: Extensive relaxing retinotomy for anterior PVR *(Video 12, Chapter 13)*

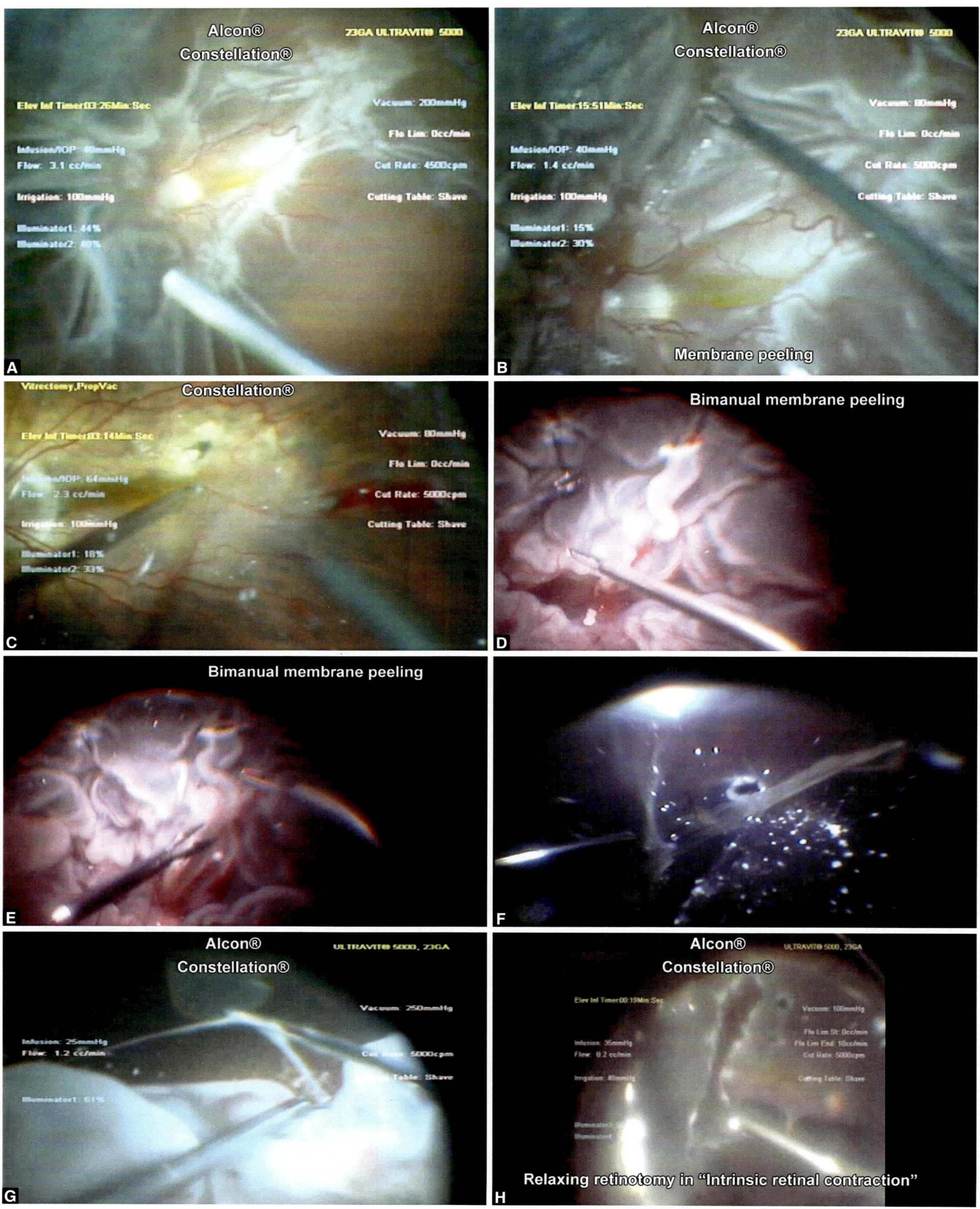

Figs 13.6A to H

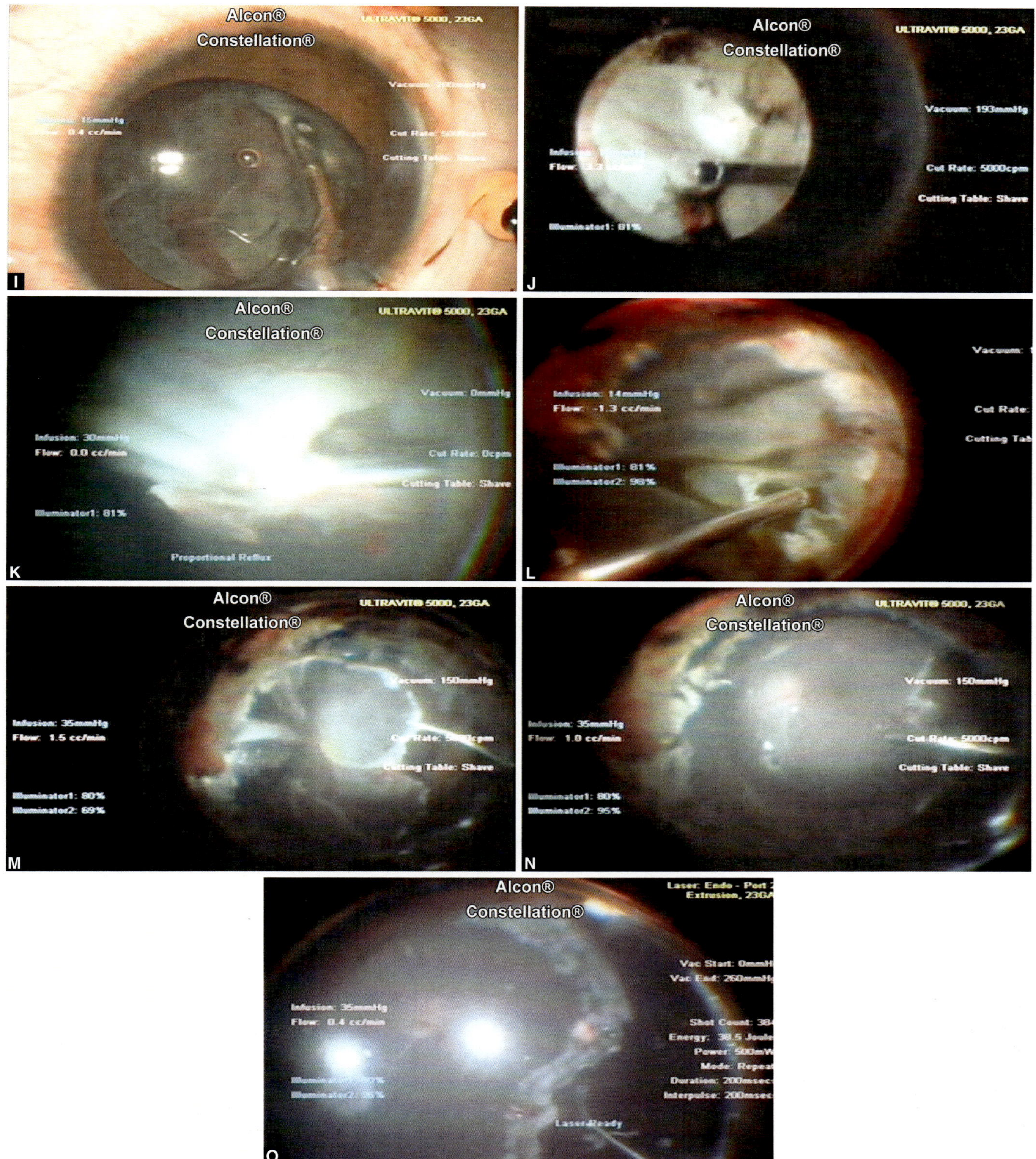

Figs 13.6A to O: (A) Intraoperative photograph in a case of old retinal detachment with starfold formation; (B) Release of strafold by forceps; (C) Sub-PFCL membrane peeling; (D and E) Bimanual membrane peeling; (F) Shows removal of subretinal band through retinotomy; (G) Shows removal of macular long subretinal band bimanually through GRT opening; (H) Shows liberal relaxing retinotomy for old retinal detachment with intrinsic retinal contraction; (I to O) Shows intraoperative steps of managing post-traumatic blood stained posterior capsule with old RD with advanced anterior PVR changes

Abbreviations: PFCL—perfluorocarbon liquid; GRT—giant retinal tear; RD—retinal detachment; PVR—proliferative vitreoretinopathy

A case of post-traumatic blood stained posterior capsule with old RD with advanced PVR changes on ultrasonography:

- Lens aspiration was done (Fig. 13.6I) and foldable PCIOL was injected
- At the time of primary posterior capsulectomy (Fig. 13.6J), detached retina was found to be attached with PC
- Vitreous hemorrhage was cleared
- Anterior PVR changes were released partially using proportionate reflux (Fig. 13.6K)
- Nearly, 270° relaxing retinotomy had to be performed to remove anterior PVR components (Figs 13.6L and M)
- PFCL was injected to flatten the retina (Fig. 13.6N)
- Laser barrage was done all around (Fig. 13.6O)
- Silicone oil was injected in one hand and PFCL was removed with other hand (Silicone oil-PFCL exchange).

5. *Posterior PVR management:* Following are some relevant facts to manage posterior PVR
   - Meticulous membrane dissection by multifunctional cutter and end grasping or ILM peeling forceps are necessary
   - In advanced posterior PVR cases, use of Chandelier's illumination helps to go bimanually
   - When preretinal PVR membranes are tough and relatively thicker than underlying thin atrophic retina (in chronic situation), it is better to stabilize the posterior pole with PFCL and to go for sub PFCL membrane dissection
   - An inability to flatten the retina during fluid-air exchange after complete membrane removal indicates there is a need for relaxing retinotomy. The surgeon should be judging this assessing the compliance of retina to reappose the concave surface of ocular wall
   - Posterior RR under silicone oil sometimes required when there is recurrent retinal detachment under silicone oil by injecting silicone oil by using silicone oil infusion pump (VFC) during active aspiration of SRF by metallic flute needle or extrusion cannula. Aspiration will be completed when silicone oil is apposed to the retina and retinotomy site.

Vitreous Base Excision

Vitreous Base Excision Without PFCL (Video 13, Chapter 13)

Vitreous base excision can be done by depressing sclera externally with a blunt tip metallic instrument or a cotton bud. If this step is done without any help of PFCL, mobile retina can often become bullous due to influx of fluid through the breaks and retina may come near the cutter port (Fig. 13.7A).

Vitreous Base Excision with PFCL (Video 14, Chapter 13)

Vitreous base excision after injecting PFCL can be done in a more controlled way. Posterior pole support by PFCL helps to flatten the mobile retina and keep the retina away from cutter to avoid additional breaks (Fig. 13.7B).

Internal Drainage of Subretinal Fluid

i. *By creating posterior retinotomy during FAX (Video 15, Chapter 13):* Creating posterior pole retinotomy in a bullous area preferably at super nasal quadrant helps in complete drainage of subretinal fluid (Fig. 13.8A). Then laser retinopexy has to start.
ii. *Through peripheral breaks using PFCL (Video 16, Chapter 13):* By injecting heavy fluid PFCL directly over the posterior pole, SRF is steam-rolled out through an anterior retinal break into the vitreous cavity (Fig. 13.8B). The intravitreal fluid then egress through the sclerotomy cannulas as the PFCL level rises. PFCL is to be injected till the posterior margin of peripheral break, then FAX has to be started for complete drainage of anterior SRF. Sometimes PFCL

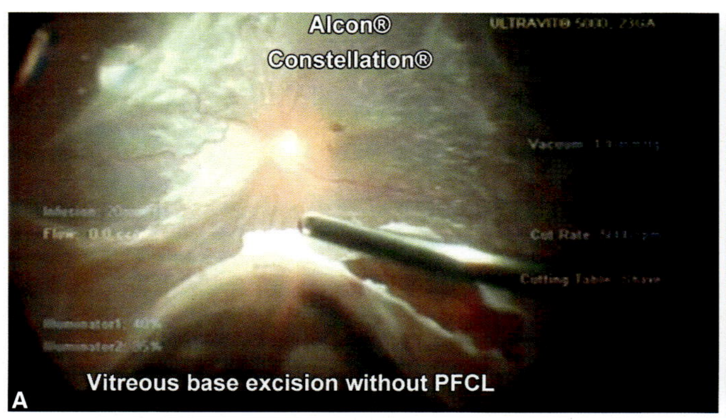

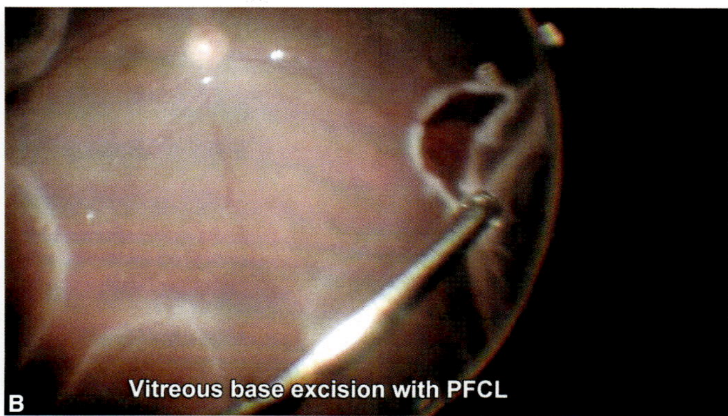

Figs 13.7A and B: (A) Vitreous base excision without PFCL; (B) Vitreous base excision with the support of PFCL

can totally fill the vitreous cavity and laser can be done under PFCL in a more controlled fashion.

RD in Special Situations

RD with Dropped Nucleus (Video 17, Chapter 13)

- In case of dislocated crystalline lens with associated GRT with retinal detachment (Fig. 13.9A), especially in postblunt trauma, PFCL has to be injected going behind the lens (Fig. 13.9B) over detached retina to keep retina away while doing lensectomy by cutter (Fig. 13.9C) or fragmatome. Here, PFCL has immense role in protecting retina.

RD with Dropped IOL (Video 18, Chapter 13)

Steps of surgery:

- A case of dropped PCIOL with total retinal detachment with multiple HSTs (Fig. 13.10A)
- Vitrectomy done
- Triamcinolone was injected to check residual vitreous adhesions with IOL (Fig. 13.10B)

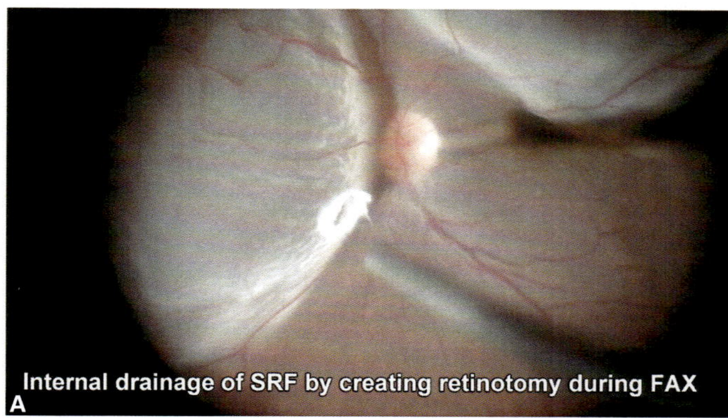

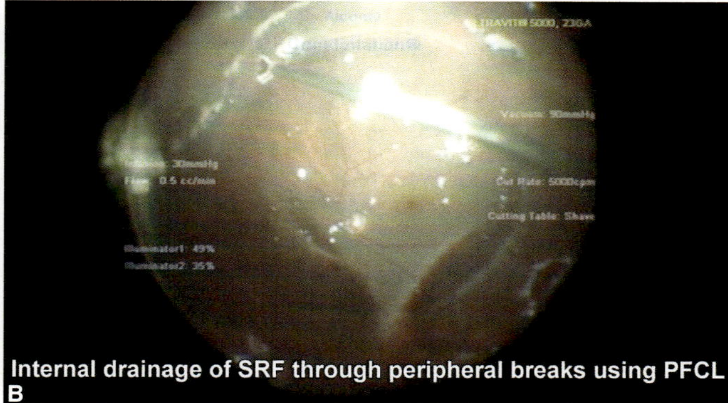

Figs 13.8A and B: (A) Internal drainage of subretinal fluid by creating posterior pole retinotomy; (B) Internal drainage of subretinal fluid through peripheral breaks by injecting heavy fluid PFCL over the posterior pole
Abbreviations: SRF—subretinal fluid; PFCL—perfluorocarbon liquid

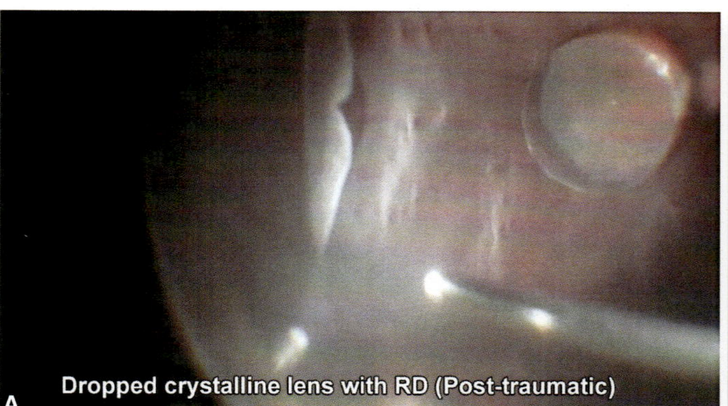

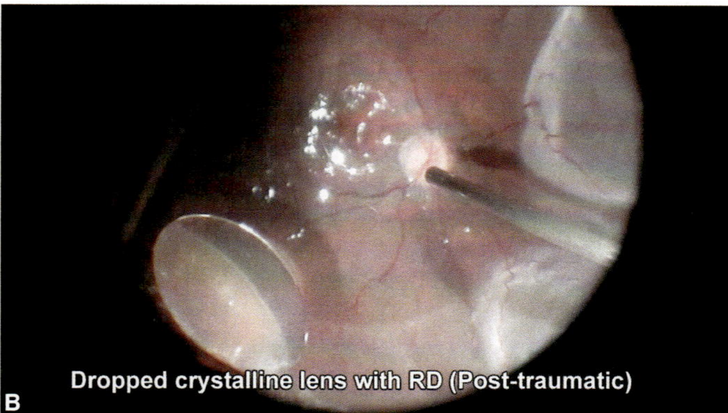

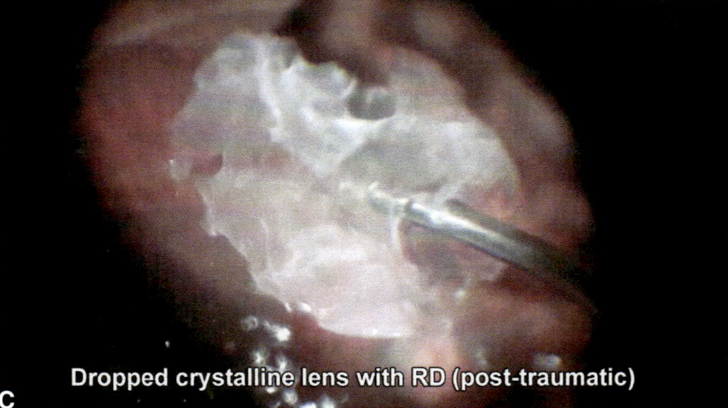

Figs 13.9A to C: Intraoperative steps of managing dislocated crystalline lens with associated GRT with retinal detachment
Abbreviations: GRT—giant retinal tears; RD—retinal detachment

- Now passive suction of a silicone-tipped backflush needle was used to lift up the IOL up to pupillary plane (Fig. 13.10C)
- Then IOL was prolapsed into the AC with the help of an end gripping forceps (Fig. 13.10D) and then removed
- PFCL injected (Fig. 13.10E)
- Vitreous base excision was done (Fig.13.10F)
- Breaks were cauterized
- Fluid-air exchange was performed
- All peripheral breaks were barraged (Fig. 13.10G) as well as 360° periphery
- Silicone oil was injected as the tamponade (Fig. 13.10H).

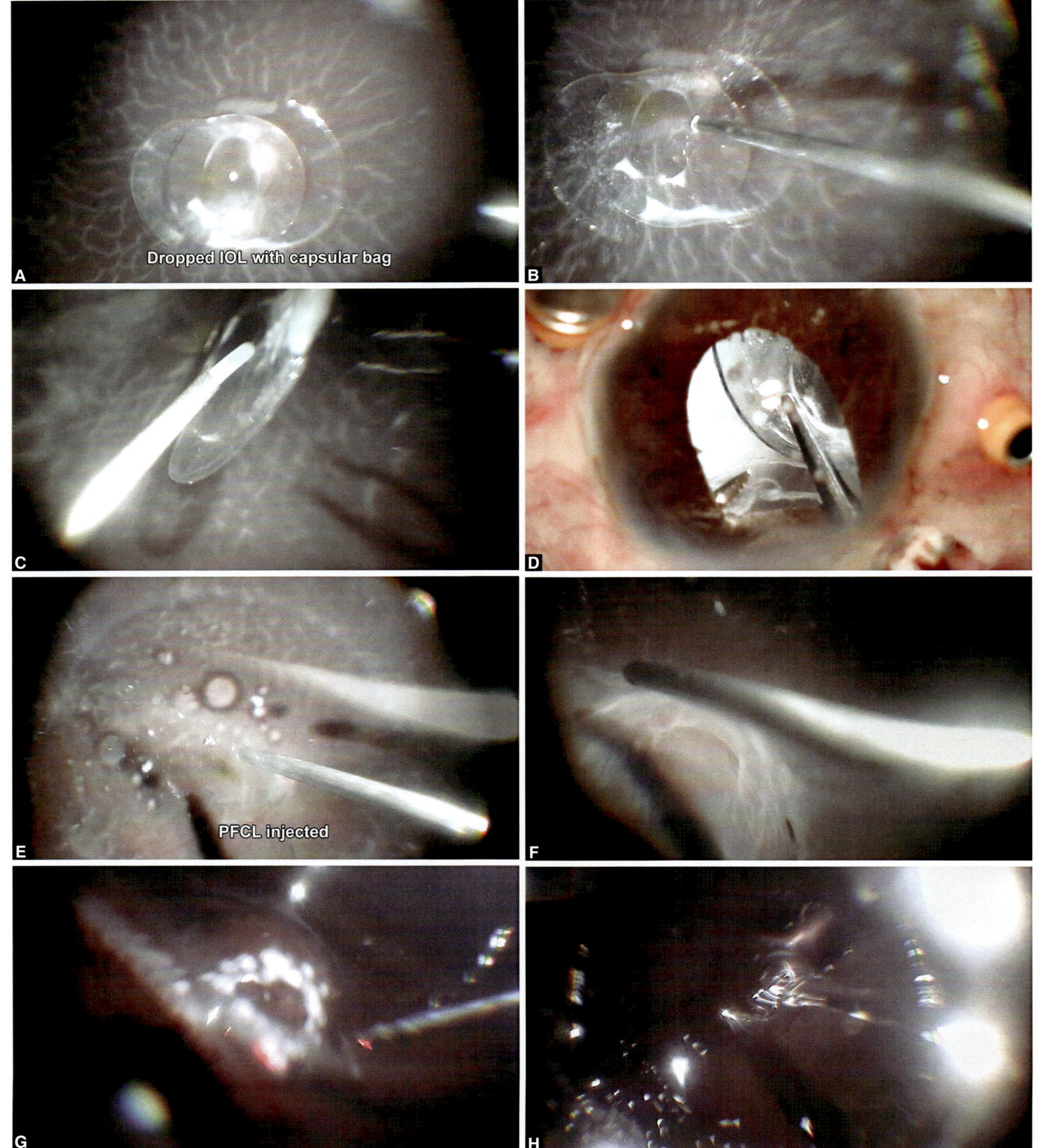

Figs 13.10A to H: Intraoperative steps of managing dislocated PCIOL with total retinal detachment

RD with Fundal Coloboma

During normal development, fetal fissure become closed by fusion of two layers of optic cup. When fusion of layers at fissure does not occur, colobomatous defect results. Dysembryogenesis of the fetal fissure thus results in a choroidal coloboma. There is hypoplastic retina overlying an area devoid of RPE and choroid.

About 40% of eyes with choroidal colobomas will develop associated retinal detachment.

Retinal tear can be at the margin of coloboma, within coloboma (within rudimentary retina) or outside the coloboma at periphery.

Treatment: Retinal detachments associated with coloboma of the choroid present a surgical challenge. The challenges are:

1. Treatment with laser or cryotherapy must be directed to the healthy tissue beyond the colobomatous area as retinopexy is impossible in the area of coloboma.
   In the colobomatous area the retinal tissue is thin and hypoplastic, the choroid and retinal pigment epithelium (RPE) are not developed and the underlying sclera is thin and ectatic, producing a staphyloma. Thus, breaks within the cobomatous area are difficult to treat. They can neither be sealed by retinopexy due to absence of choroid and RPE, nor can a buckle be placed due to the posterior location of the breaks.
2. Tears are difficult to see and difficult to treat as breaks cannot be easily detected because of the lack of contrast.
3. Other difficulties which confound the management in these cases include presence of associated ocular anomalies such as microphthalmia, cataract, lens coloboma along with nystagmus.

Treatment options:

1. *Scleral buckling:* Two radial buckles along the two edges of the coloboma two one-radial buckle extending up to the optic disc at one edge of the coloboma detected to be harboring the retinal break like U-shaped buckle.
2. Vitrectomy, internal drainage of the subretinal fluid, long-acting gas or silicone oil tamponade, endolaser photocoagulation along the edges of the coloboma posterior to the equator, trans-scleral cryotherapy along the pillars of the coloboma anterior to the equator, coupled with occasional inferior half broad scleral buckling and optional lensectomy. Meticulous retinopexy with endolaser and trans-scleral cryopexy is mandatory to isolate the area of the coloboma from the rest of the retina.

Vitreoretinal management of fundal coloboma with retinal detachment:

1. Case with breaks at margin of coloboma *(Video 19, Chapter 13)*
   Steps of surgery:
   - Fundal coloboma involved both optic disc and macula
   - Vitrectomy done
   - A break was identified within the colobomatous area near inferior coloboma margin (Fig.13.11A)
   - A separate retinotomy was made and fluid-air exchange was performed
   - Laser was done around the breaks, at the margin as well as 360° periphery
   - Silicone oil was used for tamponade.
2. Case with peripheral breaks *(Video 20, Chapter 13)*
   Steps of surgery:
   - A case of iridofundal coloboma with total RD. Fundal coloboma involved both optic disc and macula
   - TA stained vitrectomy done
   - Vitreous base excision done
   - A lattice with tears detected at superotemporal periphery (Fig. 13.11B)
   - PFCL injected to drain SRF through the holes (Fig. 13.11C)
   - Fluid-air exchange performed to drain peripheral SRF
   - PFCL removed
   - Laser done around the breaks, at the margin as well as 360° periphery (Fig. 13.11D)
   - Silicone oil has to be used for tamponade.

RD with Giant Retinal Tear (GRT)

A retinal tear that is greater than or equal to 90° of retinal circumference is called giant retinal tear.

The preoperative prognostic factors are:

- Macular detachment
- Hypotony
- Pseudophakia or aphakia
- Poor preoperative BCVA
- High-grade PVR
- GRT greater than 180 degree in extent.

Intraoperative poor prognostic factors are:

- Additional relaxing retinotomy
- Use of silicone oil.

The other eye of these patients should be examined by indirect ophthalmoscope with scleral depression.

Prophylactic treatment should be considered for:

- High myopes.
- Eyes with areas of white without pressure.
- Eyes having vitreous base condensation.

1. GRT with macula on retinal detachment *(Video 21, Chapter 13)*

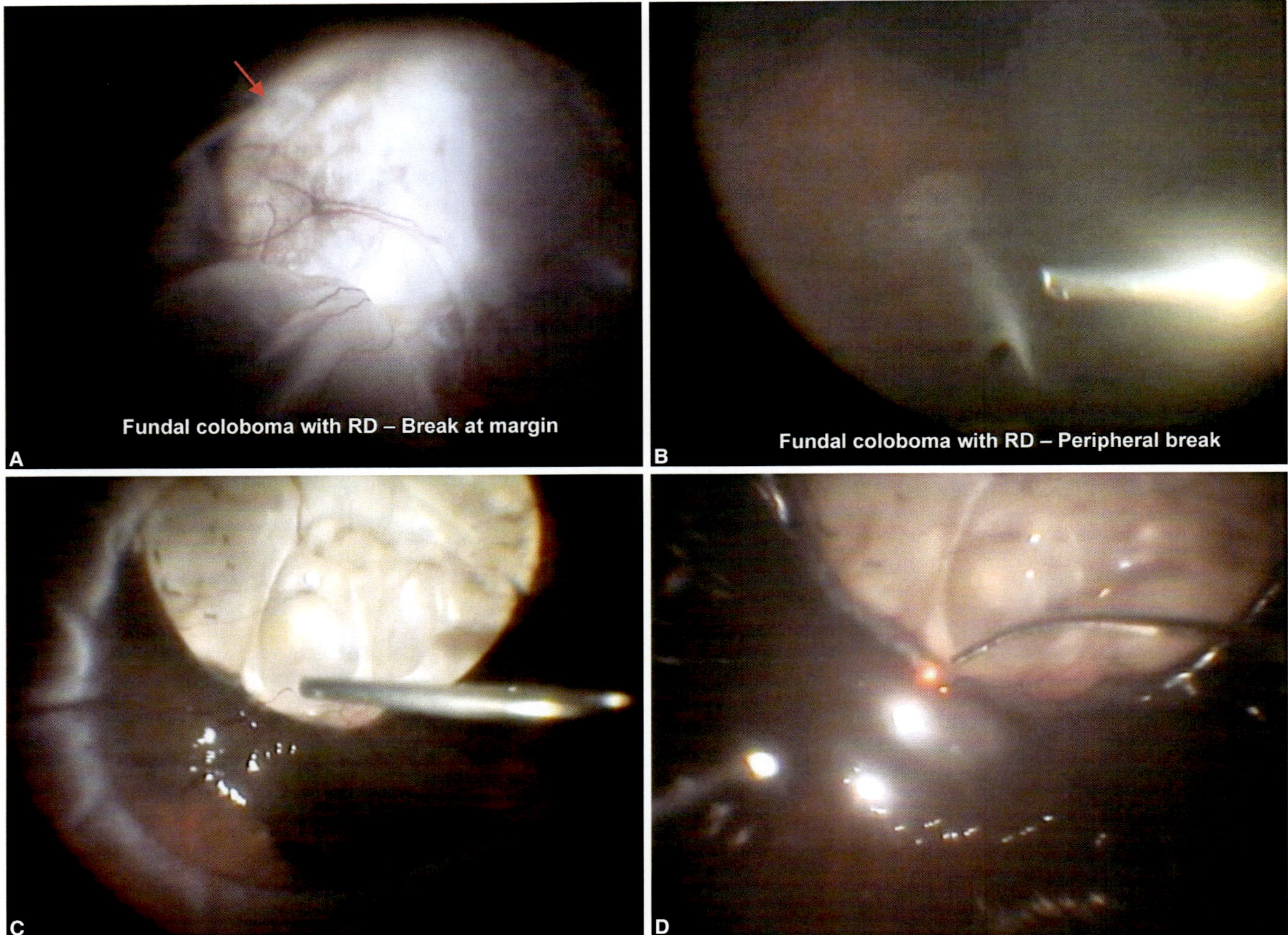

Figs 13.11A to D: (A) Fundal coloboma with retinal detachment with breaks at margin of coloboma; (B to D) Intraoperative steps in managing fundal coloboma with retinal detachment with tears at superotemporal periphery

Steps of surgery:
- A case of post-traumatic giant retinal tear with posterior extension with minimal partial retinal detachment (Fig. 13.12A)
- Vitrectomy done
- Irregular margin of the GRT trimmed (Fig. 13.12B)
- Vitreous base excision done especially at the cornus (Fig. 13.12C)
- Fluid air exchange done to drain the subretinal fluid surrounding the GRT margin (Fig. 13.12D)
- Laser done at the margin of GRT and 360 degree periphery.

2. GRT with macula-off subtotal retinal detachment *(Video 22, Chapter 13)*
   Steps of surgery:
   - A case of temporal giant retinal tear with macula-off subtotal retinal detachment (Fig. 13.12E)
   - Vitrectomy completed
   - PFCL injected up to the posterior margin of GRT (Fig. 13.12F)
   - Vitreous base excision done, trimming anterior retinal flap as well as the margin of GRT (Figs 13.12G and H)
   - Fluid-air exchange started to drain anterior SRF (Fig. 13.12I)
   - As GRT margin sagged down (Fig. 13.12J), more PFCL injected beyond the margin of GRT (Fig. 13.12K)
   - Laser started at the margin of GRT, considering the cornus (Fig. 13.12L)
   - PFCL-silicone oil exchange done, injecting silicone oil in left hand and removing PFCL with right hand (Fig. 13.12M).
3. GRT with retinal detachment with inverted flap *(Video 23, Chapter 13)*
   Steps of surgery:
   - GRT with inverted flap with total RD (Fig. 13.12N)
   - Then GRT flap lifted up passively with silicone-tipped flute needle (Fig. 13.12O)
   - PFCL injected to settle the retina (Fig. 13.12P)

- Fluid-air exchange performed and laser barrage was done at the margin of GRT extending up to periphery as well as 360° periphery
- As nasal margin of GRT sagged down, more PFCL is injected.
- Laser completed
- PFCL-silicone oil exchange done, injecting silicone oil in left hand and removing PFCL with right hand
- Last drop of PFCL removed.

4. GRT with retinal detachment with inverted flap with rolled out margin *(Video 24, Chapter 13)*
   Steps of surgery:
   - A 4 port 25G + approach in a case of GRT with inverted flap with total RD (Fig. 13.12Q)
   - Rolled out margins of inverted flap was trimmed and simultaneously cauterized bimanually
   - Then GRT flap lifted up passively with silicone-tipped flute needle
   - PFCL injected to settle the retina (Fig. 13.12R)
   - Fluid-air exchange performed to reappose the posterior flap margin
   - Laser barrage was done at the margin of GRT extending up to periphery as well as 360° periphery (Fig. 13.12S)
   - PFCL-silicone oil exchange done (Fig. 13.12T)
   - Last drop of PFCL removed.

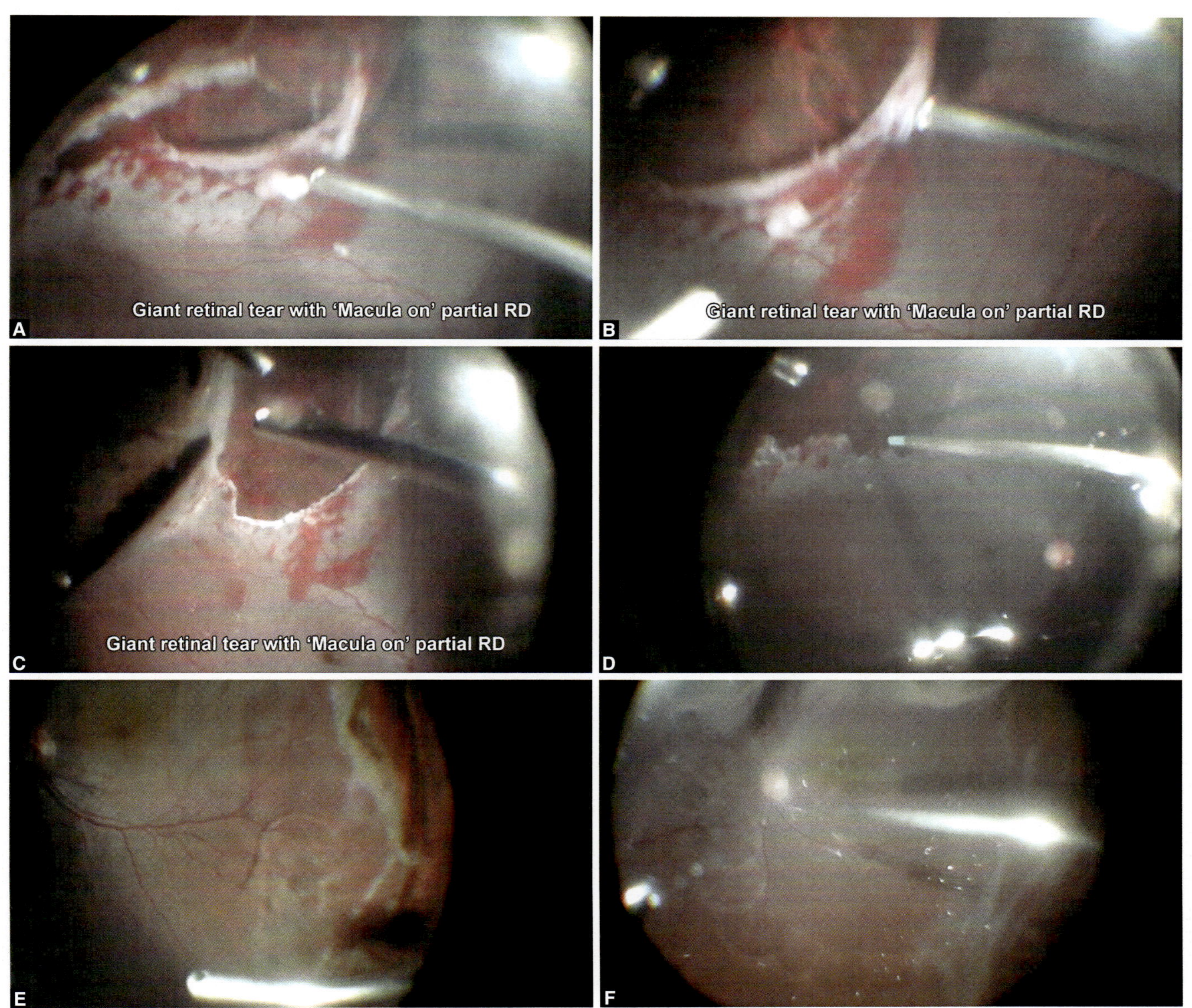

Figs 13.12A to F

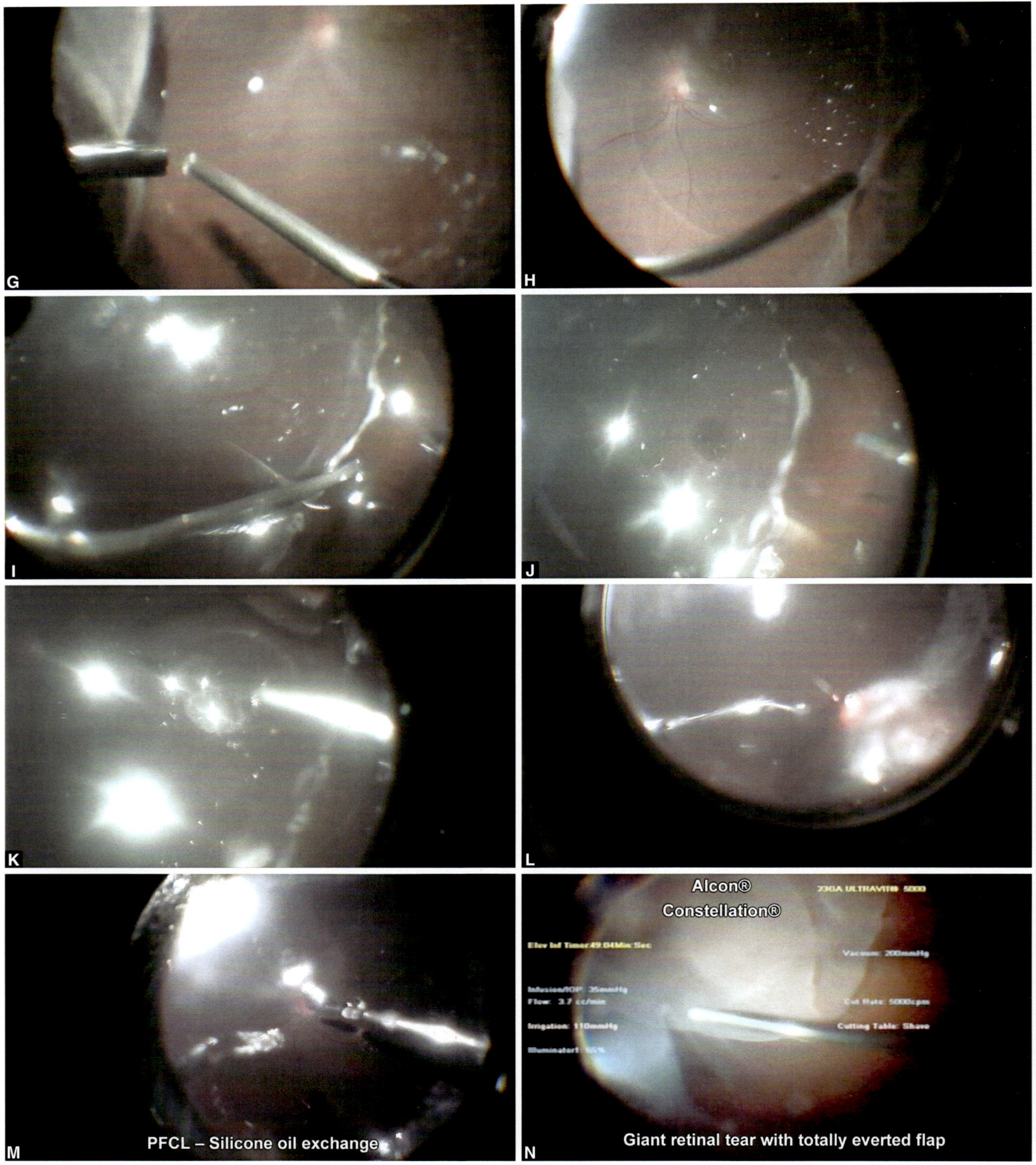

Figs 13.12G to N

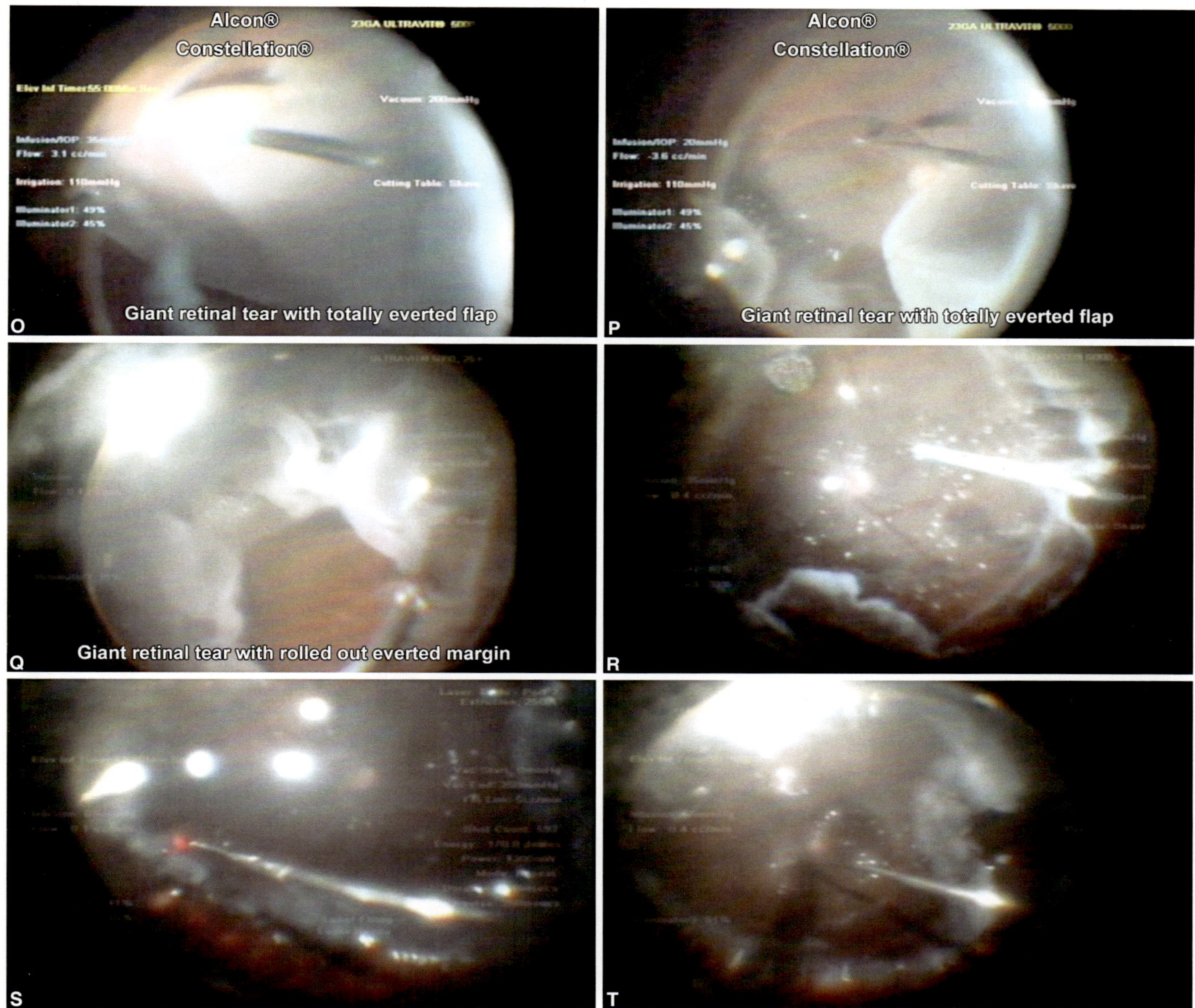

Figs 13.12A to T: (A to D) Intraoperative photographs shows post-traumatic giant retinal tear with posterior extension with minimal partial retinal detachment; (E to M) Intraoperative photographs shows temporal giant retinal tear with macula-off subtotal retinal detachment; (N to P) Intraoperative photographs shows inverted flap with total RD; (Q to T) Intraoperative photographs shows in a case of GRT with inverted flap with rolled out margin with total RD

RD with Macular Hole

To peel ILM from detached retina can be a challenging situation due to excessive mobility of retina. The use of PFCL can provide counter traction and facilitate peeling of ILM.

1. ILM peeling on mobile retina *(Video 25, Chapter 13)*
   - Without using PFCL, ILM peeling from detached retina is difficult.

   Steps of surgery:
   - Vitrectomy done (Fig. 13.13A)
   - After fluid-air exchange, BBG dye applied over macula under air
   - Infusion made on (Fig. 13.13B)
   - Dye stained ILM peeling started. Due to lack of counter support and excessive mobility of retina, ILM removal was difficult and patchy (Fig. 13.13C)
   - Then PFCL injected for internal drainage of SRF through peripheral break (Fig. 13.13D).
2. ILM peeling under PFCL *(Video 26, Chapter 13)*

- Heavy fluid PFCL provide counter traction during ILM peeling from detached retina.

Steps of surgery:

- Total RD with superior large break with macular hole
- PFCL injected to flatten BBG stained macula
- ILM flap created with Tano diamond-dusted membrane scraper and ILM peeling done under PFCL with end gripping forceps without any difficulty (Figs 13.13E to H).

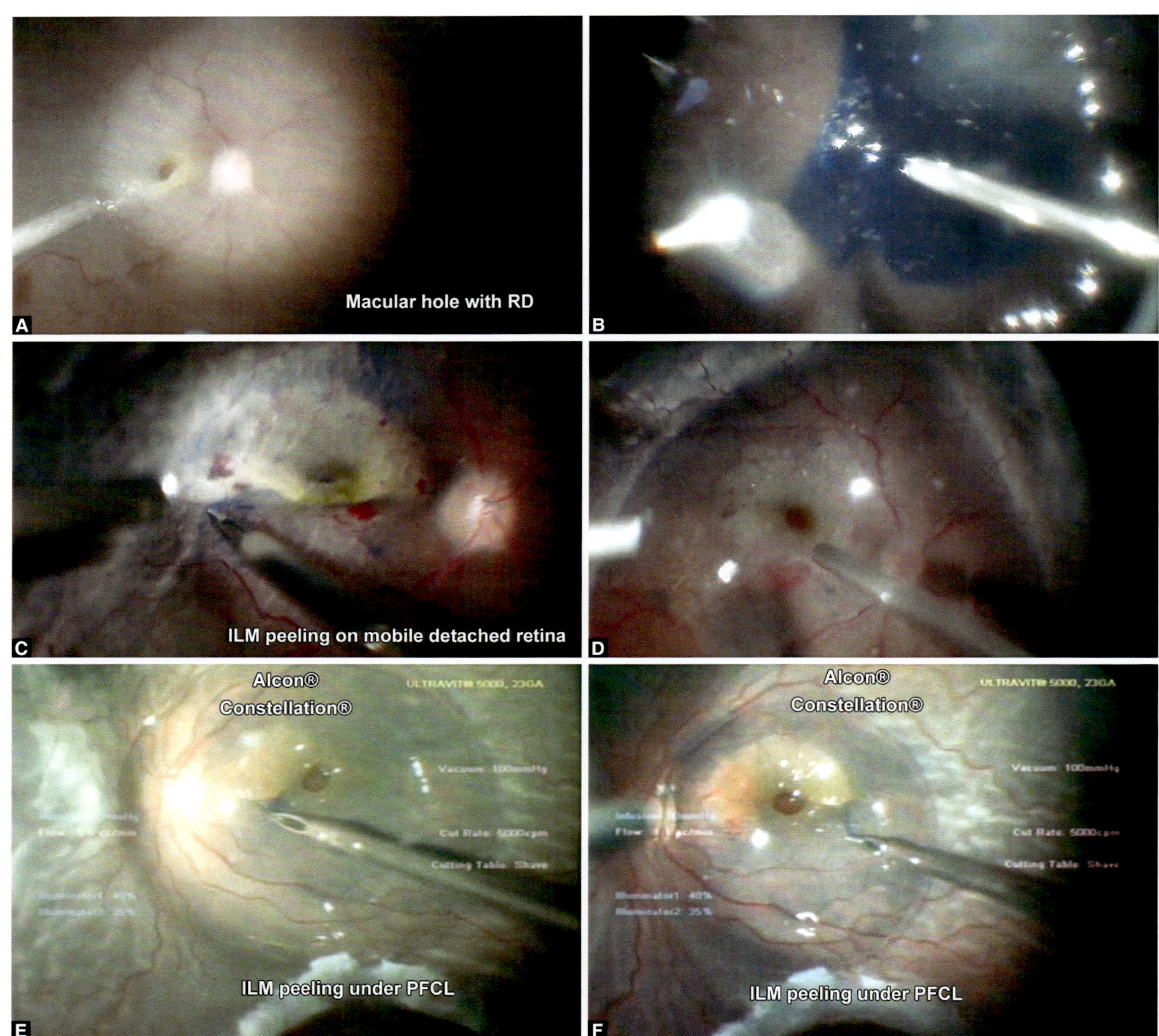

Figs 13.13A to F

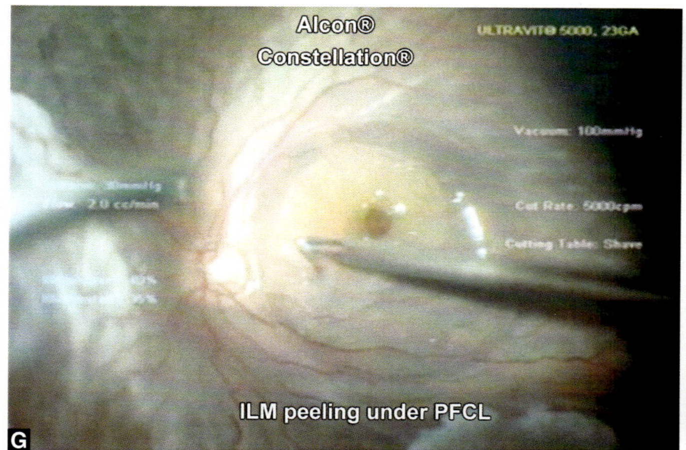

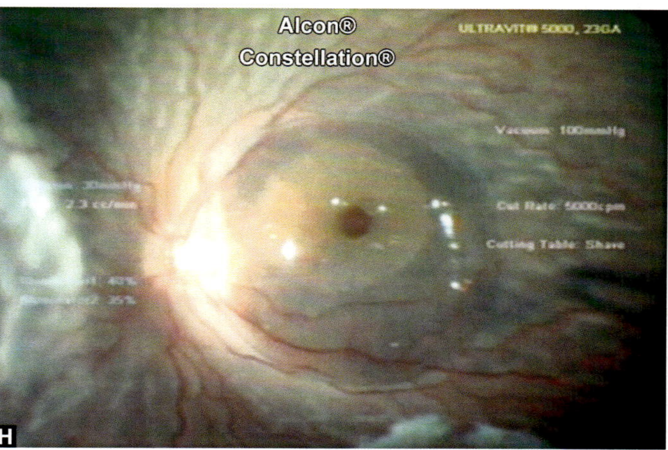

Figs 13.13A to H: (A to D) Intraoperative photographs of surgery in a case of retinal detachment with macular hole where ILM peeling was done on detached retina; (E to H) Intraoperative photographs of surgery in a case of retinal detachment with macular hole where ILM peeling was done under PFCL

RD with Choroidal Detachment

- Problem arises if RD is associated with choroidal detachment in introducing the trocar-cannula system. Due to hypotony and existing choroidal detachment, frequently the infusion port tip can be in suprachoroidal space (Fig. 13.14A). The infusion tip has to make intravitreal before turning it on *(Video 27, Chapter 13)*
- Intraoperatively, the surgery can be done setting the IOP relatively at a moderately high level (35–50 mm Hg) and this may facilitate the spontaneous micro drainage of choroidal fluid around the ports.

Steps of surgery in retinal detachment with choroidal detachment *(Video 28, Chapter 13)*:

- A case of total retinal detachment with temporal marked choroidal detachment
- TA-assisted vitrectomy done (Fig. 13.14B)
- PFCL injected (Fig. 13.14C)
- Peripheral vitrectomy along with vitreous removal around the superior break done
- More PFCL injected for complete drainage of SRF
- Fluid-air exchange started
- Anterior SRF drained
- Laser done around the break as well as all around 360 degree periphery (Fig. 13.14D)
- Choroidals aggravated during removal of PFCL (Fig. 13.14E)
- Silicone oil injected keeping IOP in higher side (Fig. 13.14F)
- Height of choroidals decreased significantly
- Sometimes, a persistent huge choroidal detachment needs to be drained. A simple method is introducing a 23/25G trocar-cannula obliquely inside the bulky choroidal space through the sclera according to the clinically maximally elevated area.

Steps of choroidal drainage during repair of retinal detachment *(Video 29, Chapter 13)*:

- A case of bullous retinal detachment (Fig. 13.14G)
- PFCL injected
- Fluid-air exchange started
- A nearly 360 degree choroidal detachment detected after drainage of subretinal fluid (Fig. 13.14H)
- Cannula plugged and IOP kept at 50 mm Hg
- A 23G trocar-cannula complex introduced obliquely through the sclera,10 mm away from the limbus according to the maximum height of choroidals into bulky engorged choroidal space (Fig. 13.14I) and trocar blade removed
- External drainage of choroidal fluid possible (Fig. 13.14J)
- Choroidal detachment nearly resolved (Fig. 13.14K)
- Blunt tip of sinsky hook used for gentle massage over the residual choroidals
- The light pipe just introduced partially into the cannula and both removed
- Barrage laser done around the inferior break as well as 360 degree
- PFCL removed
- Silicone oil injected (Fig. 13.14L)
- Postoperative fundus photograph after two weeks of surgery, shows on retina with resolved choroidals after choroidal drainage (Fig. 13.14M).

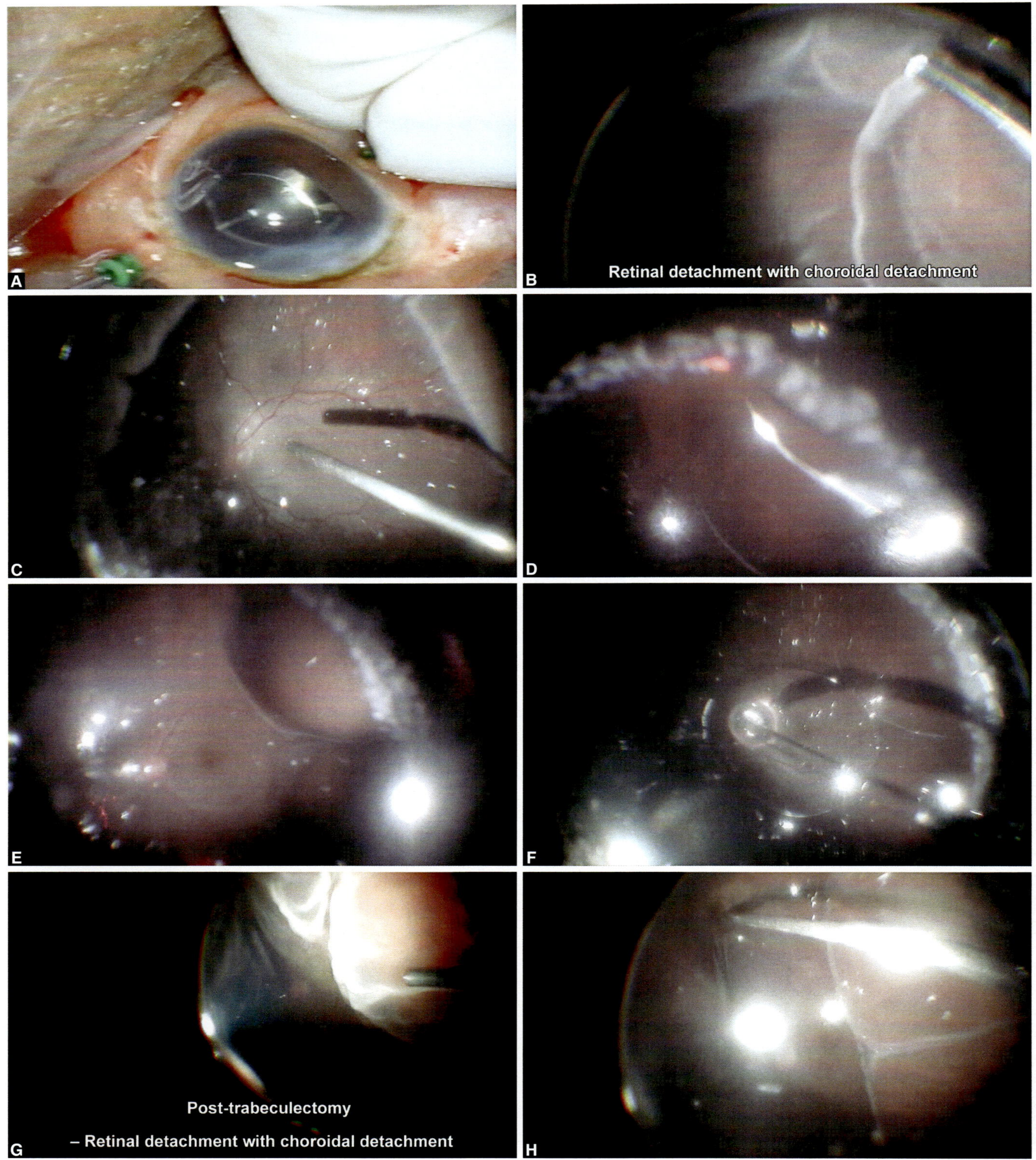

Figs 13.14A to H

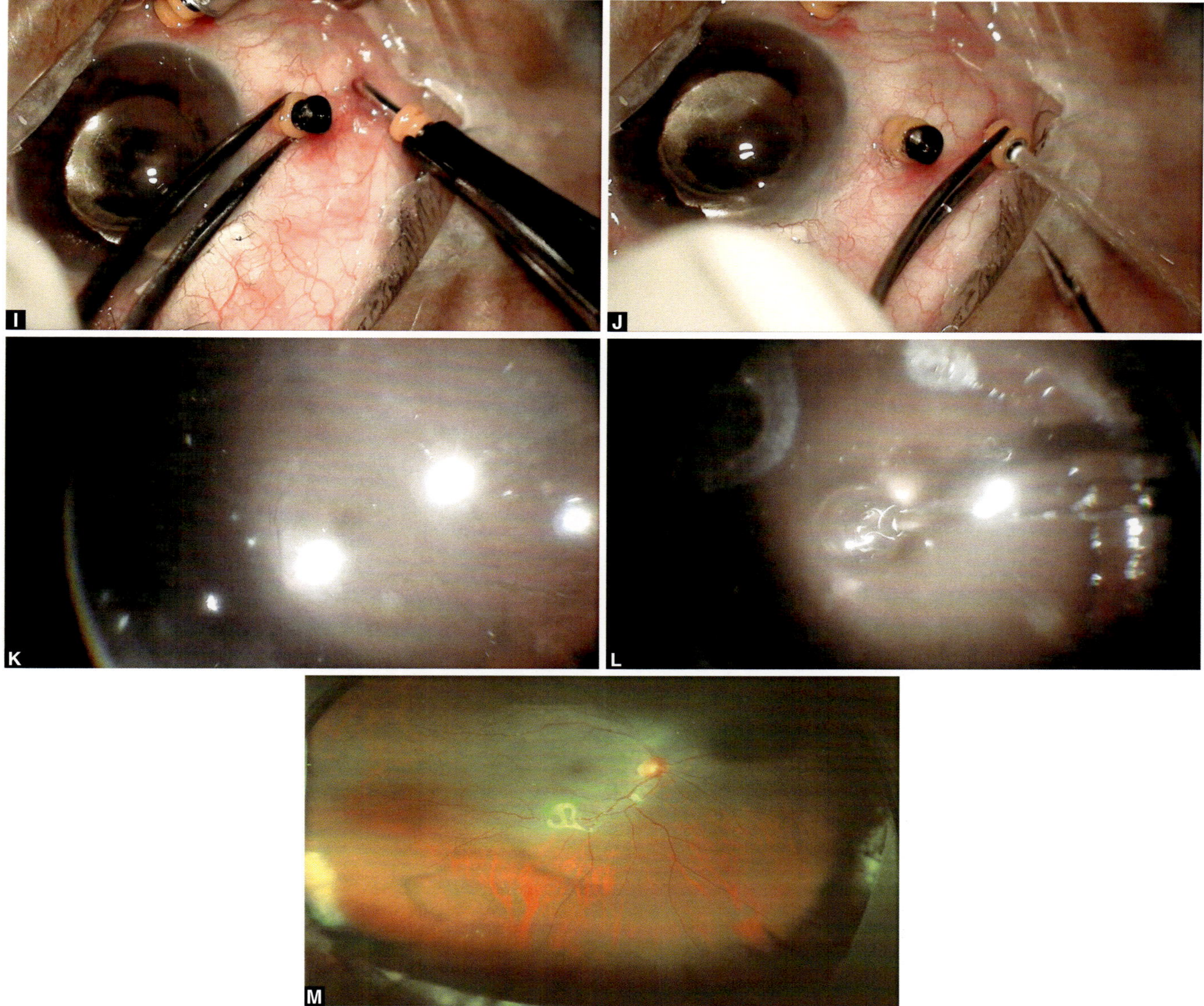

Figs 13.14A to M: (A) Infusion cannula tip in suprachoroidal space; (B to F) Intraoperative photographs of surgery in a case of retinal detachment with choroidal detachment; (G to L) Intraoperative photographs of surgery in a case of retinal detachment with 360 degree choroidal detachment where drainage of choroidal fluid performed in a suture less way; (M) Postoperative fundus photograph (after two weeks of surgery) in bullous retinal detachment with marked choroidal detachment shows on retina with resolved choroidals after choroidal drainage

Bimanual Surgeries

Bimanual vitrectomy is needed to keep both hands free to use simple or complex instruments for which one need separate light source as 4th or 5th port or with infusion cannula or illuminated cutter.

Bimanual MIVS is required in situations where we need:

- More manipulation
- Better uniform illumination
- Better peripheral tissue dissection
- Vitreous base excision in details.

The advantages it offers are:

- Better tissue respect.
- Can avoid additional complication in complex cases.

Steps where bimanual management are essential in retinal detachment:

- *For peripheral dissections of vitreous:* Peripheral vitreous fibrils around the lattices and HSTs can be dissected more carefully without any additional break formation (Fig. 13.15A)*(Video 30, Chapter 13).*
- *To use two chandelier light sources:* One can use two chandelier lights to improve illumination and to avoid

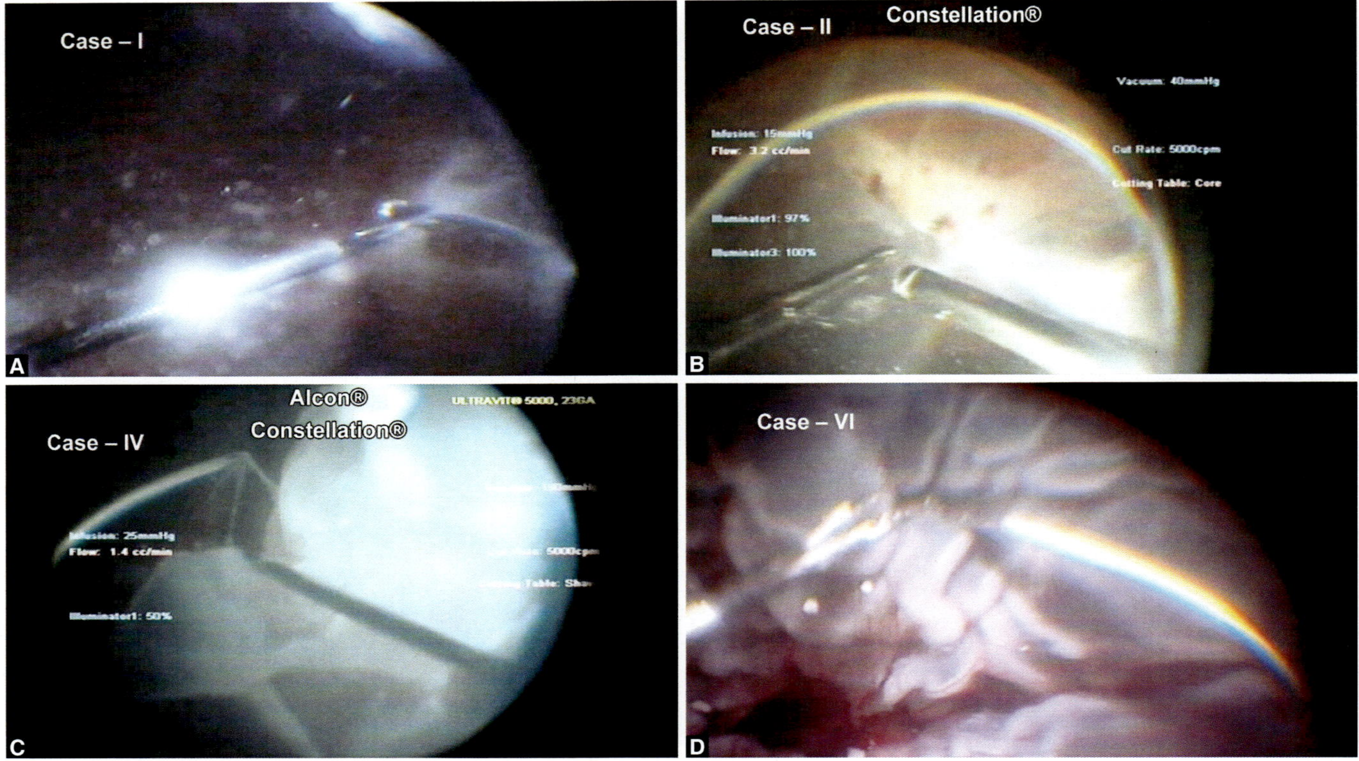

Figs 13.15A to D: (A) Bimanual peripheral vitreous dissection; (B) Bimanual vitrectomy using two chandelier lights; (C) Bimanual removal of subretinal band; (D) Bimanual release of fixed fold

instrument shadows. Peripheral tissue dissections are easier with more diffuse uniform illumination (Fig. 13.15B)*(Video 31, Chapter 13)*.

- For removal of subretinal band *(Video 32, Chapter 13)*
  - Total RD with advanced PVR with multiple sub-retinal bands
  - PFCL was injected
  - Membrane peeling was started under PFCL
  - PFCL was removed
  - Subretinal bands were identified and removed (Fig. 13.15C)
  - Again PFCL was injected
  - Now fluid-air exchange was done
  - Laser was completed
  - Silicone oil was injected.
- To release fixed folds bimanually *(Video 33, Chapter 13)*
  - Case of post-traumatic old RD with $PVRD_2$
  - A large break was detected at superotemporal quadrant
  - Triamcinolone acetonide assisted bimanual membrane peeling was started to make detached retina as much mobile as possible (Fig. 13.15D)
  - Now it is the time to inject PFCL to flatten the retina and to assess the residual traction
  - Laser was done at the margin of the break as well as 360° periphery
  - *PFCL:* Silicone oil exchange can be performed by injecting silicone oil with left hand and passively aspirating PFCL bubble. The last drop of PFCL can be removed with active suction.

Managing retinal detachment with 25 gauze Hypervit cutter: A high-speed dual-pneumatic beveled tip cutter having 20000 cuts per minute is very useful in managing a case of retinal detachment. As there is reduced peak traction force on the detached retina and reduced fluidic turbulence, fluidic stability is achieved, which reduces the pulsatility of the detached retina.

Case discussion:

- A case of total retinal detachment in a phakic eye with multiple horseshoe tears (Fig. 13.16A)
- We used 25-gauge 4 port vitrectomy system with Hypervit cutter
- Vitreous removal is faster using Hypervit cutter
- Trimming vitreous around the large HSTs is also safe
- Triamcinolone acetonide particles were injected to stain residual vitreous skirts
- PFCL was injected to secure the posterior pole (Fig. 13.16B)
- Peripheral vitreous shaving was started
- Vitreous base shaving was performed meticulously (Fig. 13.16C)

- Fluid air exchange was started, and subretinal fluid was internally drained with the help of the cutter (Fig. 13.16D)
- The laser was done around the breaks and all around the periphery (Fig. 13.16E)
- Silicone oil was used as tamponade (Fig. 13.16F)

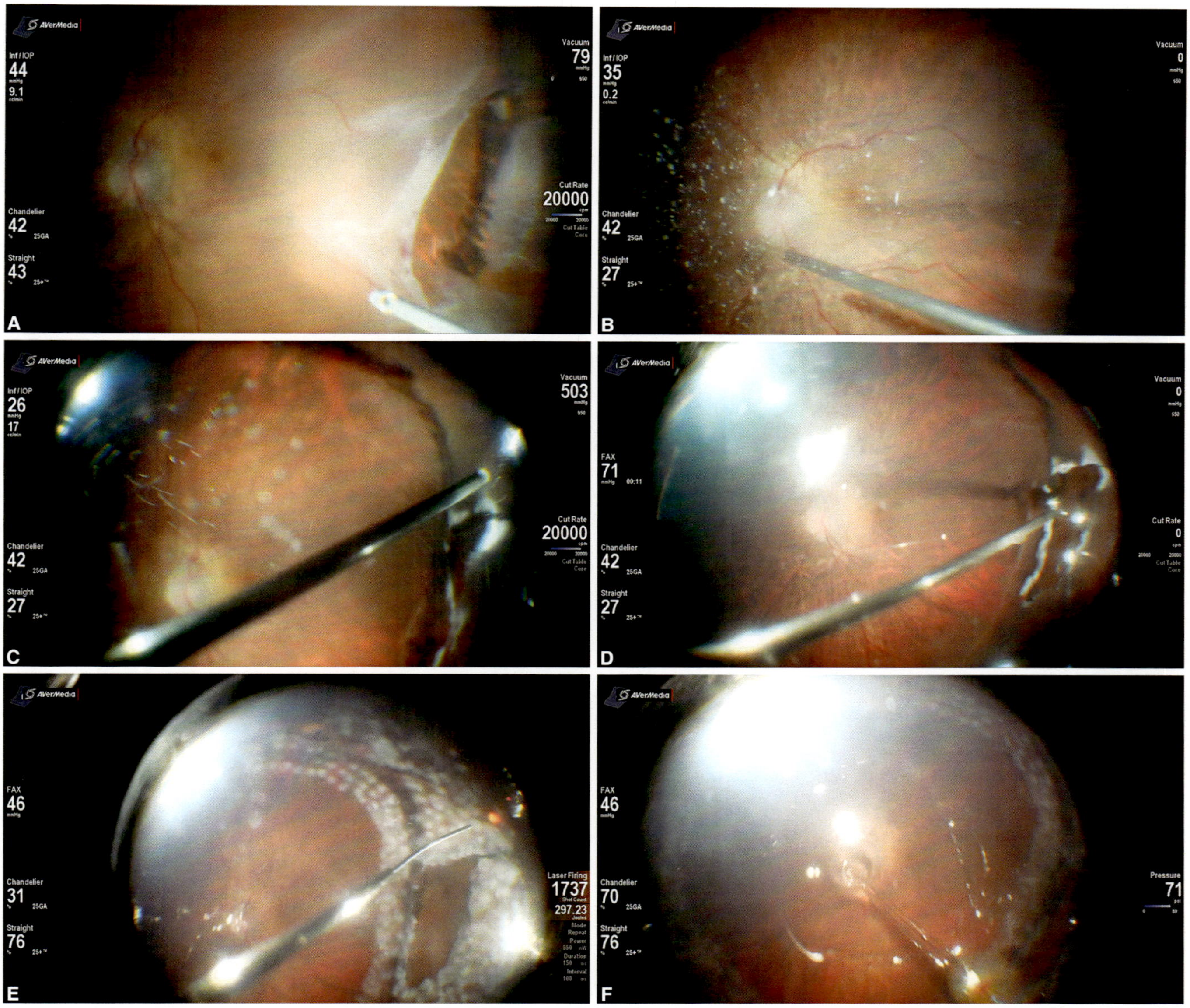

Figs 13.16A to F: Intraoperative steps of managing retinal detachment with 25-gauze Hypervit cutter.

Kindly scan the QR code below to access the online Video.

CHAPTER 14

Macular Surgeries

It is use of vital dyes to stain preretinal fine transparent tissue like epiretinal membrane (ERM), internal limiting (ILM) membranes.

Vital dyes used to stain vitreous/ERM/ILM (Table 14.1 for commonly used dyes):

- Indocyanine green (ICG 0.0125–0.025%)—stain ILM>ERM
- Infracyanine green (IFCG)—stain ILM
- Trypan Blue (0.06–0.2%)—stain ERM (0.15%), vitreous>ILM
- Triamcinolone acetonide—stain vitreous >ERM> ILM
- Sodium fluorescein (0.6%)—stain mainly vitreous
- Patent blue—stain ERM>ILM
- Eosin
- Brilliant blue (0.05%)—stain ILM>ERM>vitreous
- Bromophenol blue—for staining both ERM and ILM

Characteristics of the ideal liquid staining solution for vitreoretinal surgery:

- It should be ideal for consistent identification and visualization
- It should be easy to use for both experienced and inexperienced surgeon
- It should provide a viscous and dense solution to avoid unwanted dispersion
- Ideally, it should allow simultaneous staining of the ERM and ILM without additional air-fluid exchange
- It should be safe for intraocular use with minimal toxicity
- It should yield enhanced color-staining contrast

Combined use of 2 dyes: The rationality of the combined use of trypan blue and BBG dyes is for simultaneous staining of ERM and ILM both without any consolidated staining effect. The two dyes do not interact chemically with one another, but each dye maintains differential structures. Thus, it reflects that trypan blue has a completely different chemical action from BBG dye.

A combined solution that contains trypan blue, BBG, and polyethylene glycol:

- It offers a more viscous and denser solution
- In vitro studies show that BBG protects against trypan blue toxicity in cells
- This combined dye is less toxic to RPE cells than trypan blue alone

Methods of intravitreal dye application:

1. *Dry method/Air-filled technique:* Injecting dye after removal of fluid from the vitreous cavity by fluid-air

TABLE 14.1: Available dyes and their characteristics

	Triamcinolone	*Trypan blue*	*Indocyanine green*	*Brilliant blue*
Chemical group	Triamcinolone acetonide	Diazo	Cyanine	Triphenylmethane
Color	White	Dark blue	Dark green	Blue
Ready to use	+++	+++	–	+++
Toxicity	No	Moderate	Yes	No
Affinity to ILM	Low	Low	High	High
Affinity to ERM	High	High	Low	Moderate
Affinity to vitreous	High	Low	Low	Low
Exposure time	Short	Short	Long	Long
Fluid-gas exchange	No	Yes	No	No

exchange and then exposure of retinal surface to higher concentration of dye to vitroretinal interface.

2. *Wet method/Fluid-filled technique:* Injecting dye to fluid-filled vitreous cavity. There is possibility of unwanted staining of retinal surface elsewhere.

COMMON MACULAR SURGICAL PATHOLOGIES

Epimacular Membrane (Fig. 14.1)

- Idiopathic ERM are mostly caused by posterior vitreous detachment (90% have PVD)
- Study showed eyes with poor preoperative vision tended to improve more frequently and to a greater extent than did eyes with better preoperative vision. Retinal vascular leakage with cystoid macular edema are found to be a poor prognostic factor due to RPE atrophic change and RPE disruption. Transparent ERM carries better prognosis than opaque ERMs (Fig. 14.2)
- Postvitrectomy ERM with macular pucker (Fig. 14.3) should be operated when the membrane has matured and stopped actively contracting, especially 2 months after onset of symptoms
- Vitrectomy and PVD induction are the initial steps. Taut thick ERMs are usually associated with thick posterior vitreous. Carefully PVD induction has to be carried out as there is chance of peripheral break formation
- ERM has to be exactly delineated by staining it with trypan blue and the dye has to be applied under air after completion of fluid-air exchange. Then the extent and stained characteristics of ERM has to be assessed. *Most prominent and most thickened area or margin has to be picked up by end grasping forceps.*

OCT of macular epiretinal membrane: Macular OCT is essential not only for diagnostic confirmation, but also to prognosticate the case detecting the integrity of external limiting membrane and photoreceptor outer segment and inner segment junction junction (Fig. 14.4).

Steps of ERM Removal Surgery (Video 1, Chapter 14)

- Vitrectomy followed by TA assisted PVD induction (Fig. 14.5A)
- Fluid-air exchange and trypan blue dye application under air (Fig. 14.5B)
- Dye-stained ERM removal with end grasping forceps after washing out the dye (Figs 14.5C to G)
- Brilliant blue G application in water (Fig. 14.5H)
- Dye-assisted ILM removal with forceps (Fig. 14.5I)
- Complete or partial FAE.

OCT: Pre- and postoperative comparative OCT scans of macula showing absence of ERM and decrease in macular thickness after surgery (Fig. 14.5J).

Complications after ERM removal surgery:

1. Cataract—12–68%. Pale greenish-gray opalescence rather yellowish age-related nuclear sclerosis.
2. Retinal break 1–6%.
3. Retinal detachment—1–7% due to overlooked break.
4. Visually significant recurrent ERM—up to 5% cases.

Full-thickness Macular Hole

Idiopathic Macular Holes

Full-thickness macular holes are the defects involving all layers of retina at macula from ILM to outer segment of photoreceptors (Fig. 14.6).

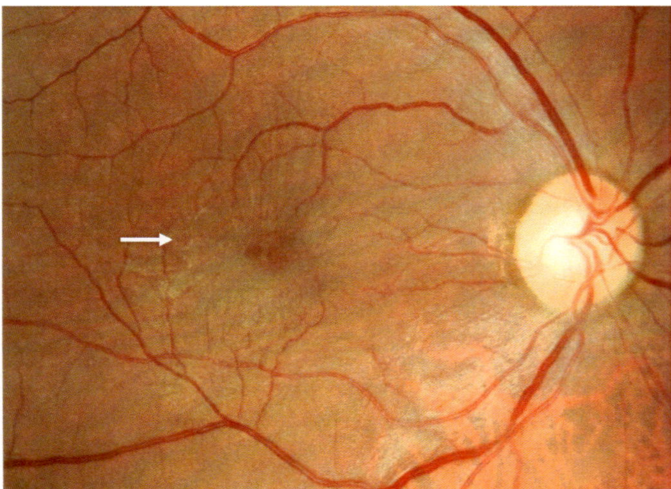

Fig. 14.1: Presence of idiopathic epiretinal membrane at macula (white arrow)

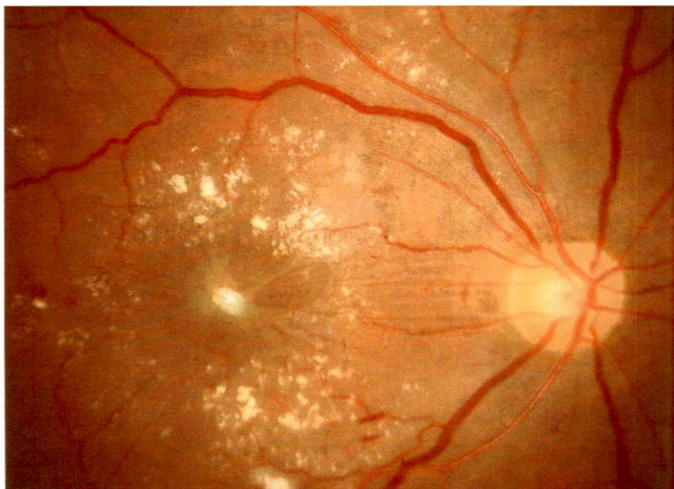

Fig. 14.2: Presence of opaque, fibrous diabetic epiretinal membrane

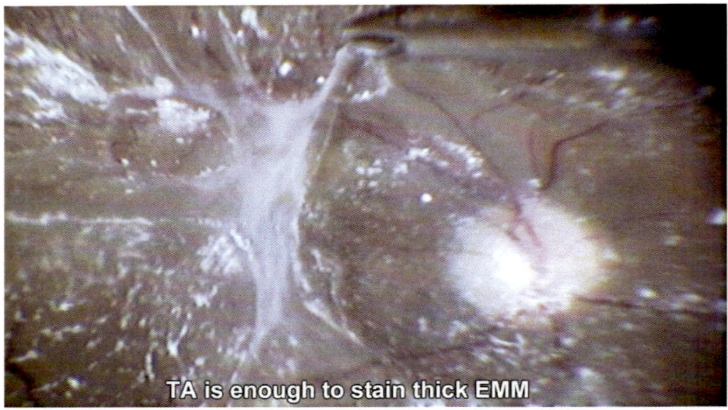

Fig. 14.3: Postvitrectomy triamcinolone acetonide-stained thick epiretinal membrane with macular pucker. (TA, triamcinolone acetonide; EMM, Epimacular membrane)

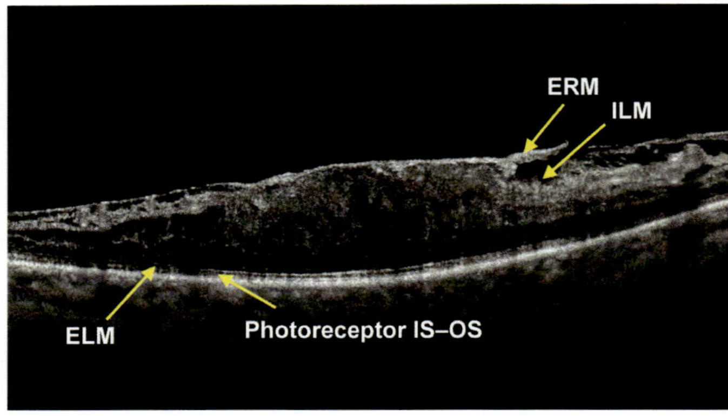

Fig. 14.4: OCT scan of macula showing thick ERM with intact ELM and intact photoreceptor IS-OS junction. (ELM, external limiting membrane; ILM, internal limiting membrane; ERM, epiretinal membrane; photoreceptor IS-OS, photoreceptor inner segment and outer segment)

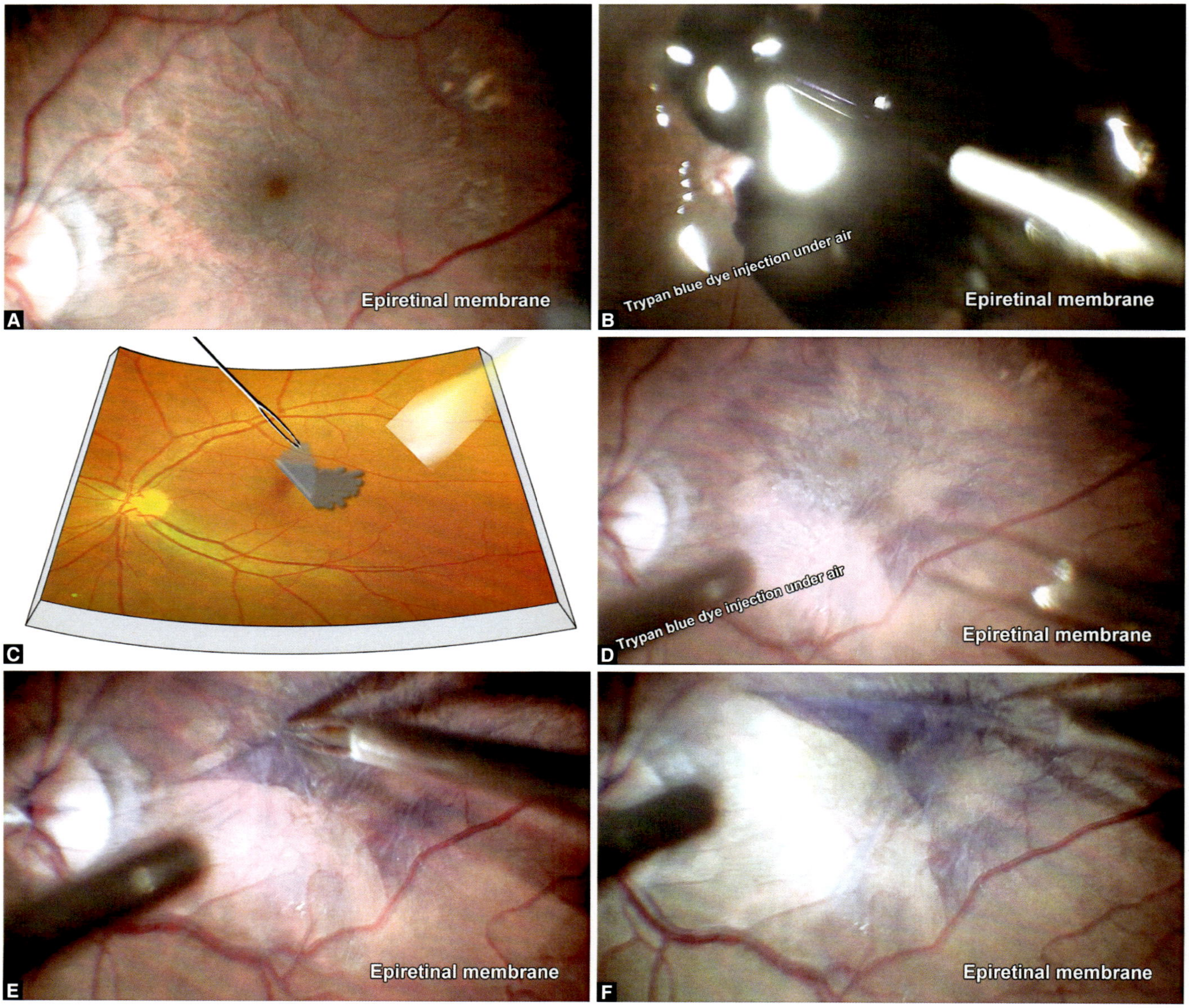

A Epiretinal membrane

B Trypan blue dye injection under air
Epiretinal membrane

C

D Trypan blue dye injection under air
Epiretinal membrane

E Epiretinal membrane

F Epiretinal membrane

Figs 14.5A to F

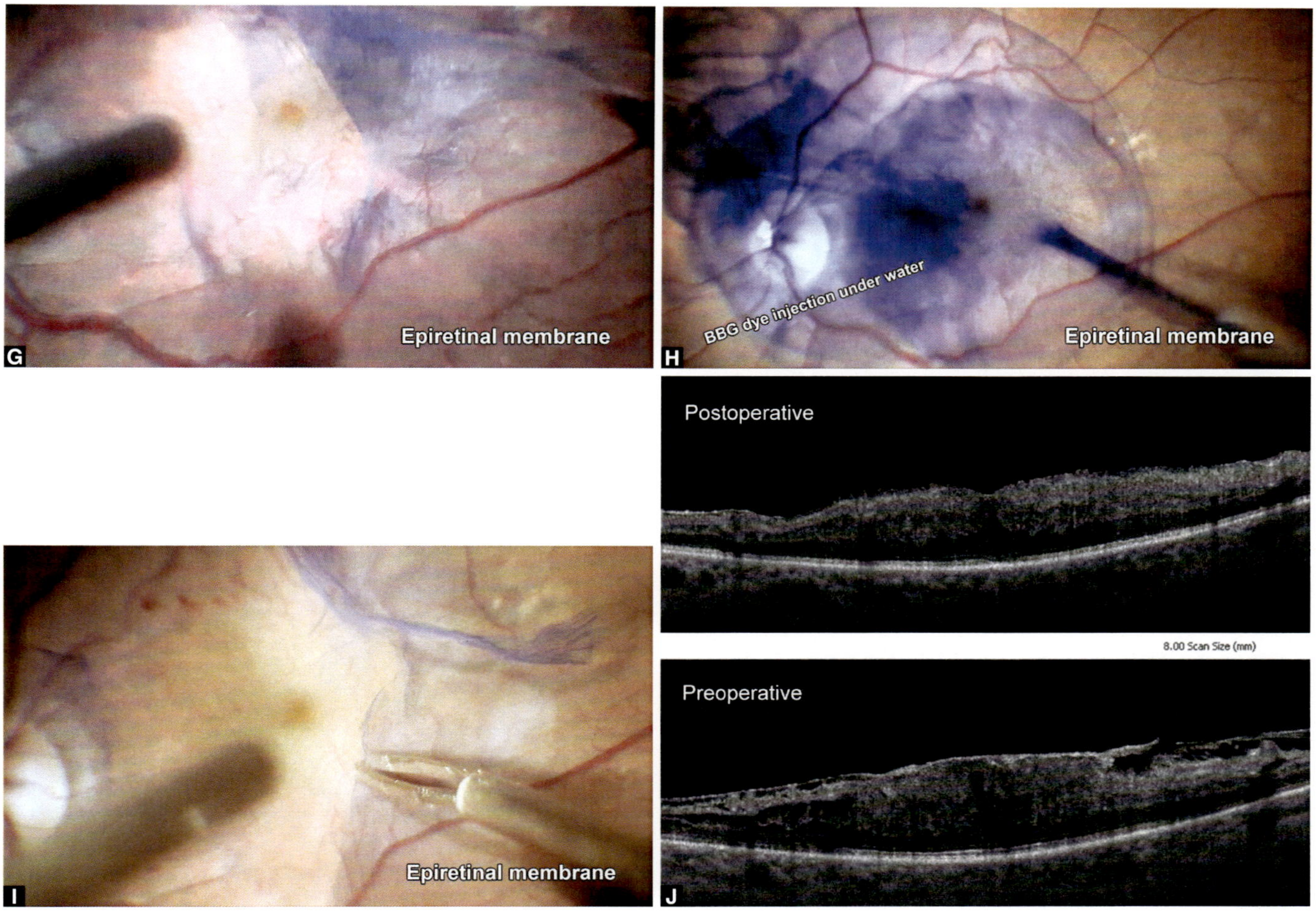

Figs 14.5A to J: (A, B and D to I) Intraoperative photographs showing steps of trypan blue dye-assisted epiretinal membrane removal surgery; (C) Illustration shows removal of epiretinal membrane by end grasping forceps; (J) Pre- and postoperative comparative OCT scans of macula showing absence of ERM and decrease in macular thickness after surgery

Pathogenesis of full-thickness macular holes are poorly understood. Vitreous traction at the vitreo retinal interface (both anterior-posterior and tangential) are the main factor. Gas's theory of pathogenesis of macular holes are the mostly accepted till now. Gas believed that tangential traction caused by shrinkage of perifoveal vitreous cortex are responsible.

Gass described four stages (Figs 14.7A to I)

Stage I: Impending macular holes—characterized by a shallow foveolar detachment resulting in a yellow spot (I-A)—Increased visibility of xanthophyll pigment secondary to foveolar detachment. It measures 100–200 micron and may be seen in other conditions like cystoid macular edema, CSR, vitreomacular traction, etc.

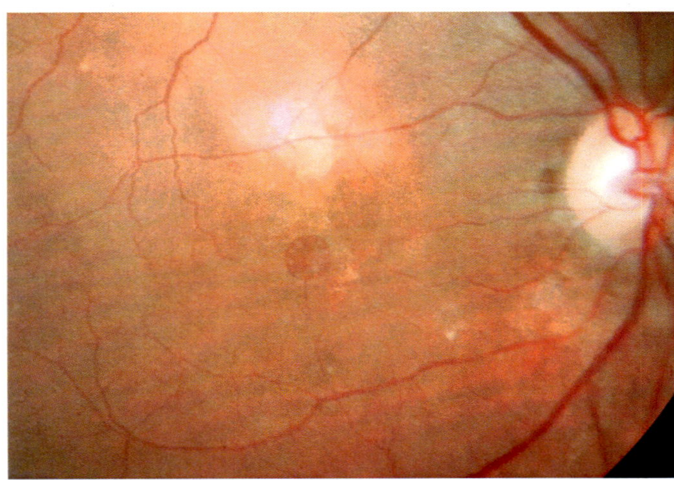

Fig. 14.6: Fundus photograph shows full-thickenss macular hole

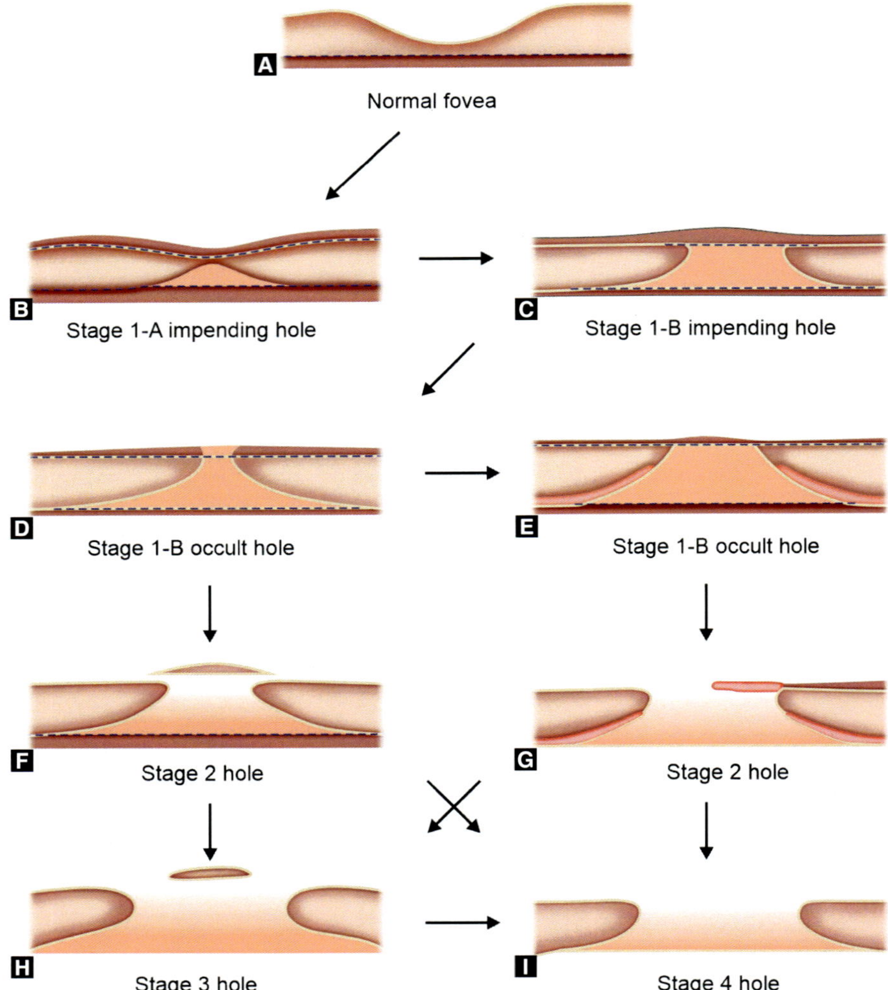

Figs 14.7A to I: Diagrammatic representation of stages of senile macular hole formation: (A) Normal fovea, with a layer of vitreous cortex lying on the ILM of retina; (B) Stage 1-A impending hole: Early contraction of the outer part of vitreous cortex, with foveolar detachment (Stage I A); (C) Stage 1-B impending hole: Further vitreous contraction and condensation of the prefoveolar vitreous cortex, with foveal detachment (Stage I B); (D and E) Stage 1B occult hole: Dehiscence of the retinal receptor layer at the umbo, with centrifugal retraction of the retinal receptors; (F) Stage 2 hole with early separation of condensed prefoveal vitreous cortex, with formation of pseudo-operculum that is larger than the hole (Stage IIA); (G) Stage 2 hole with a tear in the vitreous cortex at the junction of the prefoveal vitreous cortex and the edge of the macular hole (Stage II B); (H) Stage 3 hole with pseudo-operculum; (I) Stage 4 hole after posterior vitreous separation. (Adapted from Gass JD. Reappraisal of biomicroscopic classification of stages of development of a macular hole. American Journal of Ophthalmology 1995;119:752-9).

Yellow ring (I-B): That is occult hole. Characterized by a yellow ring from central foveal thinning and xanthophyll distribution in a ring-like configuration. There is further perifoveal vitreous contraction and condensation. 40% of Stage I macular holes progress to full-thickness macular holes.

Stage II: A full-thickness break in inner margin of yellow ring. There is early separation of condensed perifoveal vitreous cortex, forming a pseudo operculum.

Stage IIA: Condensed vitreous is still attached.

Stage IIB: Complete separation of pseudo operculum, which is still larger than the hole due to 360 degree tear of condensed vitreous cortex at the edge of retinal hole. 'Pincushion distortion' as described by the patient is due to centrifugal displacement of photoreceptors.

Stage III: Fully-developed macular hole but without complete PVD (posterior hyaloid will be attached at the disc). An operculum is seen anterior to to the macular hole, smaller in size. Watzke-Allen test (a gap in a narrow-slit beam) will be positive.

Stage IV: Full-thickness macular hole with complete separation of posterior hyaloid from both macula and optic disc.

Morgan and Schatz also implicated the theory of involutional retinal thinning or retinal degeneration in the pathogenesis of macular hole.

Risk to Fellow Eye

The reported risk of macular hole formation in the fellow eye ranges from 3 to 29%.

Preoperative Prognostic Factors

1. *Stage of MH:* Data of the Moorfields Macular Hole Study concluded that the advanced stages had a worse visual outcome
2. *Duration of symptoms:* Eyes with a shorter duration of symptoms have been well recognized to have a better visual outcome after macular hole surgery. Several lines of evidence have shown that the chance of recovering good visual acuity following macular hole surgery is decreased if the duration of symptoms is longer than 12 months.
3. *Preoperative visual acuity:* Preoperative visual acuity is one of the most important prognostic factors used in clinical practice. In general, eyes with better preoperative visual acuity have more chance to attain better postoperative visual acuity, whereas eyes with worse preoperative visual acuity are likely to gain better visual improvements.
4. *Size of the MH:* inversely correlated with visual outcomes: Eyes with a larger diameter hole have worse visual outcomes.
5. *OCT parameters and indices:*
   a. Integrity of ELM and junction of photoreceptor inner segment–outer segment (IS-OS). Intact ELM and photoreceptor IS-OS junction carry better prognosis than the cases with disrupted ELM and photoreceptor IS-OS junction (Fig. 14.8).
   b. Preoperatively macular hole surgery can be prognosticated by measuring following OCT indices:
      i. Hole form factor (HFF) (Fig. 14.9)—The HFF is the quotient of the summation of the left- and right-arm lengths divided by the basal hole diameter. The HFF is reported to be positively correlated with the postoperative visual acuity, but the correlation is weaker than those for the minimum diameter and the basal hole diameter. If a - Minimal hole diameter, b - Left arm length, c - Right arm length and d - Basal hole diameter, then HFF = (b + c)/d

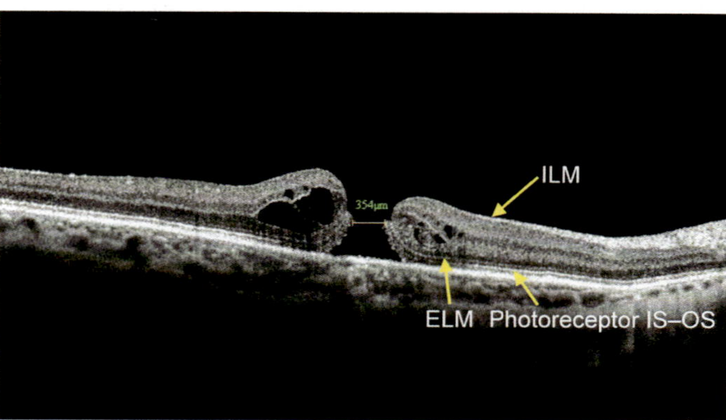

Fig. 14.8: OCT scan of macula shows full-thickness defect in foveal neurosensory retina, called macular hole with distribution of external limiting membrane and junction of photoreceptor inner segment-outer segment. (ILM, internal limiting membrane; ELM, external limiting membrane; IS–OS, inner segment-outer segment)

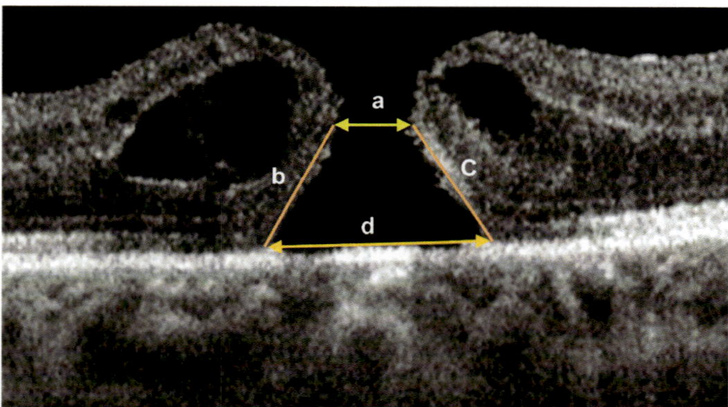

Fig. 14.9: Shows the calculation of hole form factor (HFF) from OCT

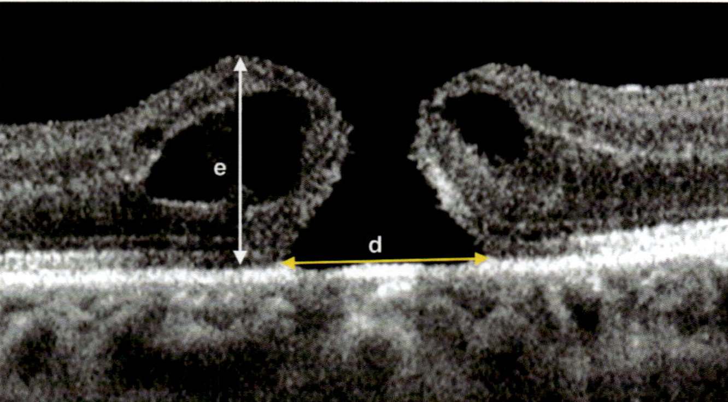

Fig. 14.10: Shows the calculation of macular hole index (MHI) from OCT

      ii. Macular hole index (MHI) (Fig. 14.10)—The MHI is defined as the ratio of the hole height to the basal hole diameter and is reported to be positively correlated to the postoperative visual acuity. Eyes with an MHI value ≥0.5 had better visual acuity than those with an MHI value <0.5, which seems to be of great help in the clinical use of the MHI.

Again if e - Hole height, then MHI = e/d

6. *Other parameters:* Pattern reversal visual evoked potential P100 latency and pattern electroretinogram N35 latency were significantly associated with visual outcomes.

Rationalities of Peeling ILM in Macular Hole Surgery

1. As contractile myofibroblasts may proliferate along the ILM causing tangential traction, removal of ILM thereby may facilitate hole closure by eliminating tangential traction.
2. The process of ILM removal may induce reparative gliosis, facilitating hole closure.
3. Removal of ILM ensures complete removal of other responsible factors for tangential traction like residual posterior hyaloid cortex strips and ERM.

Surgical steps in macular hole surgery:

1. Vitrectomy with PVD induction—Vitrectomy followed by TA-assisted PVD induction (most crucial step).
   a. *PVD induction by cutter (Video 2, Chapter 14):* Using a vacuum of 200–400mmHg or more with high intraocular pressure setting (to prevent collapse of globe), engaging the cortical vitreous with suction and creating PVD by lifting the cutter straight up until a Weiss ring is seen (Fig. 14.11A). Edges of macular hole should be observed carefully to prevent enlargement of macular hole. Care should be taken to prevent formation of retinal breaks at periphery.
   b. *PVD induction by silicone-tipped flute needle/extrusion needle (Video 3, Chapter 14):* Sweeping a silicone-tipped flute needle/extrusion needle over the retinal surface to identify the adherent cortical vitreous ('Fish strike' sign) (Fig. 14.11B).
2. ILM peeling—It ensures complete removal of all posterior hyaloid cortex and removal of all kinds of tangential traction. It removes all contractile myofibroblasts over ILM around the macular hole. It induce reparative gloss that facilitates hole closure.
   a. Brilliant blue G dye application under air or directly in water *(Video 4, Chapter 14)*. In phakic eyes dye application, it is better to apply dye directly into water, rather to apply under air, which can induce intraoperative cataract formation and that can hamper further ILM peeling (Fig. 14.11C).
      - *Initial flap formation:* By Tano diamond-dusted membrane scraper or end-gripping forceps *(Video 5, Chapter 14)* (Fig. 14.11D)
      - ILM peeling in clockwise *(Video 6, Chapter 14)* or anti clockwise direction *(Video 7, Chapter 14)* (Figs 14.11E to O)
   b. *Trypan blue-assisted ILM peeling (Video 8, Chapter 14):* Trypan blue can stain ILM, but ILM stain faintly. ILM peeling can be started anywhere in the stain macula according to the surgeon's choice and preference. (Fig. 14.11P)
   c. *Inverse flap technique (Video 9, Chapter 14) (V):* First described by Michalewska for large old macular holes. In the inverted ILM flap technique, instead of completely removing the ILM after BBG staining, a remnant attached to the margins of the macular hole left in place. This ILM remnant then inverted upsidedown to cover the macular hole. Fluid–air exchange performed and utmost care should be taken to cover the macular hole with the attached ILM by foceps or Tano diamond-dusted membrane scraper (Figs 14.11Q and R).

The logic of the inverted flap technique:
- Michalewska et al. hypothesized that the inverted ILM flap technique stimulates the proliferation of glial cells that fill the macular hole. Histopathologic findings indicate that the ILM serves as a scaffold for gliosis. This occurs because the peeled-off ILM contains Müller cell fragments capable of inducing gliosis, aiding in the closure of the macular hole. Thus, the segmented peeled-off ILM left attached may provoke gliosis both within the retina and on the surface of the ILM.
- The ILM also may be a scaffold for tissue proliferation. Michalewska et al. observed closure of the macular hole by a thin membrane with an appearance consistent with the ILM.
- In the case of a myopic macular hole, the retinal tension cannot be eliminated by ILM peeling alone, as some of the components, vascular traction and posterior staphyloma, cannot be avoided. So, ILM peeling alone may not compensate for macular hole closure in high myopia. In the case of the inverted flap technique, proliferating glial cells fill the macular hole and may compensate for retinal shortening.

3. Check vitreous base to rule out presence of any retinal break *(Video 10, Chapter 14)* (Fig. 14.11S).
4. Fluid-air exchange—Complete fluid-air exchange to be done with gentle aspiration of fluid from base of macular holes *(Video 11, Chapter 14)* (Fig. 14.11T).
5. Intravitreal gas tamponade.

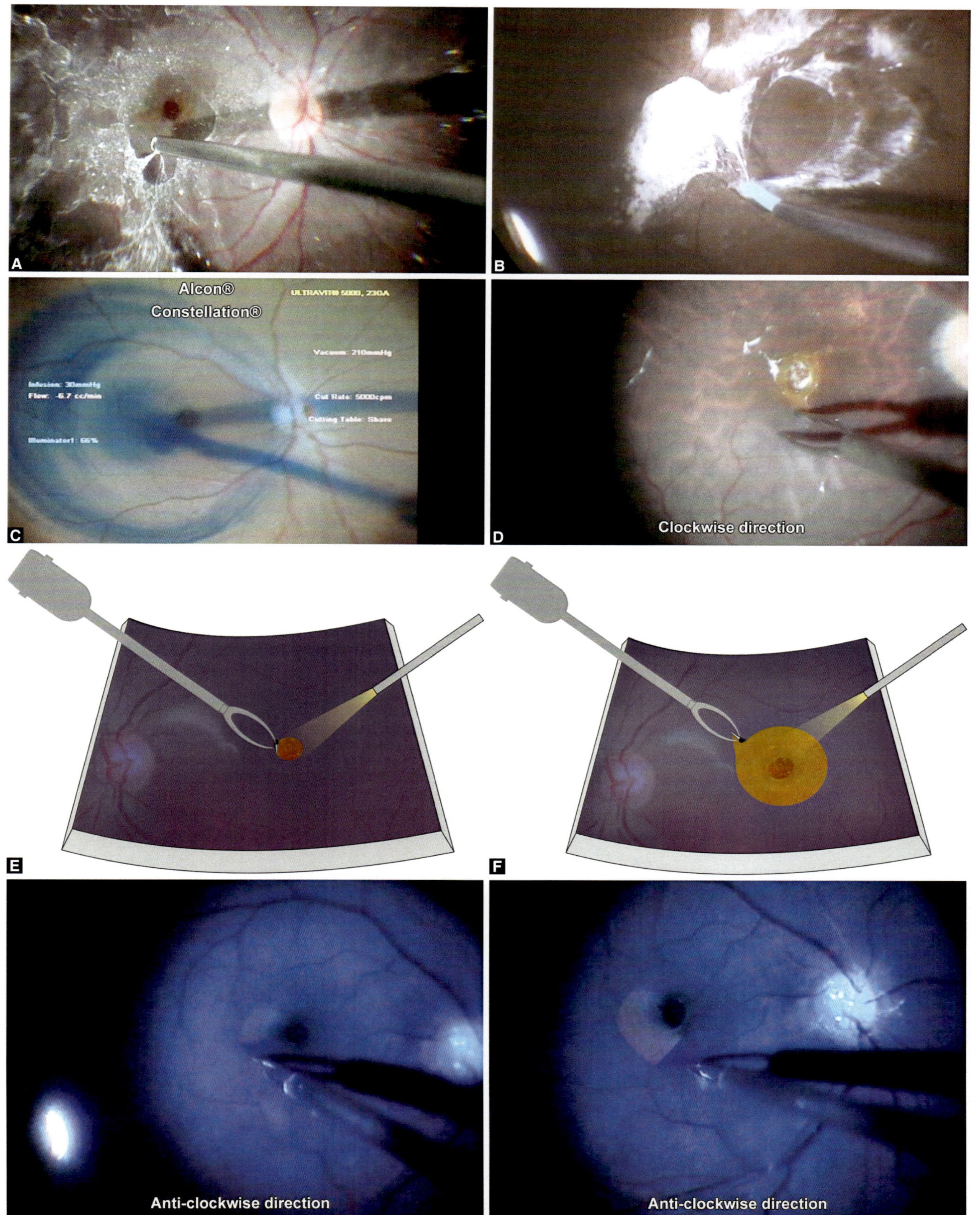

Figs 14.11A and H

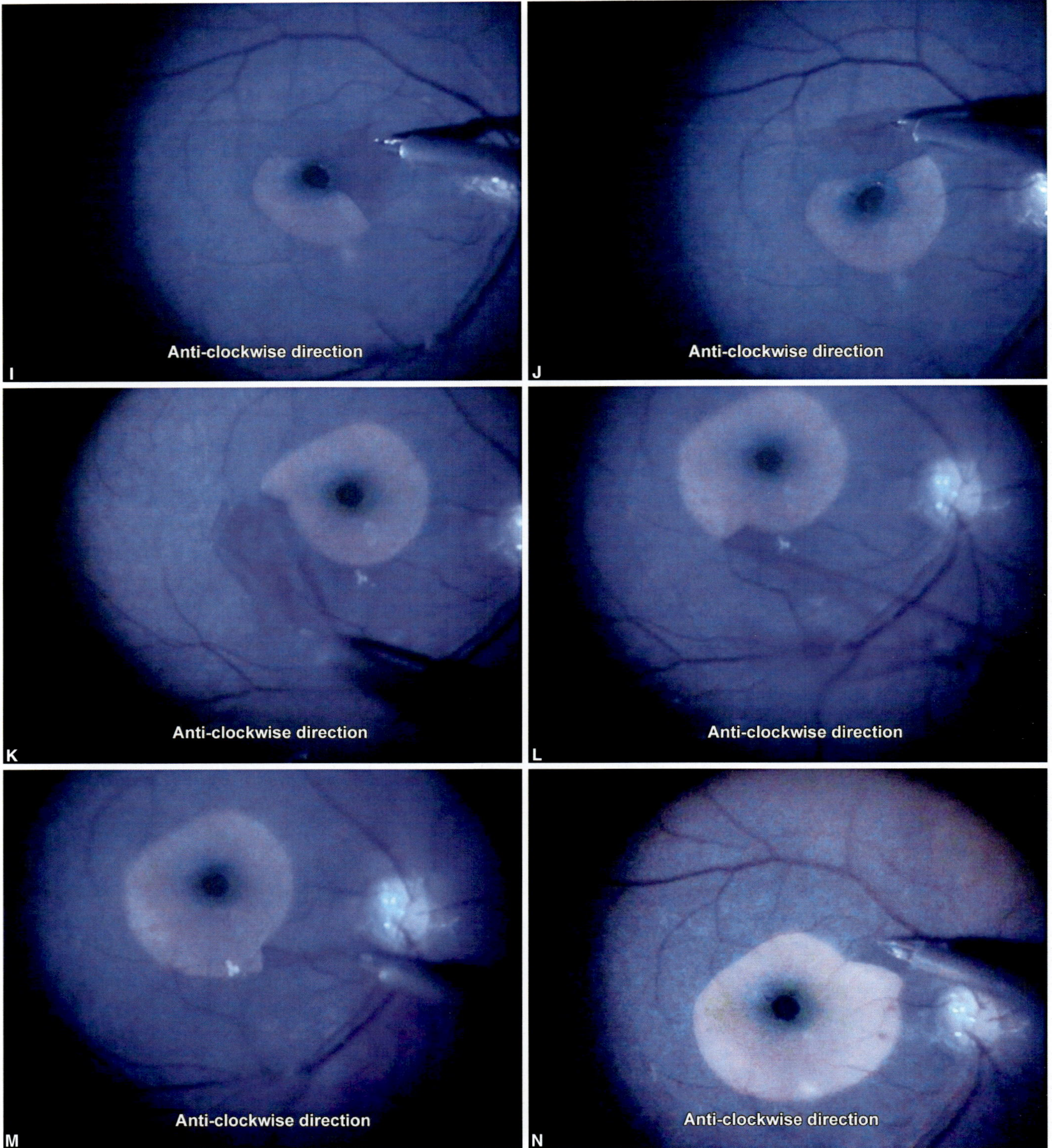

Figs 14.11I to N

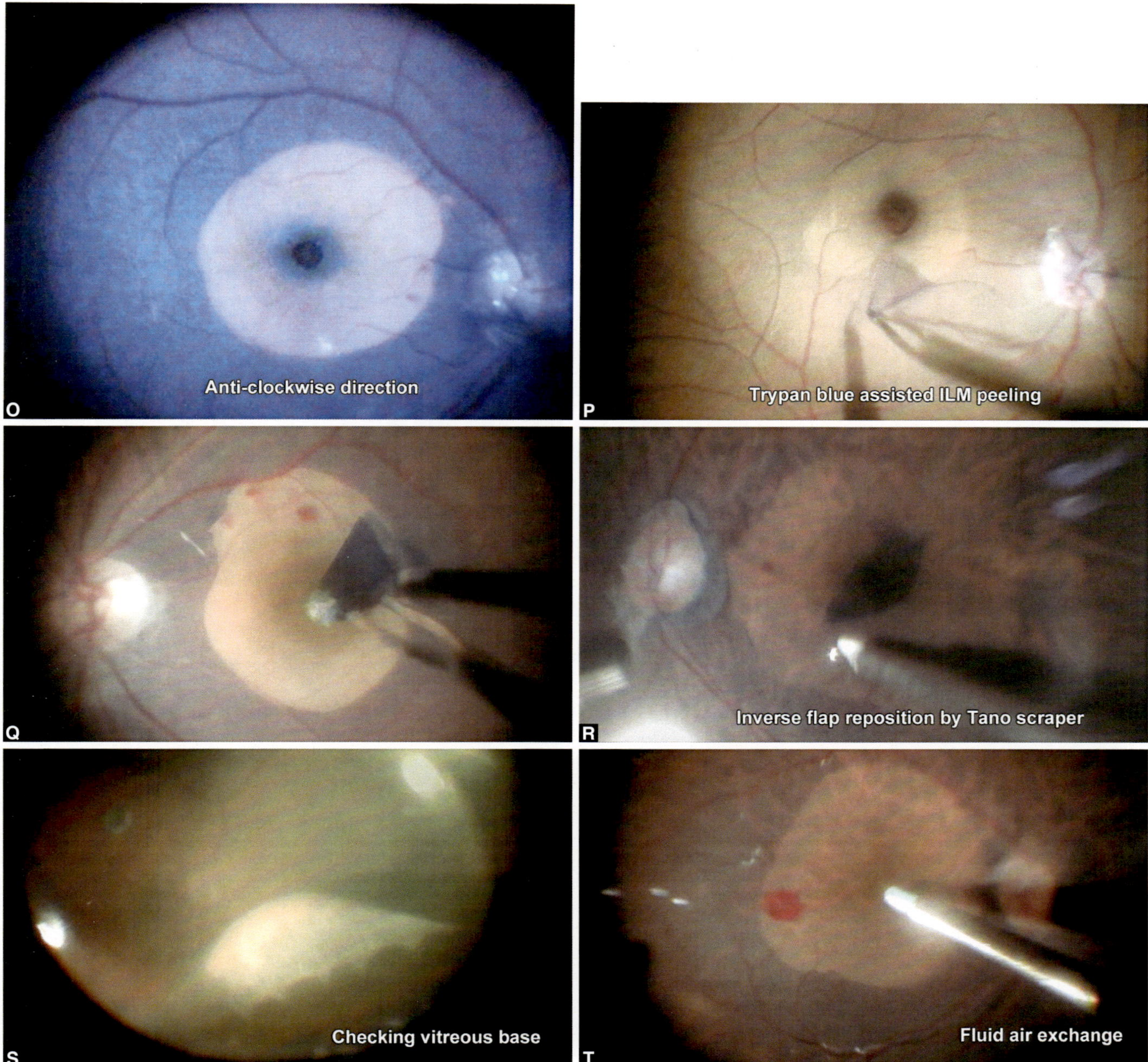

Figs 14.11A to T: (A) Shows triamcinolone-assisted PVD induction by suction of cutter; (B) Shows triamcinolone-assisted PVD induction by silicone tip flute needle; (C) Shows Brilliant Blue G dye application directly in water; (D) Creating ILM flap by tearing ILM from macular hole margin by end-grasping forceps; (E and F) Illustration shows animated form of 'onion peel technique' of ILM peel by tearing ILM from macular hole margin and then gradually enlarging it; (G to O) Intraoperative photographs shows the 'onion-peel' technique of BBG dye assisted ILM peeling by forceps in anti-clockwise direction; (P) Intraoperative photograph shows trypan Blue stained ILM peeling; (Q and R) Show intraoperative photographs of inverted flap technique by repositioning ILM tag by forceps (Q) or Tano scraper (R) keeping temporal hinge of ILM; (S) Shows intraoperative photograph of examining vitreous base by external scleral depression; (T) Shows intraoperative photograph of fluid-air exchange

Postoperative Positioning

It is important to maintain prone position postoperatively for at least seven days as holes close during this early postoperative period in more than 90% of cases.

Studies already done for macular hole surgery with long-acting C_3F_8 gas or even with simplest tamponade air. Even few studies show 'no prone positioning' with C_3F_8 gas tamponade.

Postoperative closure of macular hole: Macular hole closure pattern is variable and not predictable. It could be:

Type I closure (Fig. 14.12A) without any foveal neurosensory retinal defect.

Type II closure (Fig. 14.12B) with foveal neurosensory retinal defect.

Open macular hole (Fig. 14.12C): Persistent defect in foveal neurosensory retina with surrounding serous detachment at its base.

Kang SW et al. showed: Type I closure was 61.3% and Type II closure was 38.7% (British J Ophthalmol 2003;87:1015-19).

Secondary Macular Holes

Types

1. *Traumatic:* Due to trampoline effect of trauma, there is anterior-posterior compression and simultaneous equatorial expansion of the globe which is immediately followed by anterior-posterior decompression of the globe. Macular hole forms due to pressure necrosis at the stage of compression as well as due to PVD at the stage of anterior-posterior decompression.
2. *Postsurgical:* After surgery for optic disc pit with maculopathy, myopic foveoschisis
3. As a complication of other complicated disease pathology like PDR with multiple TRDs, from progressive thinning of neurosensory retina in parafoveal telangiectasia.

Surgical Prognostic Factors in Secondary Macular Hole Cases

1. Preoperative visual acuity—Poor preoperative vision carries poor visual prognosis.
2. Macular hole morphology—single most important factor. If it looks like idiopathic cases, it closes like it. Secondary macular holes usually larger than idiopathic cases.
3. Severity of background pathology—like retinitis pigmentosa, ischemic maculopathy in diabetics, inflammatory changes around the fovea.

Surgery for traumatic macular hole

Surgical principles *(Video 12, Chapter 14)* are same like idiopathic cases; i.e.

- Vitrectomy followed by TA-assisted PVD induction (Fig. 14.13A)
- Dye-assisted ILM peeling (Figs 14.13B to E)
- Fluid-air exchange
- Intravitreal gas tamponade.

  [Inverse flap technique (Fig. 14.13F) can be applied for large old macular holes]

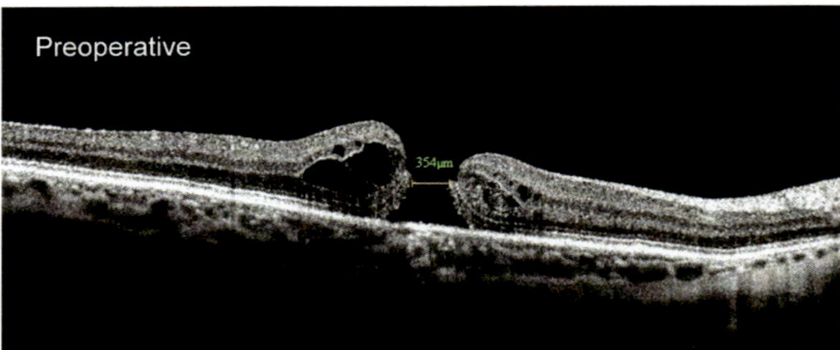

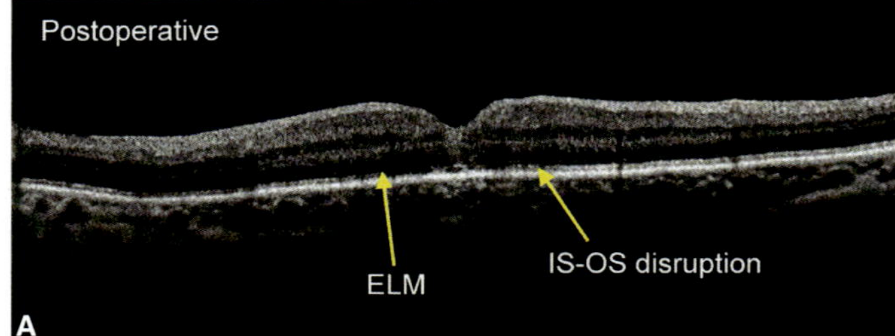

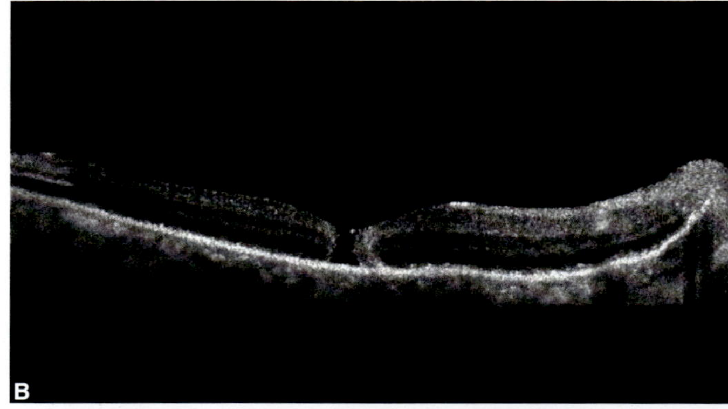

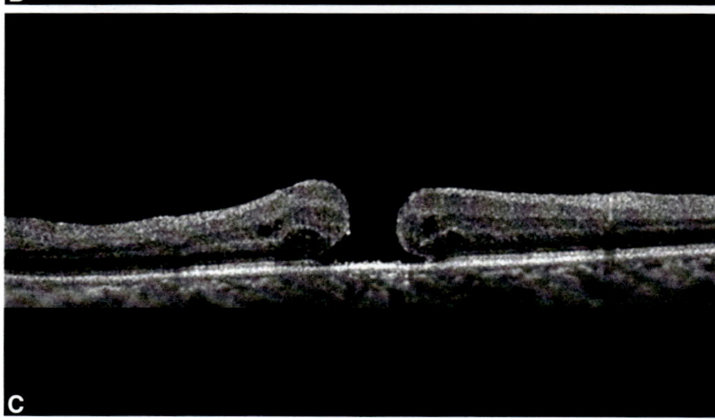

Figs 14.12A to C: (A) Pre- and postoperative OCT in case of macular hole surgery, showing Type I closure of macular hole with intact ELM but disrupted photoreceptor IS–OS junction; (B) Postoperative OCT in case of macular hole surgery, showing Type II closure of macular hole; (C) Postoperative OCT in case of macular hole surgery, showing open macular hole. (ELM, external limiting membrane; IS–OS, inner segment–outer segment)

Surgery for very large-sized macular holes: Currently available options are as follows:

1. Human amniotic membrane (HAM) graft transplantation: First described by Rizzo S et al. (*A Human Amniotic*

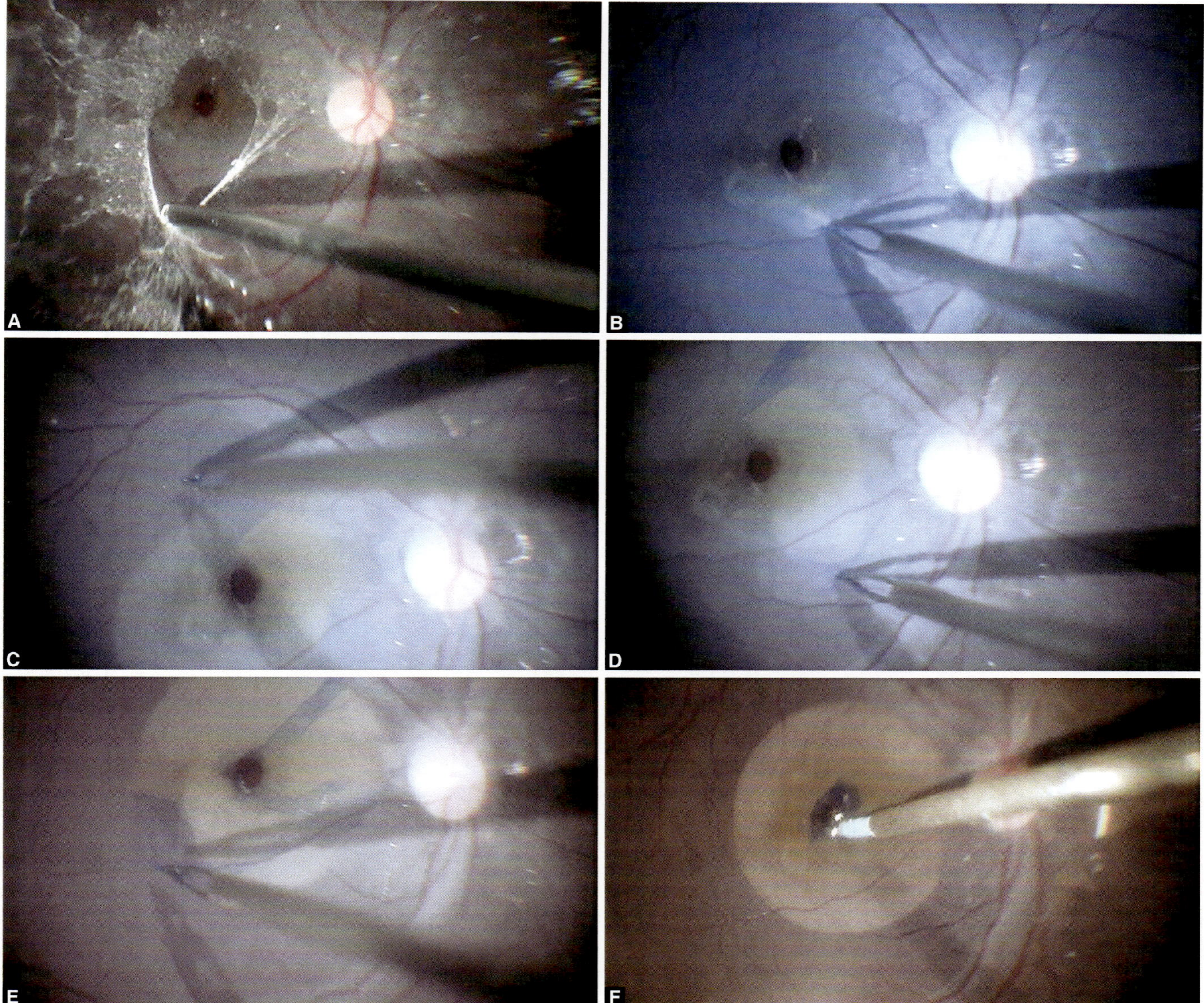

Figs 14.13A to F: Surgery for traumatic large macular hole by 'inverted flap technique': (A) PVD induction; (B to E) Dye-assisted ILM peeling with forceps; (F) Inverted ILM flaps over the macular hole

Membrane Plug to Promote Retinal Breaks Repair and Recurrent Macular Hole Closure. Retina. 2019;39 (Suppl 1):S95-S103. doi: 10.1097/IAE.0000000000002320)

Characteristic features of HAM graft are:
- Transparent human biological film—0.02–0.05 mm thick
- Nonimmunogenic
- Anti-inflammatory, antifibrotic, antiangiogenic and help in cell migration and adhesion
- Three layers (epithelial layer, middle stroma and basement membrane)
- Amniotic membrane plugs the macular hole with good functional recovery.

Case discussion (Video 13, Chapter 14):
- It was a post-traumatic macular hole with a 1046-micron diameter with BCVA 3/60 (Fig. 14.14A)
- Vitrectomy done (Fig. 14.14B)
- Triamcinolone-stained posterior vitreous detachment was performed (Fig. 14.14C)
- Then ILM was stained with Brilliant Blue dye, and ILM was peeled in an inverted flap manner (Fig. 14.14D)
- Then, an amniotic membrane graft was harvested from the preserved amniotic membrane from the nitrocellulose paper with a 2-mm trephine after staining the epithelial side over a paraffin block (Fig. 14.14E)

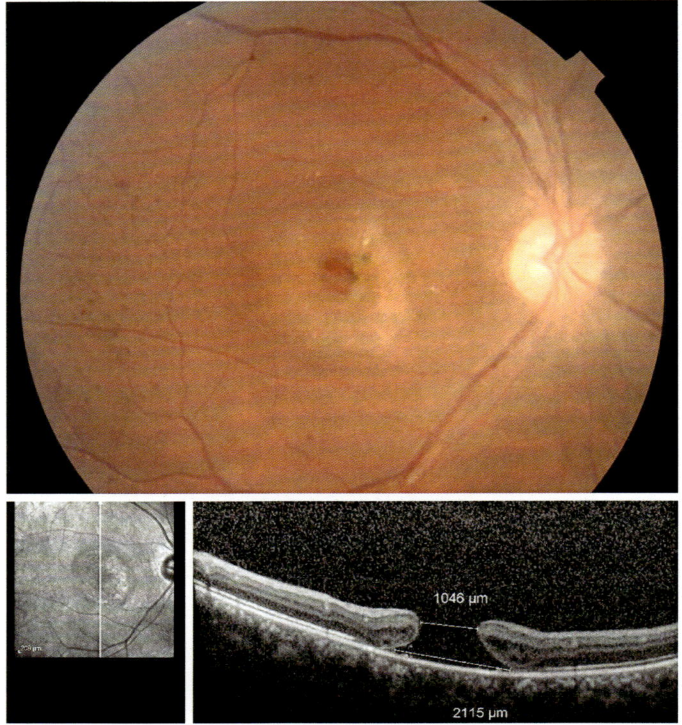

Fig. 14.14A: Post-traumatic macular hole with a 1046-micron diameter.

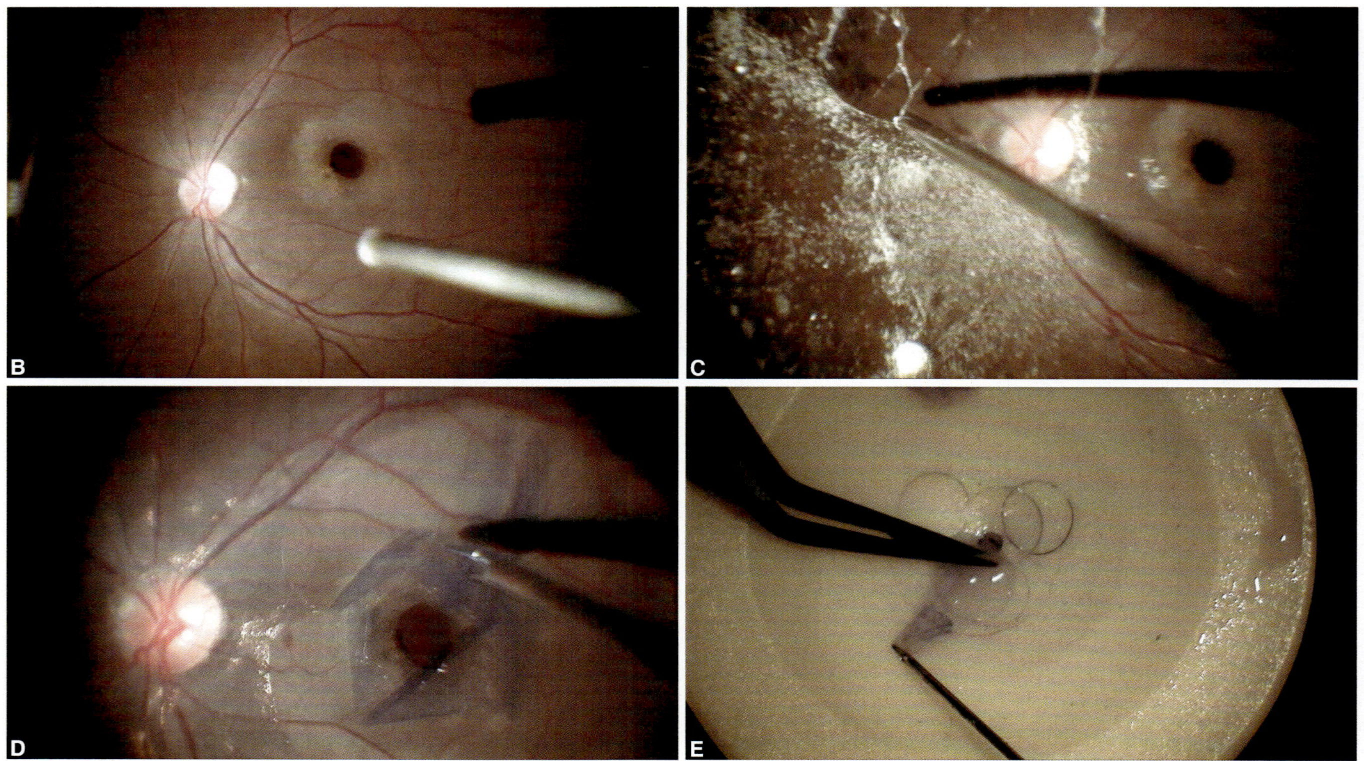

Figs 14.14B to E

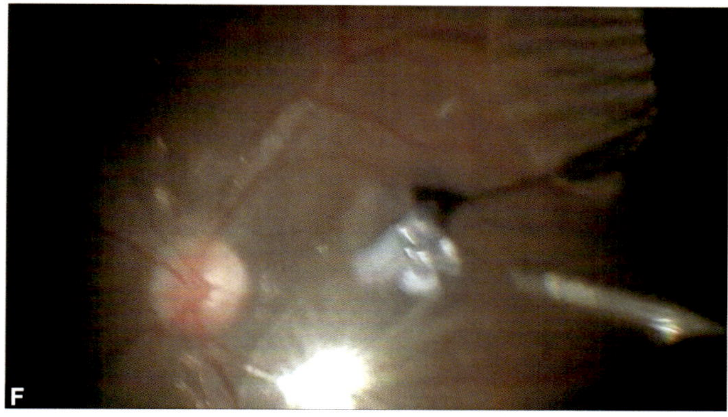

Figs 14.14B to F: Intraoperative steps of transplanting a human amniotic membrane (HAM) graft in very large post-traumatic macular hole.

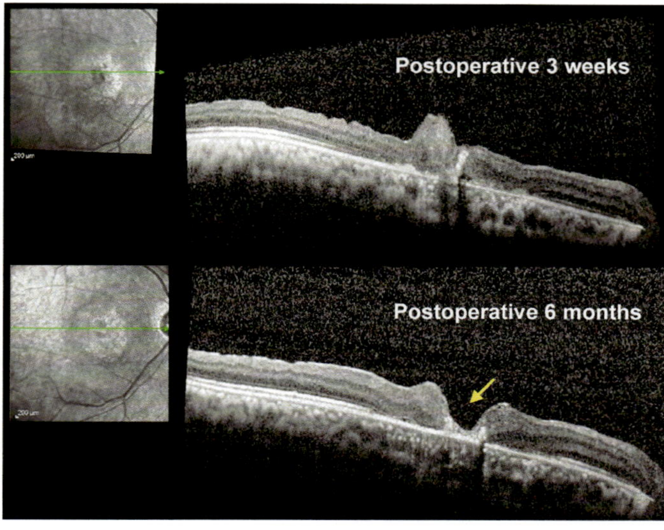

Fig. 14.14G: Postoperative OCT with closed macular hole, plugged by AMT after 3 weeks and incorporated graft within macular hole after 6 months.

- Then, the AMT graft was separated with the max grip forceps and placed over the macular hole
- The inverted flap was used to cover the graft and fluid air exchange was completed (Fig. 14.14F)
- The case was ended with gas tamponade, and the prone position was maintained for 2 weeks
- Postoperative OCT (Fig. 14.14G) shows closed macular hole, plugged by AMT after 3 weeks and incorporated graft within macular hole after 6 months.

2. Autologous retinal graft transplantation (described with failed macular hole section in Chapter 24)

Postoperative Complications After Macular Hole Surgery

1. General complications
   i. Progression of cataract.
   ii. Retinal tear and detachment—Incidence varies from 1.1% to 14%. Retinal tears are mostly temporal and inferior. Careful examination of peripheral retina and vitreous base, before fluid-air exchange, can decrease the incidence of retinal detachment.
   iii. ERM formation.
   iv. Cystoid macular edema.
   v. Endophthalmitis.
2. Specific complications
   i. Retinal pigment epithelial changes—Incidence varies from 5.7% to 75% and can be of three types—'facet lesions' (65%), 'phototoxicity lesion' (23%) and 'scattered lesions' (7%). Phototoxicity lesions are large round/oval-shaped diffuse stippling and carries poor visual prognosis.
   ii. Visual field defect—Generally seen as an absolute scotoma in inferior or temporal quadrant. There may be generalized or segmental disc pallor. Anterior ischemic optic neuropathy and branch retinal arteriolar obstruction may be responsible in some cases. There may be significant nerve fiber loss. Other responsible factors are trauma, dehydration of nerve finer layer and mechanical retinal damage from infused air during FAX (>30 mm Hg).

iii. Late reopening of macular hole—Incidence varies from 4.8% to 9.5% after ILM peeling and it is secondary to formation of ERM.

Partial Thickness/Lamellar Macular Hole

Partial-thickness macular hole or lamellar macular hole (LMH) was first described by Gass in 1975 as a macular lesion that resulted from cystoid macular edema. A lamellar macular hole is by definition a partial-thickness macular hole (Fig. 14.15A) where the inner layers of the fovea are involved with traction and detached from the underlying cellular layers of the fovea.

Lamellar macular holes typically appear as a round or irregular-shaped, well-circumscribed reddish lesion on biomicroscopy, but clinical detection of lamellar holes at an early stage can be difficult. Studies showed that 28%–37% of lamellar holes diagnosed on OCT examination were detected clinically on fundus examination. With an OCT investigation, lamellar macular holes are easily diagnosed. (Figs 14.15B to D).

Diagnostic criterias in OCT are:

1. Characteristic features of an irregular foveal contour.
2. Break in the inner fovea.
3. Intraretinal split.
4. A thin and irregular foveal floor overlying the plane of the retinal pigment epithelium.
5. An absence of a full-thickness foveal defect with intact foveal photoreceptors.

Haouchine et al. have identified foveal pseudocyst (FP) as a precursor to the development of both lamellar and macular hole formation. Lamellar holes are thought to be caused by de-roofing of the pseudocyst with preservation of the foveal base, while posterior extension of the pseudocyst leads to the formation of full-thickness macular holes.

Macular pseudo hole (MPH) (Fig. 14.15E): Lamellar macular defects with

1. A sharply punched out, well-delineated, steepened foveal contour.
2. Thickened foveal edges.
3. Small base diameter.

Morphologically on OCT scans, MPH have the smallest base diameter and thickest central foveal tissue, while LMH have the widest and deepest defects, and FP have the thinnest measured central foveal thickness.

Epiretinal membranes are a common feature associated with lamellar holes, and they have been suggested to be involved in traction on the fovea and play a role in the formation of lamellar holes. Studies showed 50–89% eyes with lamellar macular defects have ERM.

Mechanism of formation: ERM may have an important role to play in the pathogenesis of lamellar or partial thickness macular holes, but it is not responsible for the formation of all types of lamellar macular defects. It is likely that ERM exerts a centripetal force on the fovea resulting in a cleft between the inner and outer retina, leading to avulsion of the foveal tissue or the roof of a pseudocyst and that also lead to the formation of lamellar macular defect.

Surgical Steps (Video 14, Chapter 14)

1. Vitrectomy with PVD induction as the routine initial step.
2. Trypan blue dye has to be used to stain ERM (Fig. 14.15F).
3. Trypan blue dye-assisted ERM removal is necessary if PTMH is associated with ERM (Fig. 14.15G)
4. ILM peeling (brilliant blue G dye-assisted) is mandatory to ensure complete cremoval of all tangential traction (Fig. 14.15H).
5. Simple fluid-air exchange (complete or partial) is enough without any additional gas tamponade.
6. Postoperatively after vitrectomy, removal of ERM and peeling of ILM, foveal contour usually restored (Fig. 14.15I).

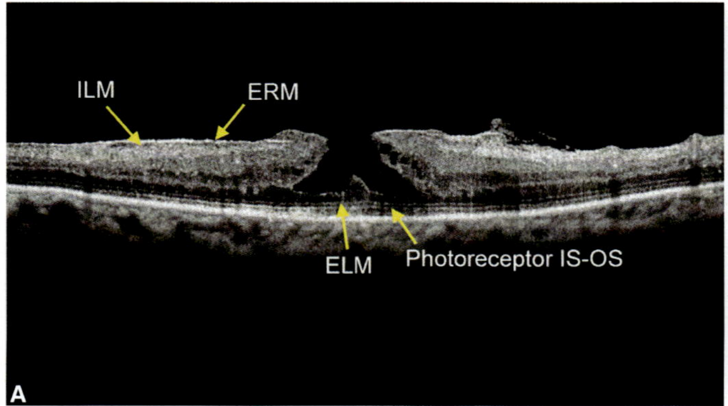

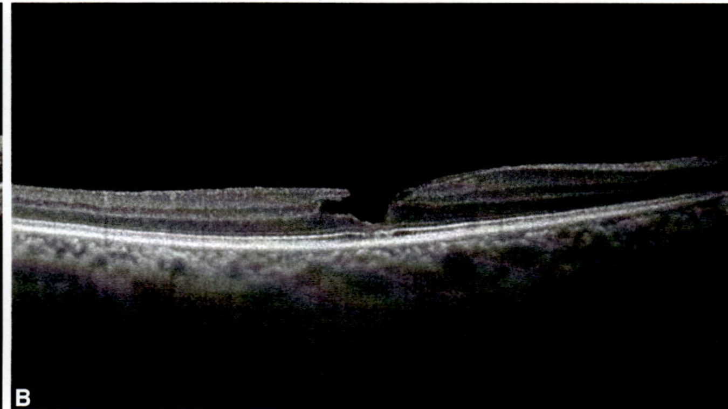

Figs 14.15A and B

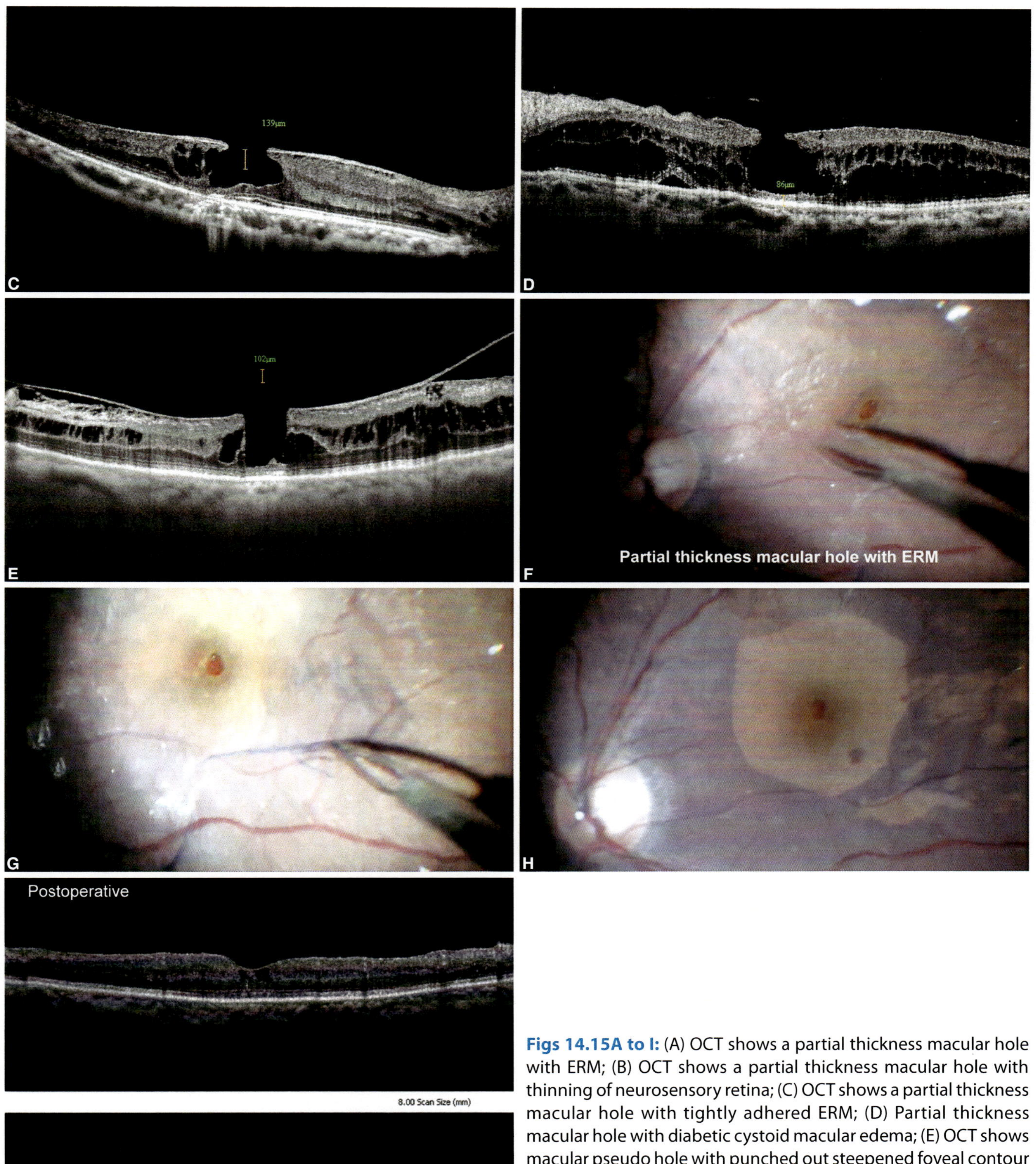

Figs 14.15A to I: (A) OCT shows a partial thickness macular hole with ERM; (B) OCT shows a partial thickness macular hole with thinning of neurosensory retina; (C) OCT shows a partial thickness macular hole with tightly adhered ERM; (D) Partial thickness macular hole with diabetic cystoid macular edema; (E) OCT shows macular pseudo hole with punched out steepened foveal contour with thickened foveal edges and small base diameter; (F to H) Shows intraoperative steps of surgery for partial thickness macular hole; (I) Shows comparative pre- and postoperative OCT scans of partial thickness macular holes after vitrectomy with ERM removal and ILM peeling. (ILM, internal limiting membrane; ELM, external limiting membrane; ERM, epiratinal membrane; photoreceptor, IS–OS, photoreceptor inner segment–outer segment)

Myopic Foveoschisis

Splitting of intraretinal layers by hyporeflective spaces on OCT of macula into outer and inner retinal layers (outer retinoschisis and inner retinoschisis) is not rare in high myopic fundus (Fig. 14.16A)

Many times lamellar macular hole, foveal detachment, preretinal hyperreflective structure like thickened posterior hyaloid membrane leading to foveal traction and rarely full-thickness macular hole can be detected on OCT.

Probable mechanism of schisis formation:

1. Thickened inner retinal layers.
2. Taut ILM.
3. Foveal traction when present.
4. May be unknown tangential tractions are the responsible factors for schisis formation.
5. Advanced tangential traction can cause serous detachment at fovea.

Surgical Steps (Video 15 , Chapter 14)

1. Vitrectomy with PVD induction as a routine step
2. Trypan blue dye-assisted ERM removal is necessary if schisis changes are associated with ERM on OCT (Fig. 14.16B).
3. ILM peeling (brilliant blue G dye-assisted) is a difficult step in presence of posterior staphyloma as tip of end gripping forceps may not reach up to ILM, but again it is mandatory to ensure complete removal of all tangential traction (Fig. 14.16C). Sometimes Tano scraper is required to remove very tightly adhered ILM (Fig. 14.16D).
4. Complete fluid-air exchange is enough without any additional gas tamponade. Postoperatively, schisis changes usually resolve with restoration of foveal contour after vitrectomy, ERM removal and ILM peeling in patients with myopic foveoschisis with ERM with partial-thickness macular hole (Fig. 14.16E).

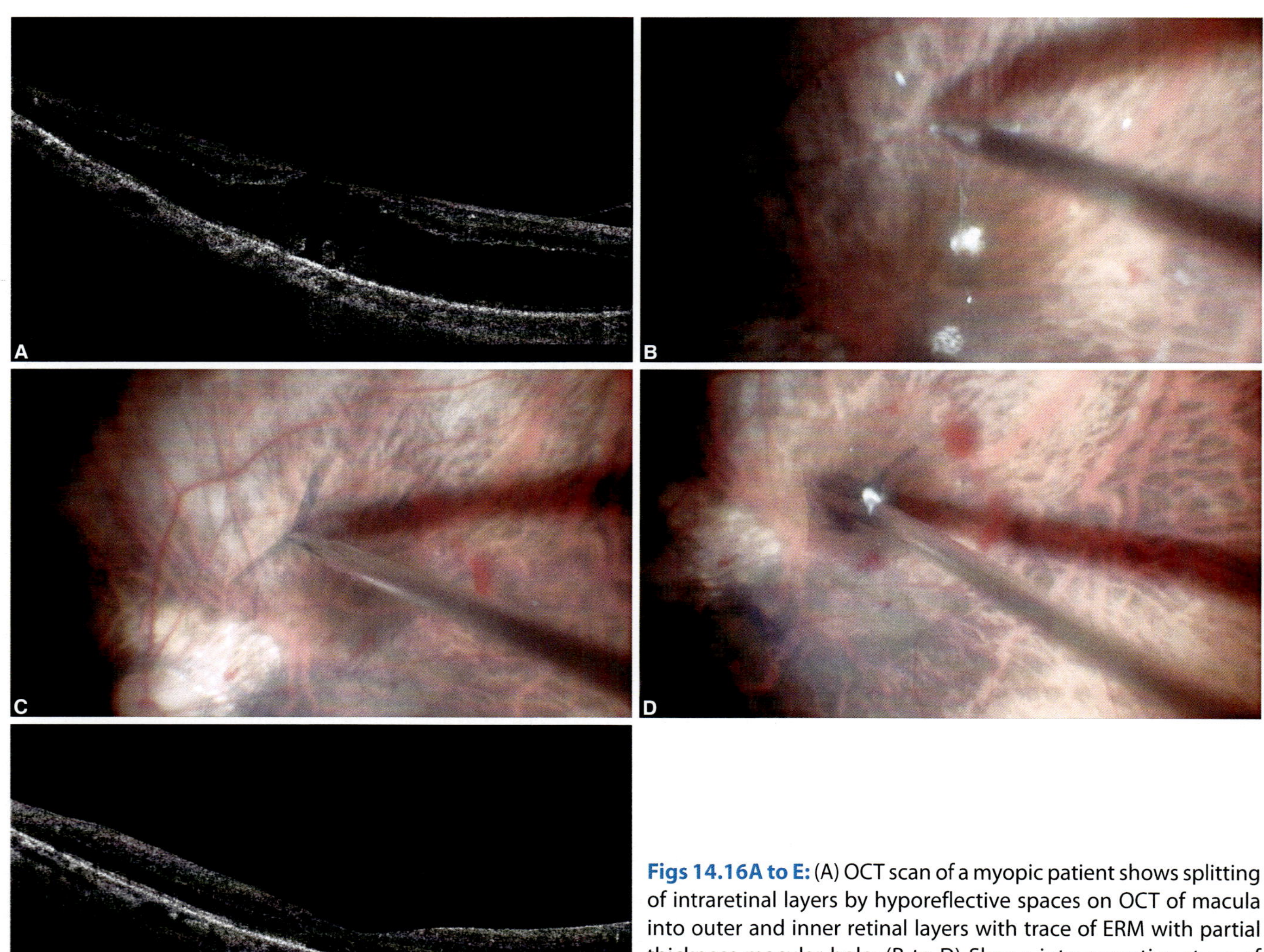

Figs 14.16A to E: (A) OCT scan of a myopic patient shows splitting of intraretinal layers by hyporeflective spaces on OCT of macula into outer and inner retinal layers with trace of ERM with partial thickness macular hole; (B to D) Shows intraoperative steps of surgery for myopic foveoschisis; (E) Postoperative OCT shows resolved schisis changes after vitrectomy, ERM removal and ILM peeling in a patient with myopic foveoschisis with ERM with partial-thickness macular hole

Optic Disc Pit with Maculopathy

First described by Wiethe in 1882, optic disc pits are small, gray-white, oval depressions found at the optic nerve head. Optic nerve pits are a rare entity, with an estimated prevalence of 1 in 11,000. Macular involvement with optic nerve pits has been reported in 25–75% of patients (Fig. 14.17A). Wide-field fundus fluorescein angiography reveals leakage tract from the disc pit to the macula (Figs 14.17B and C). OCT also confirms the characteristic serous elevation with schisis changes (Fig. 14.17D).

Visual loss in patients with optic pits may be associated with retinoschisis or serous retinal detachment involving the macula, or both.

The origin of the fluid—either vitreous or cerebrospinal fluid as the source of the intraretinal and subretinal fluid.

According to Lincoff's proposal, the fluid from optic pits forms a schisis-like cavity in the retina initially, which then progresses to an outer lamellar hole and allows fluid to track into the subretinal space.

Optic pit maculopathy can be associated with progressive visual loss and a poor visual prognosis in many patients.

Treatment option:

I. Laser photocoagulation with or without intravitreal tamponade using gas or silicone oil—Several cases of resolution of subretinal fluid after photocoagulation have been reported, but the resolution might take upto 6 months.

Possible side effects of laser photocoagulation near the disc:

- Paracentral scotomas.
- Non improvement of visual acuity.

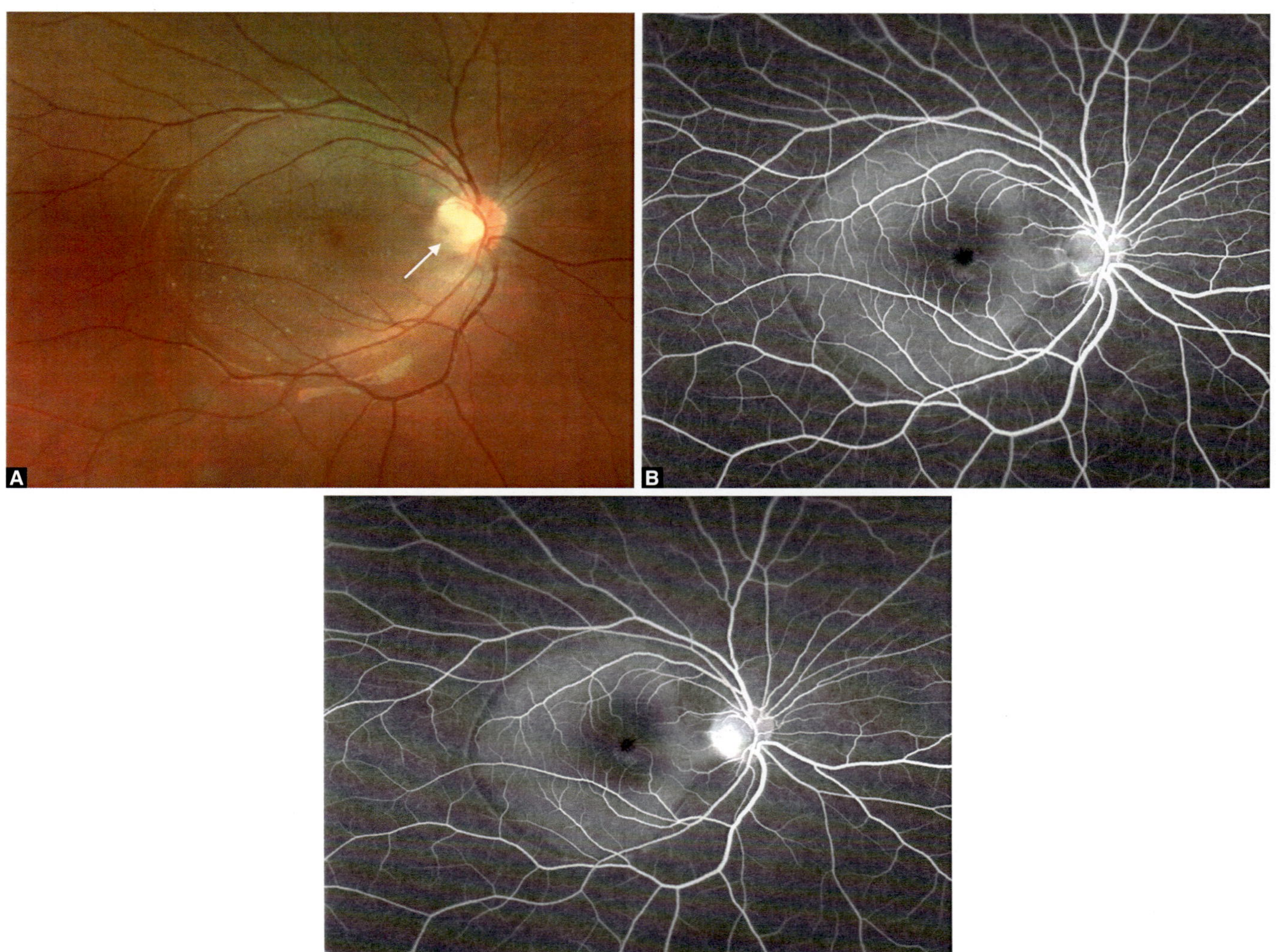

Figs 14.17A to C

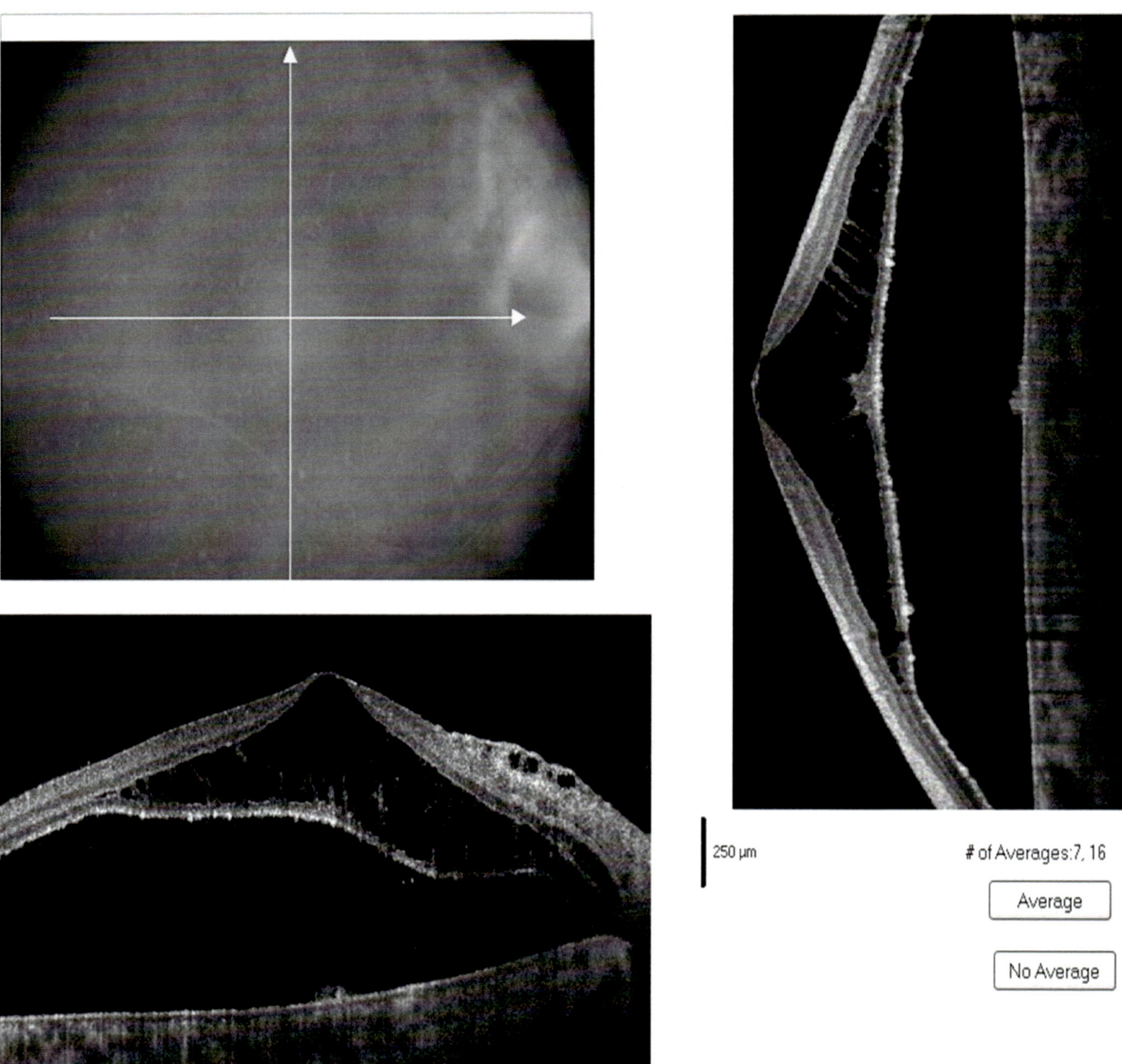
OD
8.00mm Scan Length
250 µm
# of Averages:7, 16
Average
No Average
Diagnosis:

Fig. 14.17D

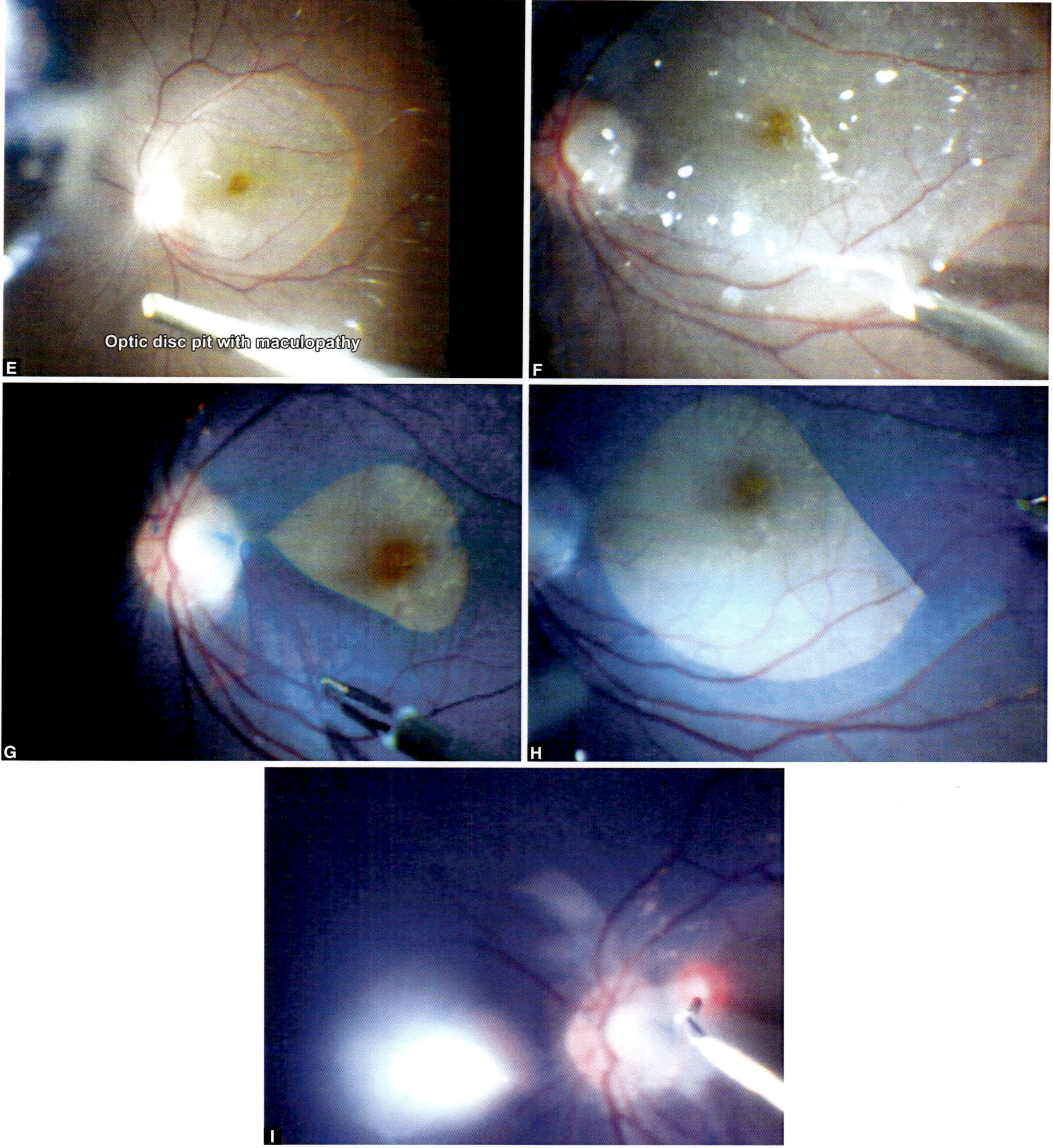

Figs 14.17E to I

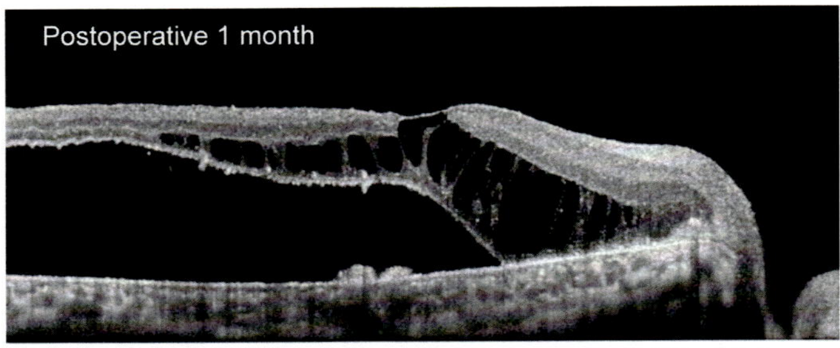

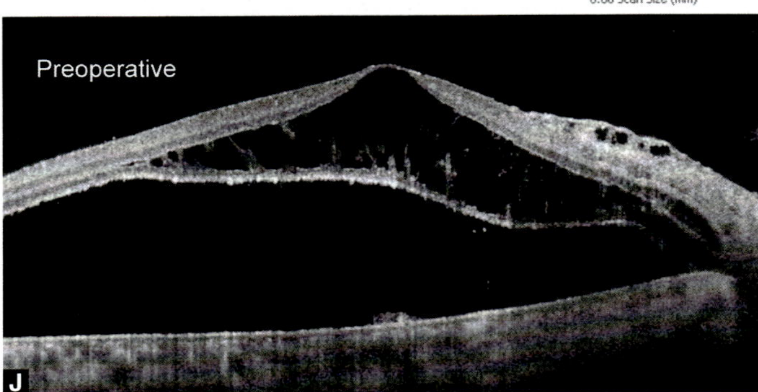

Figs 14.17A to J: (A) Optic disc pit (white arrow) with serous elevation of macula; (B) Ultrawide field fluorescein angiography (early phase) in optic disc pit with maculopathy; (C) Ultrawide field fluorescein angiography (late phase) in optic disc pit with maculopathy; (D) OCT scan macula shows large elevated neurosensory detachment with schisis changes in optic disc pit with maculopathy; (E to I) Steps of surgery for optic disc pit with maculopathy; (E) Vitrectomy; (F) PVD induction; (G and H) ILM peeling; (I) Laser barrage over the connecting tract between optic disc pit and serous detachment; (J) Pre and one month postoperative OCT of optic disc pit with maculopathy with significant reduction of serous detachment after vitrectomy with ILM peeling

- Low success rate in resolution of serous macular detachment.

Tractional forces could explain the delay of macular detachment in young adulthood and treatment failure after laser photocoagulation and gas tamponade.

II. Surgery—Vitrectomy with ILM peeling and gas tamponade without any additional laser photocoagulation—it seems to be sufficient for the treatment of optic disc pit maculopathy.

Surgical Steps (Video 16, Chapter 14)

1. Vitrectomy in optic disc pit with maculopathy (Fig. 14.17E).
2. Triamcinolone-assisted PVD induction (Fig. 14.17F).
3. ILM peeling (Brilliant Blue G dye assisted) is mandatory to ensure complete removal of all tangential traction. (Figs 14.17G and H).
4. Barrage laser at temporal margin of optic nerve head to promote collapse of the connecting tunnel between optic disc pit and macula (Fig. 14.17I).
5. Complete fluid-air exchange is required with long-acting C_3F_8 gas tamponade.

Postoperative OCT—Macular serous elevation decreases slowly after vitrectomy with ILM peeling and laser. It takes months for complete resolution (Fig. 14.17J).

Recently, sealing the optic disc pit with an autologous scleral flap, inverted ILM flap or Tisseel fibrin sealant has been tried at the end of vitrectomy with promising results.

Management of Macular Folds

It may present as:

- *Congenital retinal folds* - FEVR, Falciform folds
- *Acquired retinal folds*
  - *As a PVR component* - Macular pucker
  - Postpenetrating trauma - retinal incarceration with macula involving folds
  - Postoperative period after RD surgery, especially in treating GRTs ....due to the accumulation of residual sub-retinal fluid and improper positioning
  - After Scleral buckling Sx/Vitrectomy with gas/ Pneumatic retinopexy

Management options:

A. Premacular adhesion removal:
   i. Premacular membrane dissection
   ii. Peeling ILM
   iii. Mechanical stretching by DDMS or Finesse Flex loop

B. Submacular contraction/adhesion removal:
   i. Removal of Subretinal bands/membranes
   iv. Submacular BSS injection

Familial Exudative Vitreoretinopathy (FEVR)

- A rare inherited disorder (AD/AR/X-linked)
- Abnormal retinal angiogenesis - incomplete vascularisation of peripheral retina and retinal schema/NV
- Vitreous syneresis - vitreoretinal traction
- Temporal dragging of macula/Foveal displacement/ Falciform retinal folds/Tractional RD
- Subretinal exudation and hemorrhage
- Asymmetric
- Proposed FEVR clinical staging system in 1998 and revised clinical staging system in 2014 have been highlighted in Tables 14.2 and 14.3 respectively. But the latest staging as described by Gow & Oliver is discussed below:

Staging of FEVR (as described by Gow & Oliver):

- Stage 1 - WWP/ WWOP + Vitreous traction
- Stage 2 - + Peripheral dilated tortuous retinal vessels + Peripheral subretinal exudation + Macular dragging
- Stage 3 - Extensive TRD + Subretinal exudation & Hge

Management of FEVR

- Stage 1 - Observation
- Stage 2 - Laser/Anti VEGF for neovascularisation
- Stage 3A and above - Scleral buckling and or Vitrectomy

Management of Congenital Falciform Folds

Both long-standing pre-retinal adhesions as well as sub-retinal adhesions are responsible for the formation of congenital falciform folds :

- **For pre-retinal adhesions**, vitrectomy with removal of all membraneous adhesions along with peeling of sticky ILM and then mechanical stretching of the folded retina by Tanno scraper or Finesse Flex loop are necessary.
- **To remove sub-retinal adhesions**, sub-retinal injection of BSS is necessary to stretch the folded retina from behind. It should be done away from the retina to avoid the formation of a macular hole.

Case discussion:

The steps of an innovative option are as follows:

- Video 17, Chapter 14
  - A 43-year-old male presented with dimness of vision since childhood, but in his left eye for 1 month
  - His RE vision was finger counting 2ft, and LE vision was 5/60 with normal IOP in both eyes. There was macula involving long falciform fold extending up to periphery in RE and fovea threatening RD in LE. (Fig.14.18A)
  - Our plan was vitrectomy with ILM peeling with submacular SF6 gas injection in RE and vitreoretinal intervention with silicone oil injection in LE.

TABLE 14.2: Shows the proposed FEVR clinical staging system in 1998.

Stage	*Clinical features*
1	Avascular retinal periphery without extraretinal vascularization
2	Avascular retinal periphery with extraretinal vascularization
2A	Without exudate
2B	With exudate
3	Extramacular retinal detachment
3A	Primarily exudate
3B	Primary tractional
4	Macula-involving retinal detachment, subtotal
4A	Primarily exudative
4B	Primary tractional
5	Total retinal detachment
5A	Open funnel
5B	Closed funnel

TABLE 14.3: Shows the revised FEVR clinical staging system in 2014.

Stage	*Clinical features*
1	Avascular periphery or anomalous intraretinal vascularization
1A	Without exudate or leakage
1B	With exudate or leakage
2	Avascular retinal periphery with extraretinal vascularization
2A	Without exudate or leakage
2B	With exudate or leakage
3	Extramacular retinal detachment
3A	Without exudate or leakage
4	Macula-involving retinal detachment, subtotal
4A	Without exudate or leakage
4B	With exudate or leakage
5	Total retinal detachment
5A	Open funnel
5B	Closed funnel

- Vitrectomy is done along with the removal of all pre-retinal adhesions around the falciform fold (Fig.14.18B)
- Triamcinolone assisted all membranous attachment around the falciform fold was removed (Fig.14.18C)
- Macula was stained with Brilliant Blue G dye (Fig.14.18D)
- Peeling of ILM was possible in a patchy manner to remove invisible tractional components (Fig.14.18E)
- Macular folded retina was gently stretched with Tannos' scratches (Fig.14.18F)
- Balanced Salt Solution (BSS) was injected subretinally around the falciform fold to remove all subretinal adhesions (Fig.14.18G)
- Fluid air exchange was completed (Fig. 14.18H)
- SF6 Gas tamponade was used at the end of surgery.
- Post-operatively, after 3 months, the patient gained 20/80 vision with flattened fold on macular OCT with on retina (Fig. 14.18I)

In a nutshell, the overall management of any retinal fold involving macula:

- If retina is ON - Vit + ERM removal + ILM peeling + Subretinal BSS inj + Gas
- If retina is OFF - Vit + ERM removal + ILM peeling + peripheral retinectomy + PFCL+FAX+EL +SOI
- If in the post-operative period, with ON retina - Preretinal membrane removal + Subretinal BSS injection + Stretching by DDMS + FAX
- If Post-operative PVR, under SO with ON retina - SOR+ Preretinal membrane removal + FAX+ Long-acting gas tamponade

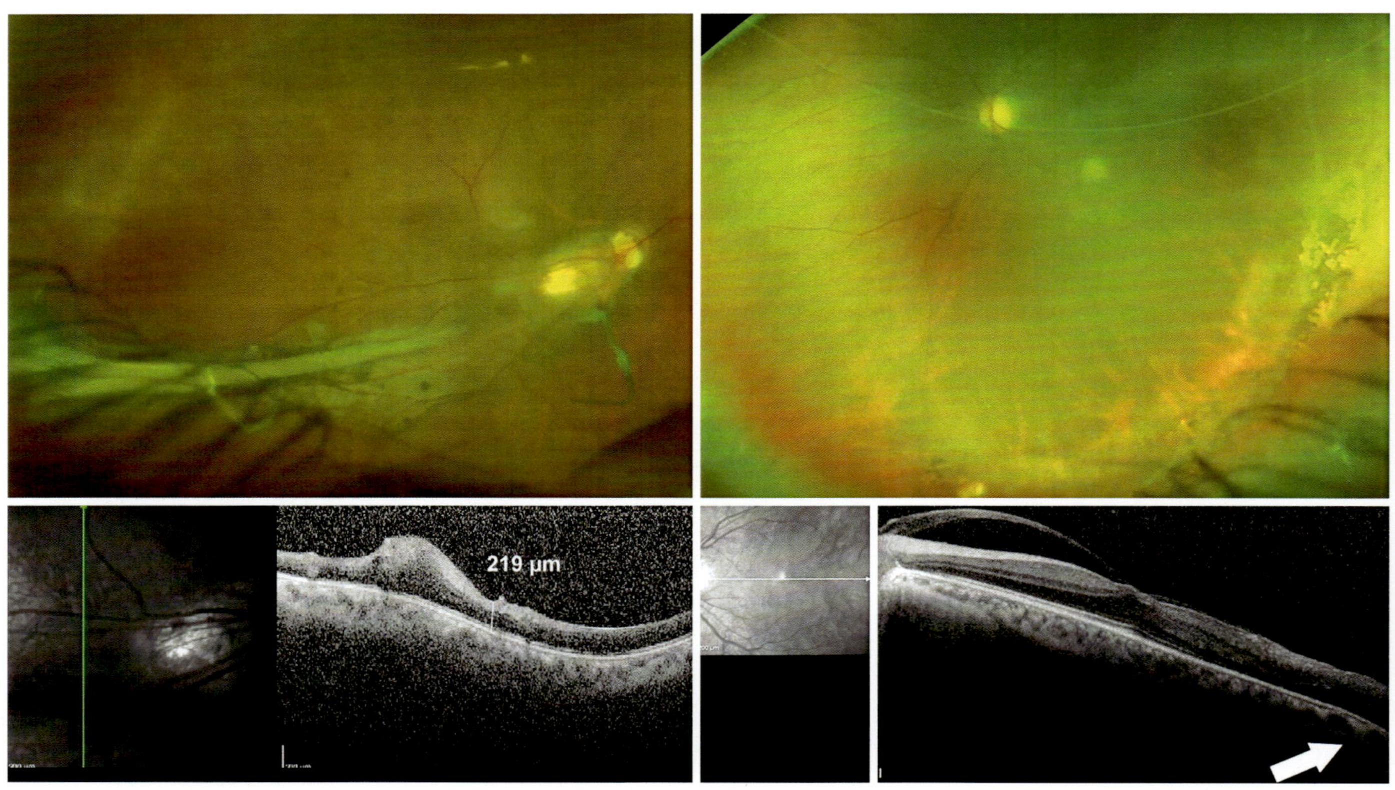

Fig. 14.18A: Wide-field fundus photo and macular OCT scan show macula involving a small fundal coloboma with a long congenital falciform fold extending up to the periphery in RE and fovea threatening temporal RD in LE.

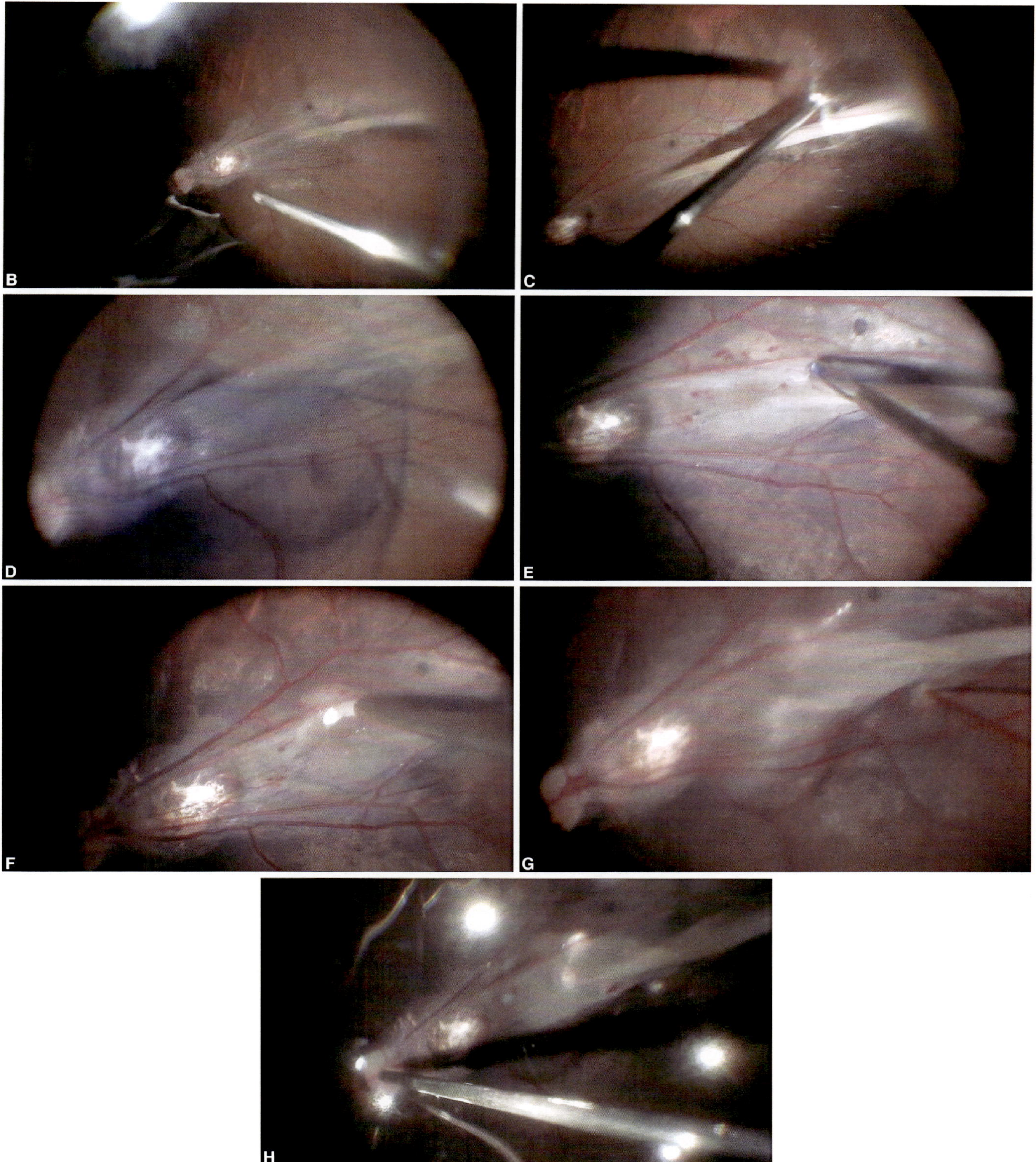

Figs 14.18B to H: Shows intraoperative steps of managing a case of congenital falciform fold

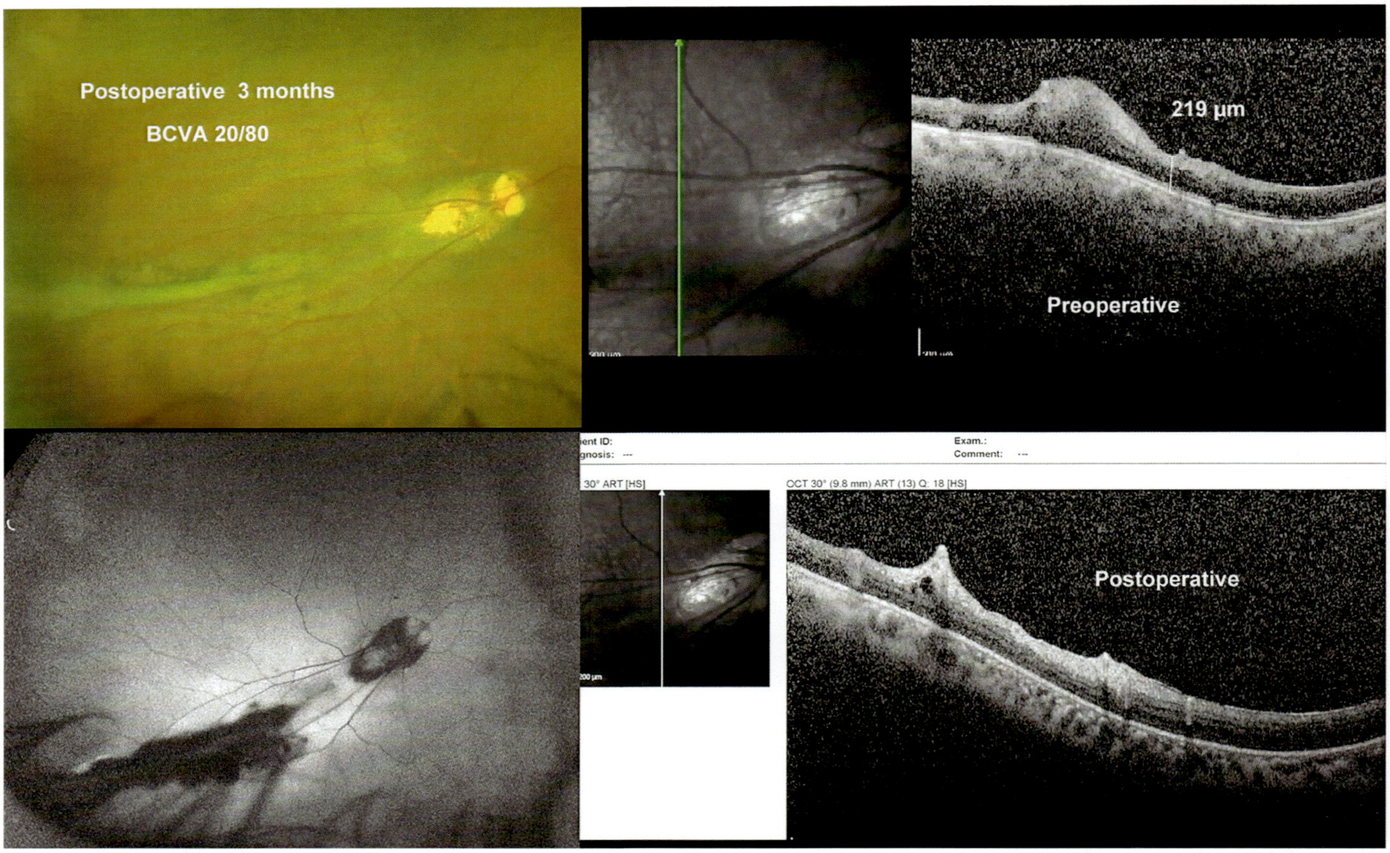

Fig. 14.18l: Postoperative wide-field fundus photo and macular OCT show a decrease in falciform fold after 3 months.

Kindly scan the QR code below to access the online Video.

CHAPTER 15

Managing Complications After Cataract Surgeries

MANAGEMENT OF DROPPED CATARACTS

Retained lens fragments including nuclear and cortical remnants, occur more frequently with phacoemulsification than any other types of cataract extraction. Incidence vary from 0.3% to 1.1%. Risk factors are elderly patient with hard cataract, pseudoexfoliation, loose zonules, posterior polar cataract, postvitrectomy cataract. Even vertically positioned phacoemulsification probe can catch posterior capsule and result in posterior capsular tear (Figs 15.1A and B). Liquified vitreous or previously vitrectomized eye with minimal vitreous support can result in subsequent posterior drop of remaining lens matters.

Clinical Features

Clinically, the eyes present with signs of marked intraocular inflammation and secondary glaucoma, sometimes with hypopyon mimicking endophthalmitis.

Ultrasonography is mandatory to rule out retained intraocular lens fragments.

Sometimes small amount of retained flocculent cortical matters may be reabsorbed in many cases.

Important Points to be Considered

- Preoperatively topical anti-inflammatory and antiglaucoma medications should be started
- Vitrectomy should be planned urgently if possible on the very same day, if vitreo retinal setup is available
- Vitrectomy can be delayed for a few days only to allow corneal edema to clear
- Adequate core vitrectomy should be performed before phacofragmentation
- One should start with low fragmentation power (5–10%) for more efficient removal of nucleus
- PVD induction is to be completed whenever possible
- Vitreous base examination with scleral depression is necessary to find out any additional missed small fragments and to rule out presence of retinal tear or retinal detachment
- Now, one should check for capsular support to place secondary IOL.

If coexisting retinal detachment and retained lens fragment are present, vitreous gel removal with induction of PVD is required first, followed by stabilizing the posterior pole with heavy fluid PFCL and floating the nuclear fragment anteriorly.

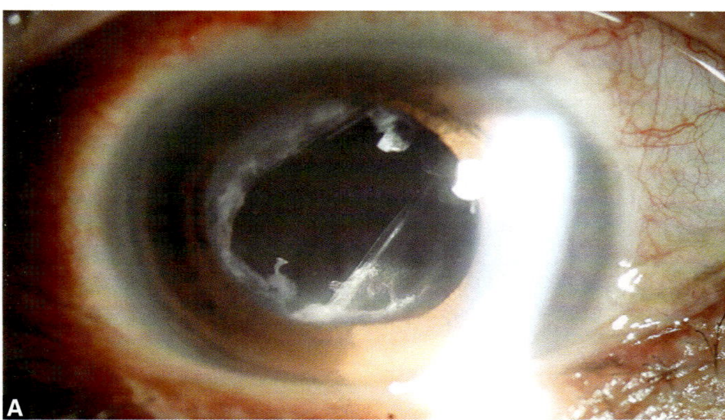

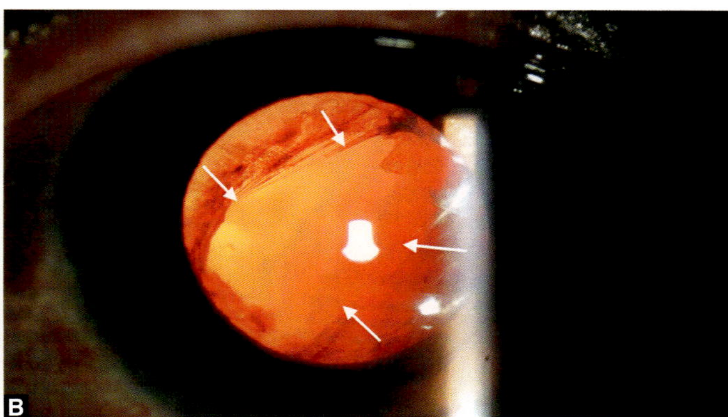

Figs 15.1A and B: (A) Posterior capsular tear (white arrows) with absence of crystalline lens in diffuse; (B) Retro-illumination

Then one should start fragmentation over the PFCL. Retina has to be attached by starting fluid air exchange and then laser around the break, removal of PFCL and end up the case using proper tamponade. IOL insertion should be planned as a second stage surgery after the retinal reattachment.

Risk of retinal detachment after vitrectomy for retained lens fragment varies from 0–19.2%.

Common Entities

Dropped Cortex

Case discussion (Video 1, Chapter 15):

- There was capsular remnant with retained cortical materials
- Anterior vitrectomy was done first
- Retained cortical materials were removed
- Vitrectomy was started
- Posterior polar cataract was well-visualized on the back surface of dropped cortex chunk (Fig. 15.2A)
- Lensectomy was done
- Triamcinolone-assisted PVD induction was done
- Residual vitrectomy was completed
- Vitreous base was checked
- Viscoelastic injected underneath the iris to expand the sulcus
- Now foldable multipiece IOL was placed in sulcus over the intact rim of anterior capsulorrhexis (Fig. 15.2B).

Dropped Epinuclear Fragments

Case discussion (Video 2, Chapter 15):

- A case of anterior chamber IOL with dropped retro IOL cortex with dropped epinucleus with vitritis (Fig. 15.3A)
- Retro IOL cortex removed with cutter
- Opaque vitreous along with cortical matters removed
- Epinuclear fragments were over the macula and they were removed keeping cutting rate 1000–2000 cpm and suction 500–600 mm Hg (Fig. 15.3B)
- Peripheral vitrectomy completed and periphery checked.

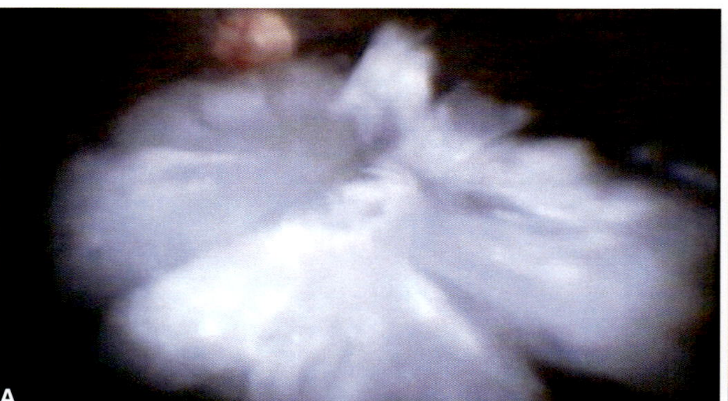

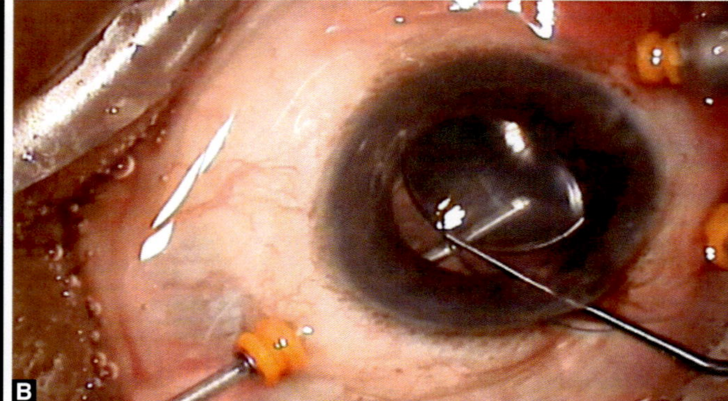

Figs 15.2A and B: Intraoperative steps of surgery for managing dropped cortex

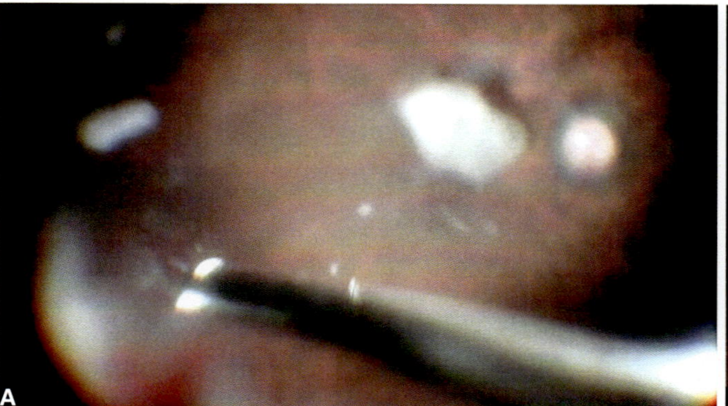

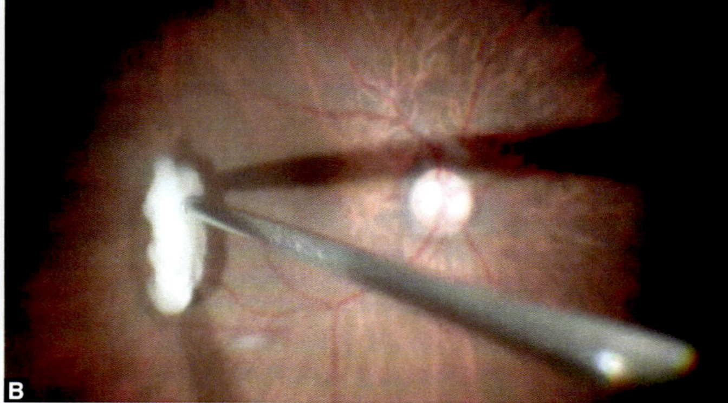

Figs 15.3A and B: Intraoperative steps of surgery for managing dropped epinucleus with vitritis

Dropped Nucleus

Case discussion (Video 3, Chapter 15):

- A case of status postcataract surgery with aphakia with preoperative dropped nucleus (Fig. 15.4A)
- It was a whole nucleus with surrounding cortex with vitritis
- 25G vitrectomy done surrounding the nucleus
- Triamcinolone-assisted residual vitreous fibrils were checked
- Now, PFCL was injected to up the whole nucleus up to the mid-virtual plane to protect retina (Fig. 15.4B)
- Right-handed port to a 20G port (Fig. 15.4C)
- Now phacofragmentation of the nucleus started (Fig. 15.4D)
- PFCL removed (Fig. 15.4E)
- Vitreous base checked
- Capsular extensions were checked
- Now IOL was placed in the sulcus (Fig. 15.4F)
- 20G port sutured (Fig. 15.4G)

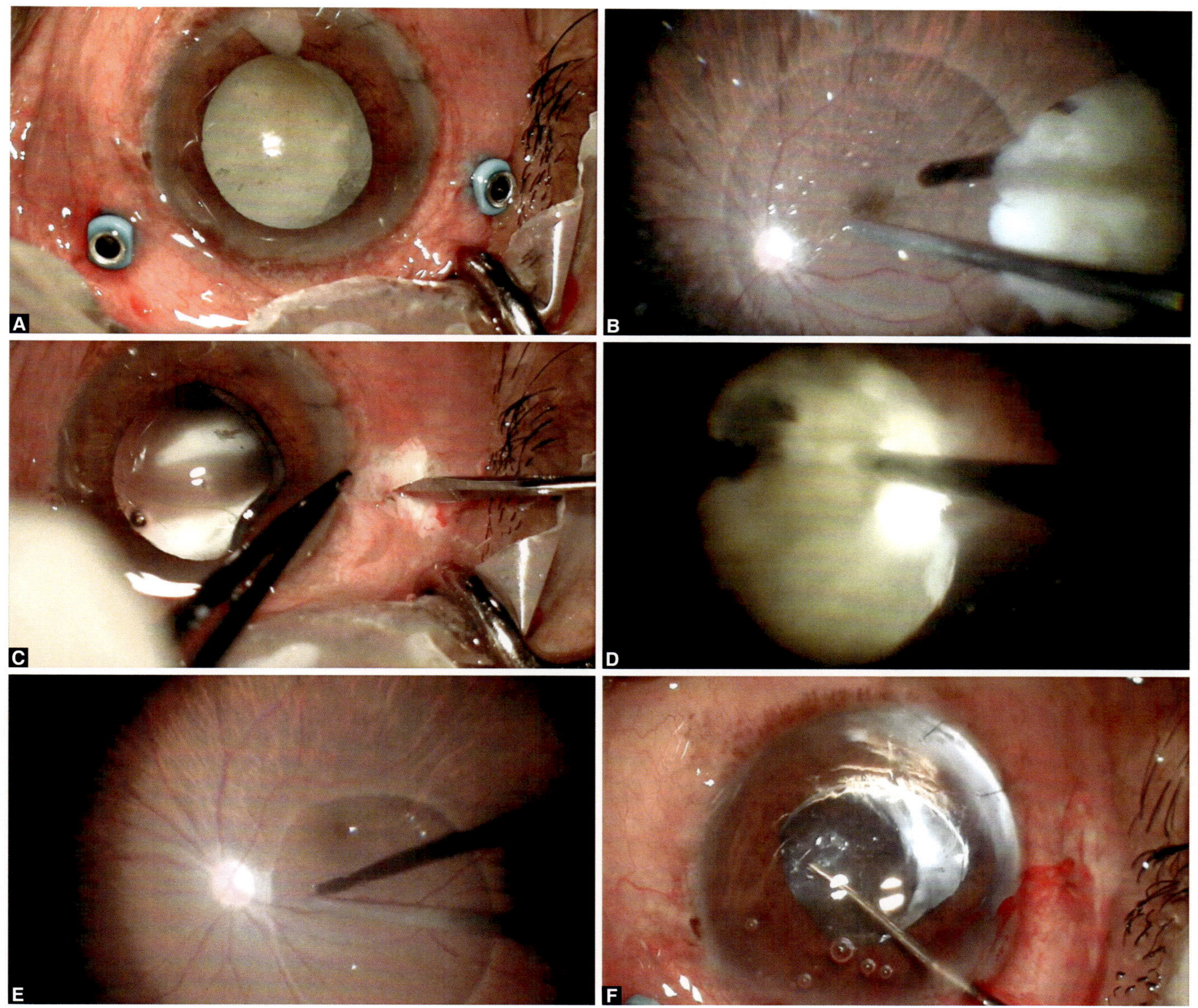

Figs 15.4A to F

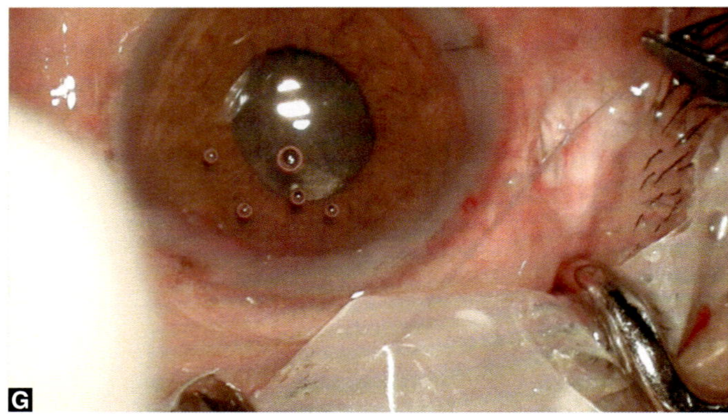

Figs 15.4A to G: Intraoperative steps of surgery for managing dropped nucleus (PFCL assisted)

MANAGEMENT OF DROPPED IOLs

Intraocular lens (IOL) dislocation occurs due to lack of optimal posterior capsular support.

- Most frequently if happens due to insertion of IOL in presence of posterior capsular tear. PC tear may get extended during insertion of leading haptic or there is already a large unrecognized tear
- Lack of intact anterior vitreous face also makes IOL unstable. Liquified vitreous or absent vitreous (vitrectomized eye) cause immediate dislocation of IOL
- Tenacious vitreous around the IOL or in anterior chamber cause slow delayed dislocation of PCIOL in postoperative period.

Presenting symptom—Related to the degree of malposition of IOL. IOL can be severely luxated. IOL removal is necessary in this situation also.

- A completely dislocated IOL inside the vitreous cavity always necessitates IOL removal. Presenting symptoms are blurred vision after surgery and floater of a particular shape of an IOL. Sometimes, these symptoms may be tolerated by many eyes, so the vitreoretinal intervention can be delayed.

Risk of retinal break formation and subsequent development of retinal detachment is more in eyes with liquified vitreous. But increased inflammation, cystoid macular edema or retinal detachment necessitates early intervention.

Before removal of IOL, capsular support should be always assessed, especially inferior part. At least inferior six clock-hours of residual posterior capsular support should be present to place a multipiece or a rigid IOL. An IOL with damaged or broken haptic should be removed and anterior chamber IOL should be placed in absence of adequate capsular support.

Techniques of Dislocated IOL Removal

Conventional Technique of IOL Removal

Dropped IOL removal by end gripping forceps:

Steps of surgery *(Video 4, Chapter 15):*

- 23G vitrectomy done removing all vitreous adhesions surrounding the rigid IOL
- Scleral tunnels were made
- Capsular support was checked and found insufficient
- Triamcinolone was injected to check for residual vitreous
- Now end gripping forceps was used to lift up PCIOL by holding at the junction of it's haptic and optic (Fig. 15.5A)
- Then IOL was supported from back surface by endoilluminator and prolapsed in AC
- Superior haptic was broken and broken part was removed
- Rigid PCIOL was explanted
- Residual vitrectomy was completed
- ACIOL was implanted
- Cannulas were removed.

Dropped IOL removal with PFCL:

Steps of surgery *(Video 5, Chapter 15):*

- A case of dropped single piece PCIOL because of large PC rent (Fig. 15.5B)
- 23G cannula was introduced
- Scleral tunnel was made
- Vitrectomy was started
- Injected triamcinolone
- PVD induction was done with the suction of the cutter (Fig. 15.5C)
- Residual anterior vitrectomy was done
- Dropped PCIOL was free of any vitreous adhesions
- Now PFCL was injected to float up the IOL (Fig. 15.5D)

- Haptic was held with end gripping forceps (Fig. 15.5E) and brought at pupillary plane
- Anterior chamber entry was done and IOL was removed through scleral tunnel (Fig. 15.5F)
- PFCL was removed
- Last drop of PFCL was removed with silicone-tipped backflush needle
- Vitreous base was checked
- Viscoelastic were injected behind the iris to form sulcus
- Multipiece PCIOL was placed in sulcus, keeping the haptics vertically as nasally PC support was absent (Fig. 15.5G).
- Centrally posterior capsulectomy was done
- All cannulas were removed.

New Simple Safe Technique of IOL Removal

Dropped PCIOL removal by passive suction:

Steps of surgery *(Video 6, Chapter 15):*

- Three 23G pars plana ports were placed
- Scleral tunnels were made
- Started with vitrectomy
- All vitreous adhesions surrounding the rigid IOL was removed
- Now PCIOL was lifted up with the help of passive suction of a backflush needle up to just behind the pupillary plane (Fig. 15.5H)
- Then IOL margin was held with end gripping forceps and one haptic followed by optic were prolapsed in AC
- AC entry was done through sclera tunnel and IOL was removed
- Triamcinolone-assisted residual vitrectomy was completed
- Vitreous base was checked
- PI was done, keeping pupil in miotic stage with pilocarpine solution
- ACIOL was implanted
- Cannulas were removed.

Dropped PCIOL removal by active suction

Steps of surgery *(Video 7, Chapter 15):*

- There was dropped PCIOL with intact capsulorrhexis margin with inferior zonular dialysis
- Vitrectomy was started to remove vitreous attachments surrounding the PCIOL
- Triamcinolone was injected to remove residual vitreous attachments
- Central capsulectomy was performed in posterior capsule
- Vitreous base was checked
- Now active suction was applied over IOL optic with flute needle and IOL was bring at pupillary plane (Fig. 15.5I)
- IOL haptics and optic was prolapsed through the PC opening

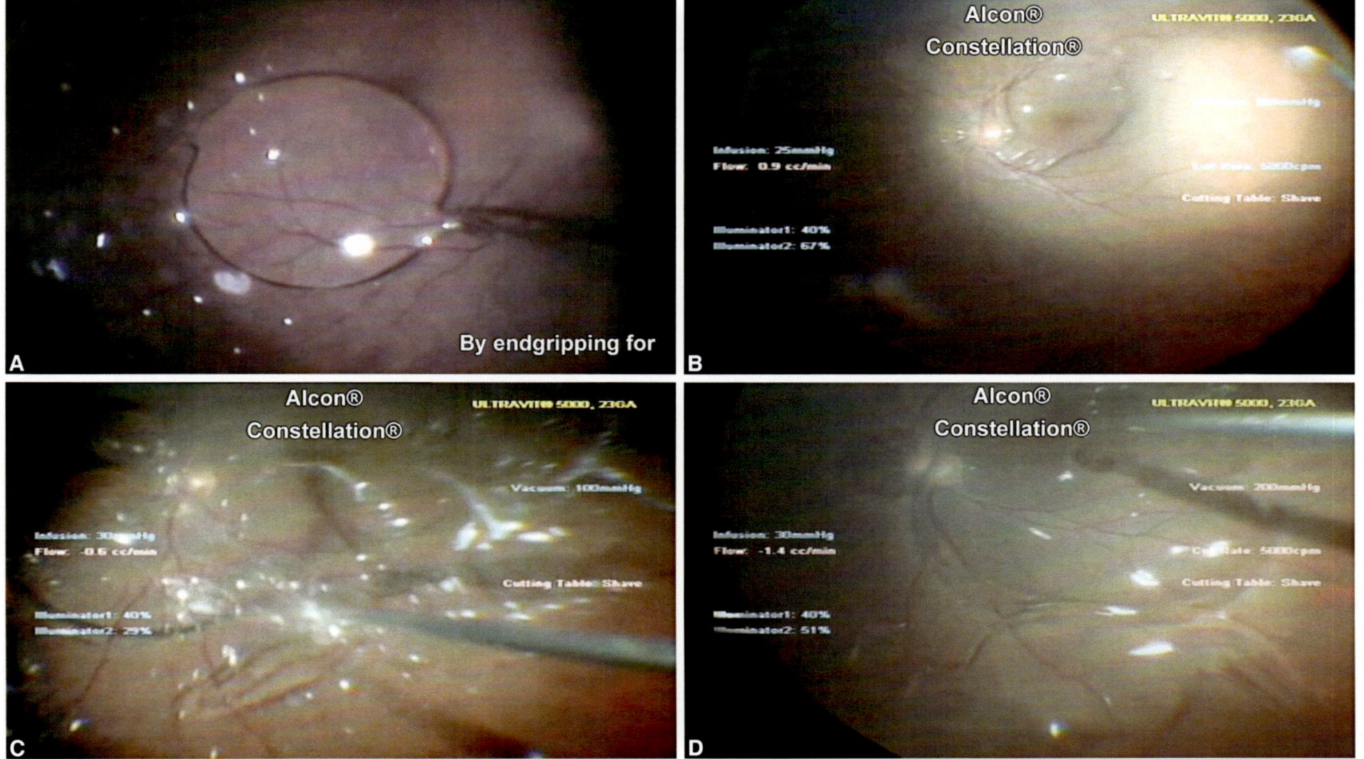

Figs 15.5A to D

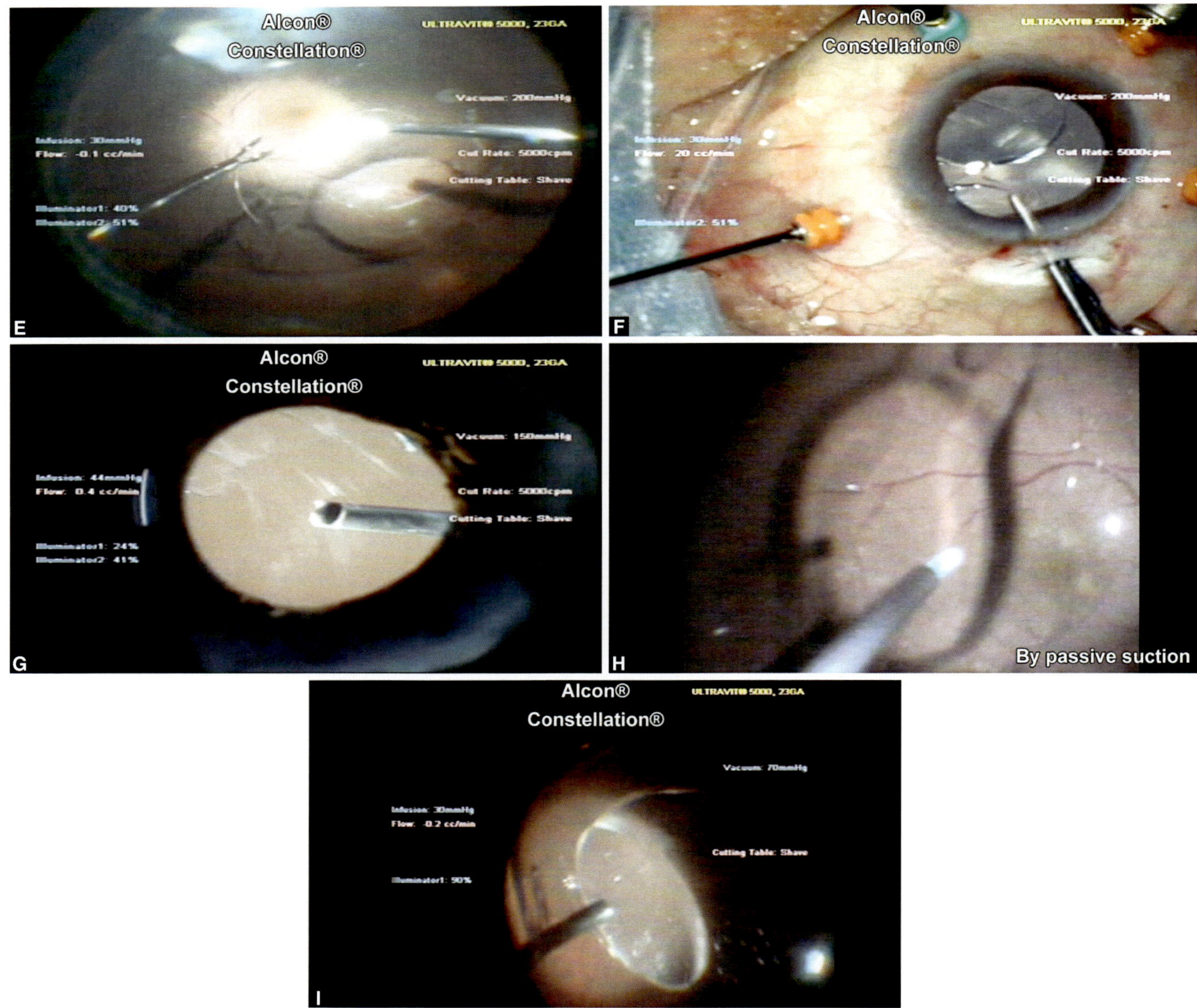

Figs 15.5A to I: (A) Dropped IOL removal by end gripping forceps; (B to G) Intraoperative steps of surgery for managing dropped PCIOL (PFCL assisted); (H) Retrieval of PCIOL with the help of passive suction of a back-flush needle; (I) Retrieval of PCIOL with the help of active suction of a back-flush needle

- Foldable IOL was explanted out by extending corneal tunnel
- A multipiece IOL was implanted over capsulorrhexis margin in the sulcus—23G cannulas were removed.

Postoperative complications: The postoperative complications are usually difficult to separate from those associated cataract surgery. Complications are as follows:

- Cystoid macular edema
- Retinal detachment—It occurs in about 2% of cases.

MANAGEMENT OF SUPRACHOROIDAL HEMORRHAGE

Suprachoroidal hemorrhage (SCH) is a rare condition, defined as blood in the suprachoroidal space, i.e. there is collection of blood in between sclera and choroid (Fig. 15.6A). The potential space between sclera and choroid, the suprachoroidal space, is actually virtual, and normally contains approximately 10 microliter of fluid.

A SCH can be categorized with respect to size, extent of hemorrhage, relationship to intraocular surgery, or precipitating event.

It is the most feared intraoperative or postoperative complication in every intraocular surgery, including cataract, glaucoma surgery, penetrating keratoplasty, scleral buckle and vitrectomy and always have poor visual outcome. For an anterior segment surgeon this is almost once in a lifetime scenario.

It is as a consequence to rupture of the short or long posterior ciliary arteries or vortex veins or their tributaries.

Causes

Reports revealed following are etiological factors:

1. Spontaneous onset SCH
2. Traumatic etiology
3. As complication of ocular surgery.

The incidence of SCH after ocular surgery varies, ranging between 0.04% and 1%, for different procedures, depending on ocular and systemic risk factors. Factors reported to predispose one to SCH include advanced age, glaucoma, increased axial length, systemic cardiovascular disease, nonphakic status, and a history of vitreous loss.

Indications of Drainage of SCH

Surgical drainage of the SCH has been advocated for patients with

- Extreme pain
- A flat anterior chamber
- Uncontrolled elevated intraocular pressure
- Retinal detachment (RD)
- Kissing suprachoroidal hematoma
- Retinal or vitreous incarceration in the wound.

Timings of Drainage of SCH

Decision of timing for secondary drainage of SCH by a vitreoretinal surgeon depends on duration of SCH as well as ultrasonographic evidence of liquefaction of SCH. Thus, B-scan ultrasonography is important both for diagnosis and management of SCH. Besides determining the extent and location of a SCH, vitreoretinal status can be determined. Liquefaction of blood in the suprachoroidal space can be seen echographically and it usually occurs between 7 and 14 days. So it is always better to drain SCH during this period.

Management Options

Surgical management described earlier are radial sclerotomies combined with vitrectomy and use of per fluorocarbon liquid and silicone oil. The standard surgical technique for serous/hemorrhagic choroidal drainage requires conjunctival opening, a 2–3 mm sclerotomy (Fig. 15.6B), and sometimes the introduction of a cyclodialysis spatula into the suprachoroidal space to facilitate further outflow.

Use of anterior chamber maintainer and SCG drainage through anteriorly placed 23G cannula followed by vitrectomy with PFCL and ending with silicone oil have been described by Rossi T et al. in three cases.

Sutureless Technique to Drain SCH

Steps are described below *(Animation, Video 8, Chapter 15):*

- A 23G trocar-cannula complex introduced obliquely 10–15 mm posterior to the limbus into suprachoroidal space according to the maximum height of elevation on USG and trocar removed to drain blood
- 23G vitrectomy done and heavy fluid PFCL injected to push suprachoroidal hematoma from inside
- IOP was kept high
- External passively blood drainage through 23G cannula was possible in a sutureless way (Fig. 15.6C)
- Multiple 23G sclerotomies made for more complete removal of SCH. Silicone oil was used for constant endotamponade
- PFCL removed
- Fluid-air exchange done
- Silicone oil was used for constant endotamponade (Fig. 15.6M).

Case Discussions

Case I (Video 9, Chapter 15):

In a case of postcataract surgery suprachoroidal hemorrhage—

- 23G vitrectomy done (Fig. 15.6D) and heavy fluid PFCL injected to push suprachoroidal hematoma from inside
- A 23G trocar-cannula complex introduced obliquely 10–15 mm posterior to the limbus into suprachoroidal space according to the maximum height of elevation on USG (Fig. 15.6E) and trocar removed to drain blood (Fig. 15.6F)
- IOP was kept high from 40 to 70 mm Hg
- External passively blood drainage through 23G cannula was possible in a suture less way (Fig. 15.6G)
- Multiple 23G sclerotomies made for more complete removal of SCH
- PFCL removed
- Fluid-air exchange done
- Silicone oil was used for constant endotamponade (Fig. 15.6H).

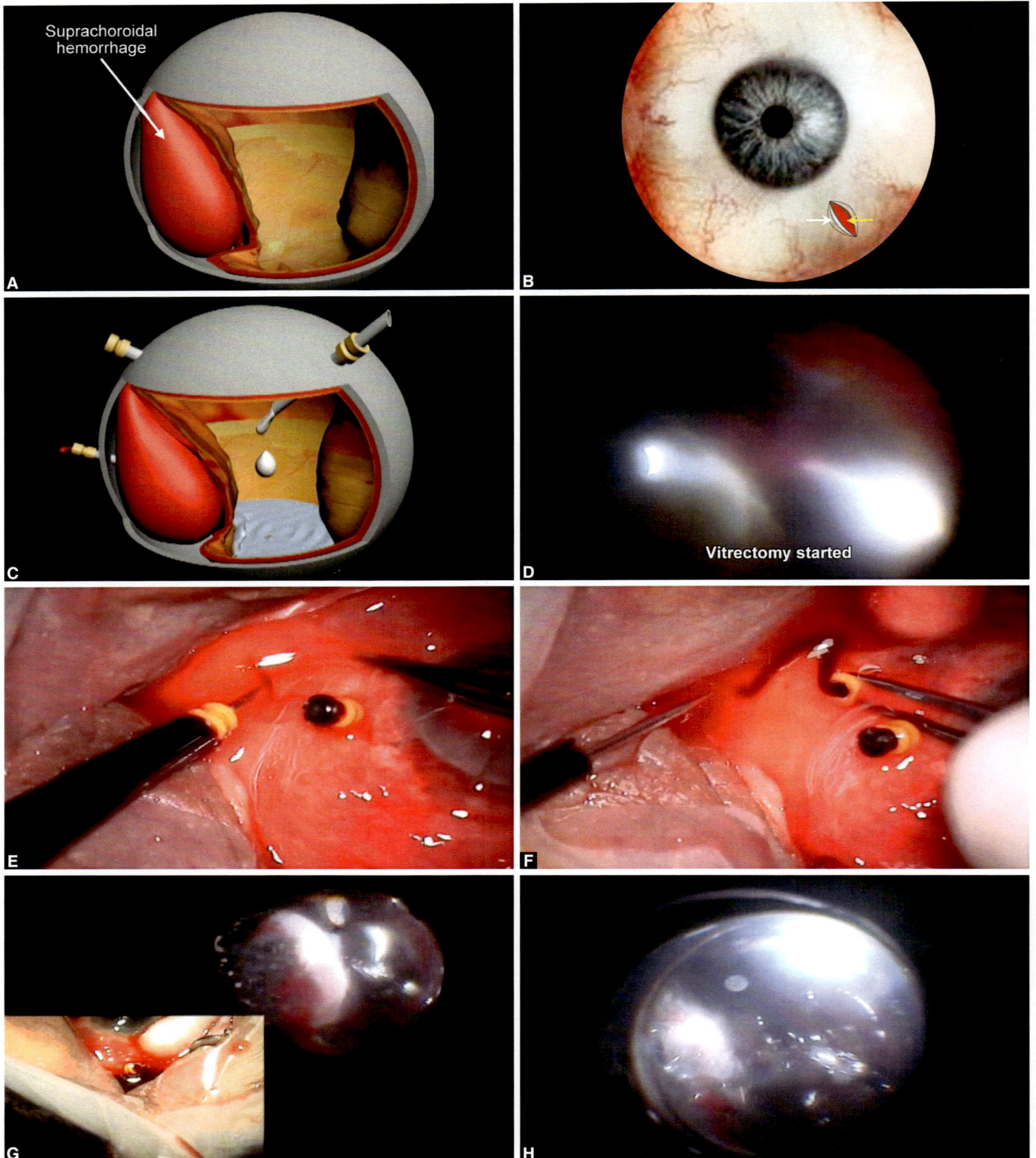

Figs 15.6A to H

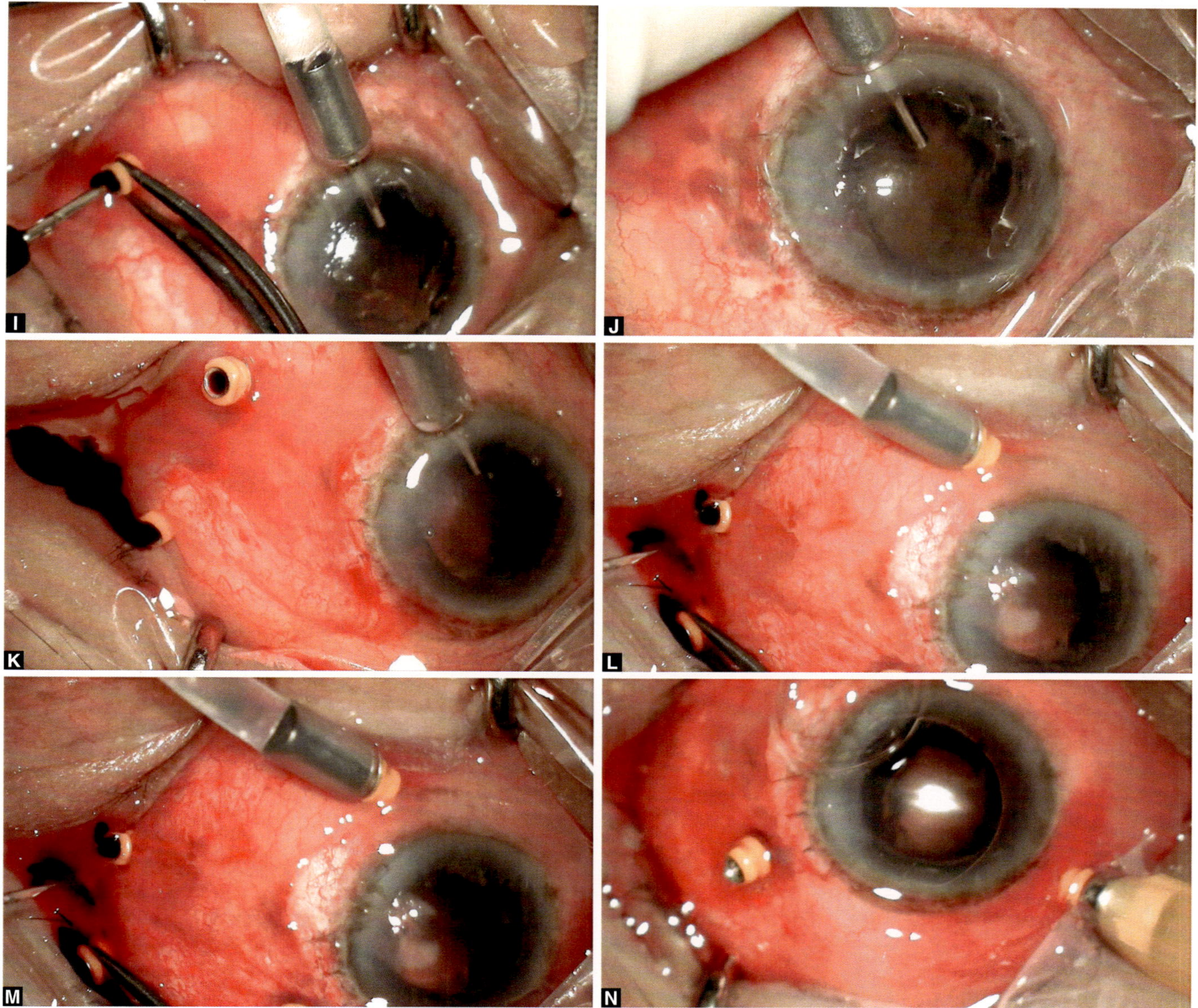

Figs 15.6A to N: (A) Animated form of suprachoroidal hemorrhage (SCH); (B) Drainage of supra choroidal hemorrhage (yellow arrow) by radial sclerotomy (white arrow); (C) New sutureless technique to drain suprachoroidal hemorrhage by oblique insertion of 23G cannula; (D to H) Intraoperative steps of surgery for managing postcataract surgery suprachoroidal hemorrhage (Case I); (I to N) Intraoperative steps of surgery for managing postcataract surgery suprachoroidal hemorrhage (Case II)

Case II (Video 10, Chapter 15)

- In a case of postcataract surgery suprachoroidal hemorrhage, anterior chamber maintainer used initially as infusion (Fig. 15.6I)
- Then a 23G trocar-cannula complex was introduced obliquely into suprachoroidal space according to the maximum height of suprachoroidal blood and trocar blade removed to drain blood partially (Fig. 15.6J)
- Multiple sutureless sclerotomies made (Fig. 15.6K)
- Then three pars plan ports placed. PFCL injected and higher intravitreal pressure kept high (Fig. 15.6L)
- Multiple sutureless sclerotomies made for more complete external drainage of blood smoothly aided by the pushing effect of PFCL from inside (Fig. 15.6M)
- Silicone oil used for constant endotamponade (Fig. 15.6N).

25-gauge cannula-assisted posterior passive drainage of suprachoroidal blood in a sutureless way [*Boral SK, Agarwal D. Modified posterior drainage of postoperative suprachoroidal hemorrhage. Indian J Ophthalmol. 2021;69(12):3584-90. doi: 10.4103/ijo.IJO_3533_20. PMID: 34827000; PMCID: PMC8837346.*]:

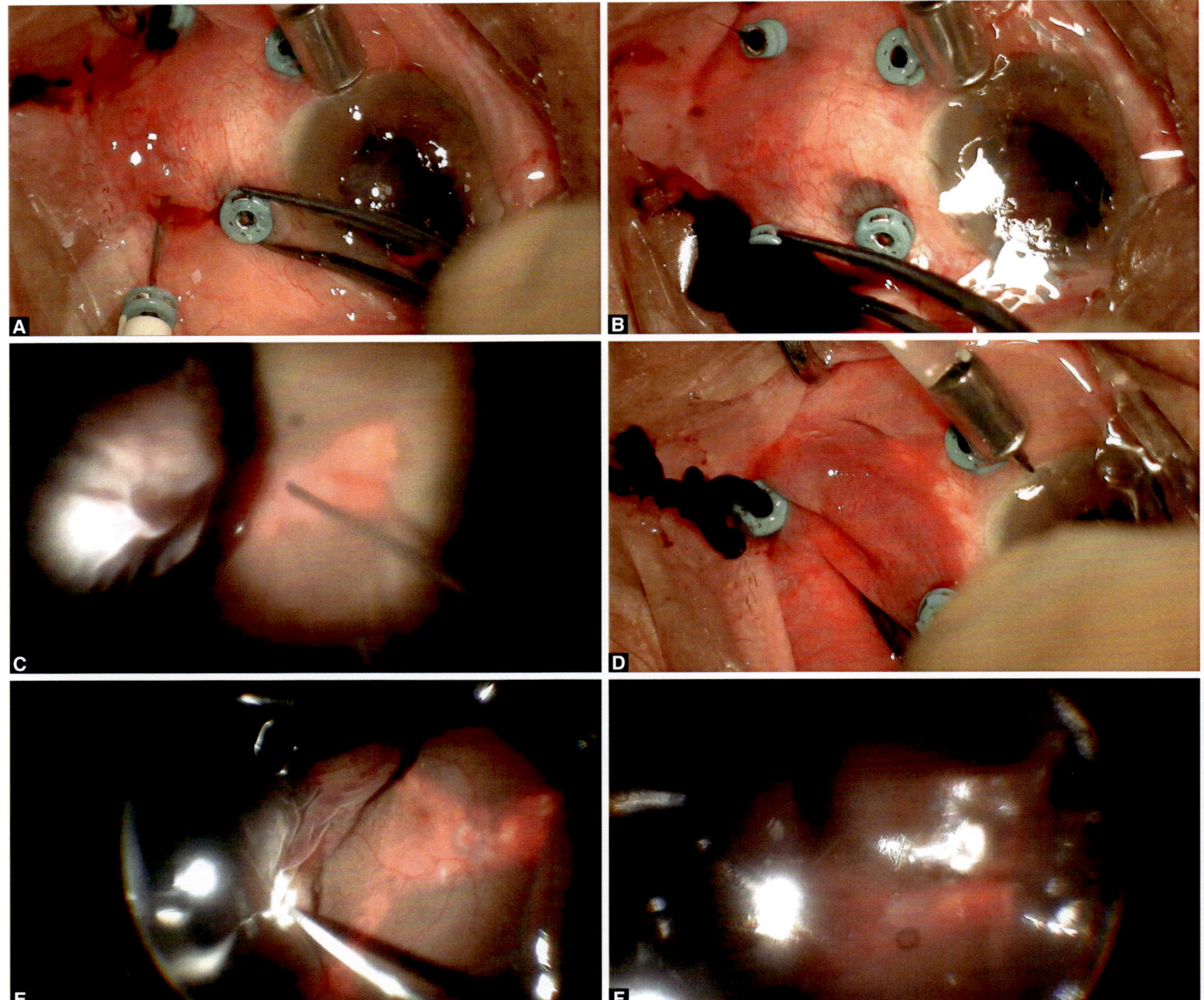

Figs 15.7A to F: Intraoperative steps of 25-gauge cannula-assisted posterior passive drainage of suprachoroidal blood.

Case III (Video 11, Chapter 15)

- This is a case of retained lens matters with kissing suprachoroidal hematoma after an attempt of phacoemulsification
- The suprachoroidal hematoma was decided to drain after 10 days of primary intervention after adequate clot lysis
- Preoperative anterior segment photo shows retained lens matters and ultrasonography revealed kissing suprachoroidal hematoma (Fig. 15.8 Preoperative ASP and USG)
- An anterior chamber maintainer was introduced after the failed attempt to introduce an infusion cannula
- 25-gauze vitrectomy started
- There was marked kissing suprachoroidal hematoma
- Then a 25-gauze nonvalved trocar-cannula was inserted obliquely into the suprachoroidal space, 11 mm behind the limbus and the trocar blade was removed (Fig. 15.7A)
- Dark-colored altered lysed blood was drained through the nonvalved cannula, keeping the intraocular pressure at 50 mm Hg (Fig. 15.7B)
- Then, again nonvalved trocar-cannula was introduced at multiple sites, superior and inferior to the initial drainage sites. The gentle scleral massage was applied externally for more drainage of suprachoroidal blood.
- Then, triamcinolone particles were injected and PFCL was introduced to push the suprachoroidal

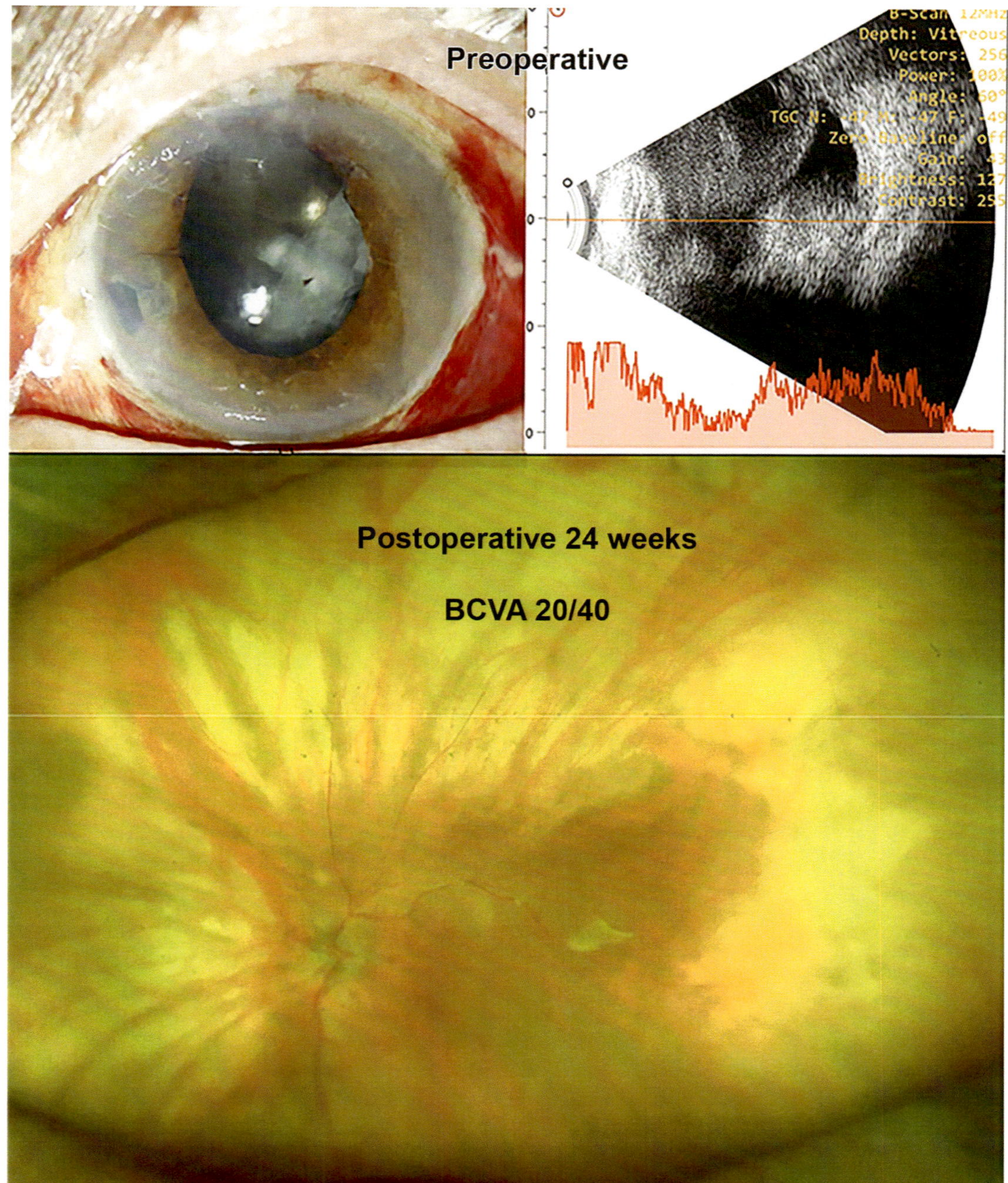

Fig. 15.8: Preoperative anterior segment photo and ultrasonography, revealing kissing suprachoroidal hematoma. After 24 weeks of intervention, the patient gained BCVA 20/80 and the wide-field fundus photograph shows on retina after removal of silicone oil.

elevations from inside and external passive drainage of suprachoroidal blood (Figs. 15.7C and D)

- Now a 6-mm 23-gauze infusion port was introduced
- The retina was detached and subretinal fluid was drained through the retinotomy (Fig. 15.7E)
- PFCL was removed after adequate drainage of blood
- The laser was done around the retinotomy site
- Silicone oil with 5000 cSt viscosity was used for constant long-term endotamponade (Fig. 15.7F)
- After 24 weeks of intervention, the patient gained BCVA 20/80 and the wide-field fundus photograph shows on retina with nearly resolve SCH after removal of silicone oil (Fig. 15.8).

This sutureless method is less traumatic than the radial sclerotomies, as described earlier.

Use of silicone oil is essential as it is a noncompressible fluid and provides a constant endotamonade and minimize risk of rebleed.

Kindly scan the QR code below to access the online Video.

CHAPTER 16

Penetrating Injuries and Retained Intraocular Foreign Bodies

OCULAR INJURY

Ocular injury can be of two types:

A. *Blunt trauma:* It cause transmission of external force to the globe with resultant distortion. Since sclera and cornea are relatively inelastic, the globe cannot stretch in response to the deformation. The net effect is change of shape of the globe, not the volume. Sudden change in shape can exert tractional forces, especially at the vitreous base, resulting in formation of peripheral tears and dialysis. An after blunt trauma by a projectile can cause four phases of globe deformation:
   1. Compression (Fig. 16.1A).
   2. Decompression (Fig. 16.1B).
   3. Overshooting (Fig. 16.1C).
   4. Oscillation.

   Due to trampoline effect of trauma, there is anterior-posterior compression and simultaneous equatorial expansion of the globe (Fig. 16.1A) which immediately followed by anterior-posterior decompression of the globe (Fig. 16.1B). Induction of posterior vitreous detachment usually occurs at this stage of decompression.

   Macular hole also sometimes forms due to pressure necrosis at the stage of compression as well as due to posterior vitreous detachment at the stage of anterior-posterior decompression.

B. *Penetrating trauma:* Penetrating injuries can result in smaller self -sealed wounds by uveal tissue or vitreous or a large-sized corneal/scleral tear that result in hypotony and expulsive choroidal hemorrhage.

Essential Roles of Vitrectomy in Penetrating Ocular Traumas

1. Vitrectomy eliminates the scaffold for fibrovascular ingrowth of tissues at entry and exit wounds and that may reduce the risk of development of retinal detachment.
2. Vitrectomy allows the removal of intraocular debris like traumatic cataract, disrupted lens matters, vitreous-lens admixture, vitreous hemorrhage to clear visual axis and any retained intraocular foreign bodies (RIOFB).
3. Removal of formed vitreous relieves traction and allows the use of laser photocoagulation and intraocular tamponade to treat retinal injury and retinal detachments.

Indications of Vitrectomy in Ocular Traumas

1. Traumatic cataract with disrupted posterior capsule.
2. Lens-vitreous admixture in anterior chamber or in vitreous cavity.
3. Severe vitreous loss.
4. Nonresolving vitreous hemorrhage.
5. Retinal detachment or retinal tear, dialysis, incarceration.
6. Retained intraocular foreign bodies (RIOFB).
7. Post-traumatic endophthalmitis.

Clinical and Slit Lamp Examination

1. BCVA—Most important factor and predictive factor for visual recovery.
2. Presence of overt or occult scleral and corneal rupture, associated uveal tissue prolapse and presence of vitreous at the wound.
3. Corneal clarity.
4. Pupillary reaction to detect relative afferent pupillary defect (RAPD) to rule out optic nerve damage.
5. Anterior chamber—For hyphema or vitreous prolapse.
6. Lens—To note cataractous changes, any subluxation, if present then degree of subluxation. If aphakic, intravitreally dislocated lens is to be ruled out.
7. Examination of fundus—To detect vitreous hemorrhage, choroidal and retinal detachment or presence of any RIOFB.

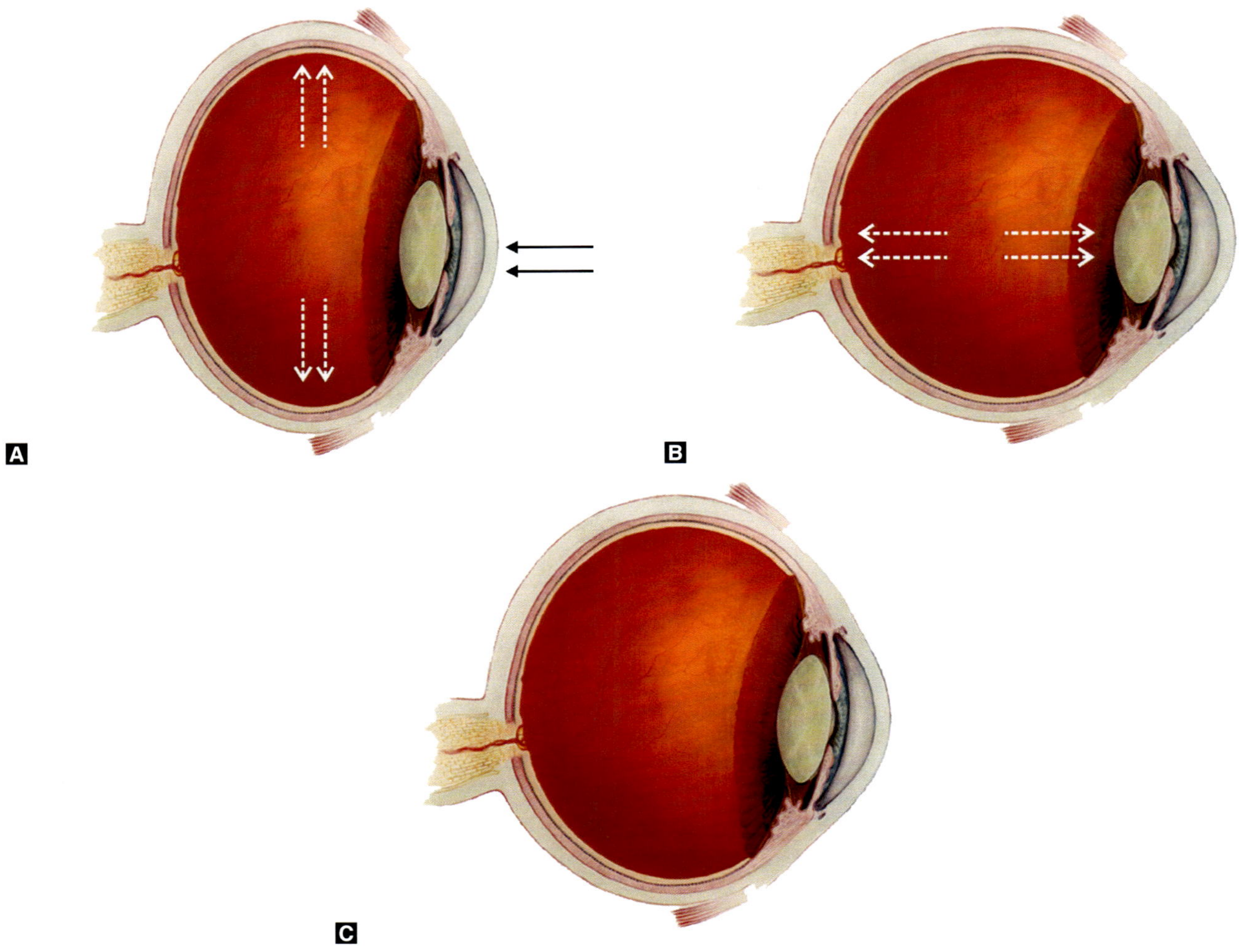

Figs 16.1A to C: (A) Stage of compression; (B) Stage of decompression; (C) Stage of overshooting

Ultrasonography

It is required when media is opaque due to edematous cornea, traumatic cataract, ruptured lens materials in pupillary area, hyphema, vitreous hemorrhage.

1. It can assess for choroidal or retinal detachment.
2. To detect both radiolucent or radiopaque RIOFBs.
3. It can detect and precisely localize the site of of RIOFB (which gives high-amplitude spikes on A scan). It is particularly helpful to detect radiolucent RIOFBs.
4. It can assess for posterior exit wound in suspected globe rupture cases.

Typical USG Picture (Vide Chapter 8)

On A scan: Irregular shape with very high reflectivity spikes.

On B scan: Very bright signal that persist at low gain settings with marked shadowing of ocular and orbital structure just posterior to RIOFB.

(RIOFB less than 0.5 mm in diameter does not produce shadowing; one should do A scan with oblique sound beam procedure).

RIOFBs Difficult to Detect on USG

- Very small FB
- Located in anterior segment (especially within lens capsule)
- Located in the plane of iris
- If it is embedded in the pars plicata.

Magnetic Property of Metallic RIOFBs on USG

By Ossoing's method: It utilizes standard A scan to detect small vertical movements of FB spikes as a pulsed magnet is slowly advanced towards the eye. These slight pulsatile movement of FB indicate that it is metallic.

Spherical RIOFB (like gun-shot pellet): Sound wave reverberate within the object and each time reverberation occurs.

X-ray orbit: Orbital plane film X-rays (AP and dead lateral view) confirm presence of metallic RIOFBs (Figs 16.2A and B).

CT scan orbit: For more accurate localization of RIOFBs. Thin radiographic cuts (2 mm or less) may help in localization, whether the RIOFB is intraocular or inside ocular coats or external to the ocular coat (Figs 16.2C to F). The indications of CT scan orbit in cases of RIOFB are:

- When there is suspicion of multiple foreign bodies
- To localize the RIOFB, whether intraocular or extraocular.

MRI: It is to be avoided in presence of metallic RIOFBs as there is a risk of intraocular damage from migration of ferromagnetic RIOFB.

Electrophysiological tests: To assess visual potential in severely injured eyes with absent or questionable light perception.

- *Bright-flash Visual Evoked Potential (VEP):* It can assess macular and optic nerve integrity, i.e. central visual function
- *Flash Electroretinogram (ERG):* It reflects function of mass photoreceptors, not only central visual field.

Timing of Intervention

Some studies says intervention within first 72 hours is associated with favorable outcome. But, delay of several days, sometimes helps to reduce the severe intraocular bleeding from uveal congestion and helps in spontaneous separation of posterior hyaloid face.

Iron RIOFB

Intraocular degenerative changes is called 'Siderosis'. Reactions can be—Direct-iron deposited in immediate neighborhood of the RIOFB like subconjuctival tissue, cornea, sclera, iris, lens, retina and optic nerve or Indirect-iron is diffused widely throughout ocular tissue.

Pathogenesis

1. Electric dissociation by constant current in posterior to anterior direction.
2. Simple diffusion.

Clinical Changes of Siderosis

Cornea: Rusty staining of epithelium (not involving stroma, Descemet's membrane and endothelium).

Iris: Moderately dilated pupil—yellowish-brown staining.

Angle: Heavily stained trabeculae and secondary glaucoma.

Ciliary body: Accommodative failure, marked staining of epithelium (musculature is little affected).

Cataract: Unique subcapsular brownish dots, characteristic yellowish tint of the lens capsule in slit lamp examination, sometimes atrophic changes leading to iridodonesis.

Vitreous: Clouds of brown spots due to degenerative changes.

Choroid: Involved only in advanced stage when retina and choroid are indistinguishable.

Retina: Initially peripheral pigmentary changes, perimacular pigment deposition with loss of foveal reflex, sclerotic changes in arteries, retinal detachment and endophthalmitis.

Optic nerve: Yellowish rusty color.

Chalcosis

Intraocular copper RIOFB
Pure copper RIOFB cause suppurative reaction.

Clinical Changes

Cornea: Deposition of tiny, closely packed granules in descemet's membrane. Brilliantly glittering greenish-blue segmental or complete ring in peripheral cornea at the level of descemet's membrane.

Lens: Sunflower cataract, spokes run from centre to periphery till equator like petals of a flower.

Aqueous humor: Packed with brightly refringent, greenish-brown colored microscopic particles.

Vitreous humor: Copper deposition gives a red coppery tint immediately behind the lens.

Iris: Greenish coloration.

Retina: Rarely affected. If deposited in retina, brilliant highly reflective deposites arranged along the main trunks of both arterioles and venules.

Other metallic RIOFBs with their effects are given in Table 16.1.

Chemically inert RIOFBs

Following RIOFBs are inert and does not give result in any intravitreal reaction—

- Precious metals like gold (pure), silver, platinum
- Stone, rock, clay, coal
- Glass, quartz, porcelain, plastic
- Organic materials like rubber.

These RIOFB cases can be followed-up without any kind of intervention.

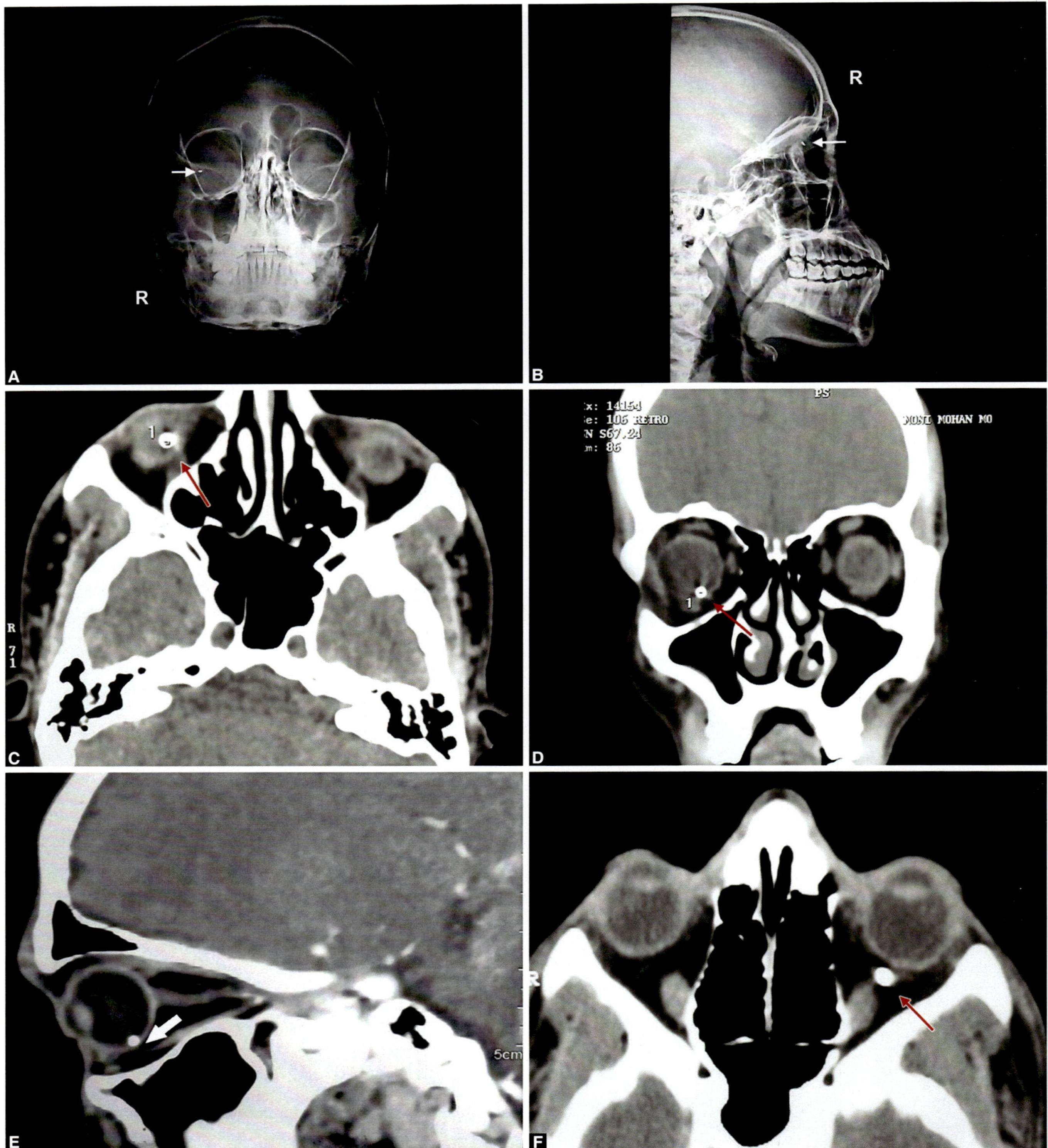

Figs 16.2A to F: (A and B) Digital anterior-posterior (AP) and lateral view of orbital X-ray with radiopaque RIOFB; (C) Axial view of CT scan orbit shows intraocular hyperintense metallic foreign body; (D) Coronal view of CT scan orbit shows hyperintense metallic foreign body inside the inferior ocular coat; (E) RIOFB within scleral coat in sagittal view of CT orbit; (F) Axial view of CT scan orbit shows hyperintense extraocular (retro orbital) metallic foreign body

The dictum is—All penetrating injury with suspected retained intraocular foreign bodies should underwent orbital X-ray (for metallic RIOFBs) or CT Scan Orbit (for both metallic and nonmetallic RIOFBs).

Metallic RIOFBs, not visible in Orbital X-ray—Aluminium (Bone density index is less with metals like aluminium, thus it cannot be separated from the bone shadows).

The clinical situations:

1. Metallic RIOFB with clear lens—
   Case discussion *(Video 1, Chapter 16)*:
   - A case of encapsulated iron RIOFB with clear lens with vitreous haze (Fig. 16.3A)
   - TA-assisted Vitrectomy done

TABLE 1: Other metallic RIOFBs with their effects

RIOFBs	*Clinical features*
Aluminium	Punctate, striate, irregular lental opacities
Mercury	Active purulent inflammation which rapidly develop phthisis bulbi
Nickel	Purulent inflammation
Zinc	Little reaction
Lead	Most inert metallic RIOFB, as it covered with a layer of insoluble carbonate, preventing it's diffusion

   - RIOFB was at superonasal periphery
   - One port was converted to 20G by MVR blade (Fig. 16.3B)
   - PFCL injected to protect posterior pole (Fig. 16.3C)
   - RIOFB was made free
   - A 20G magnet was used to bring the RIOFB from the retinal surface (Fig. 16.3D)
   - An end grasping forceps was used to hold the RIOFB (Fig. 16.3E)
   - A 20G forceps was again used to hold the RIOFB and tried to remove
   - Magnet was again used to dislodge the RIOFB from the port and held by foreign-body holding forceps and removed (Figs 16.3F and G)
   - Laser done around the site of RIOFB
   - PFCL removed
   - Fluid-air exchange done
   - 20G port sutured (Fig. 16.3H).
2. Metallic RIOFB with cataract—The principles to with deal this kind of situation are as follows:
   - IOL implantation should be avoided immediate after cataract extraction (Fig. 16.4A)
   - Intravitreal RIOFB should be brought out by the suction of cutter through the pre-existing posterior capsular tear or by creating tear in posterior capsule (Figs 16.4B and C)

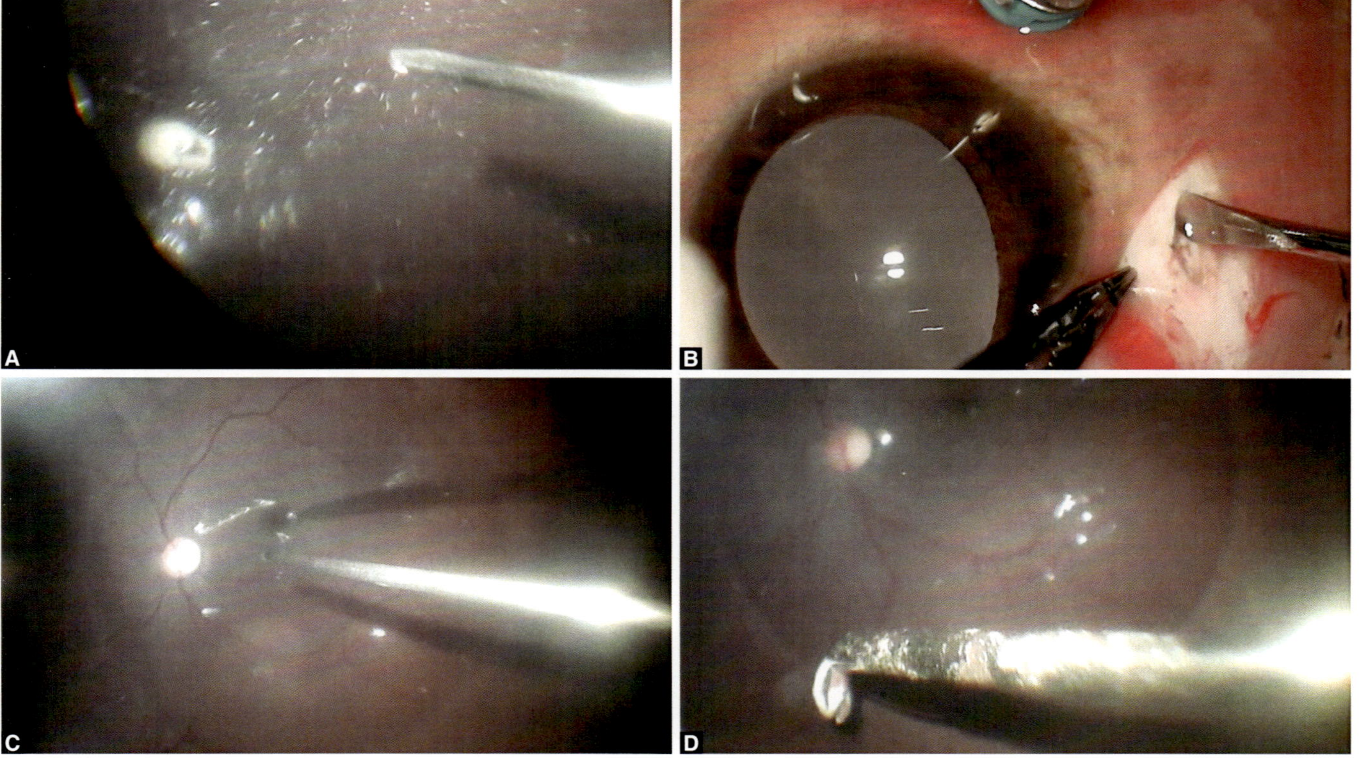

Figs 16.3A to D

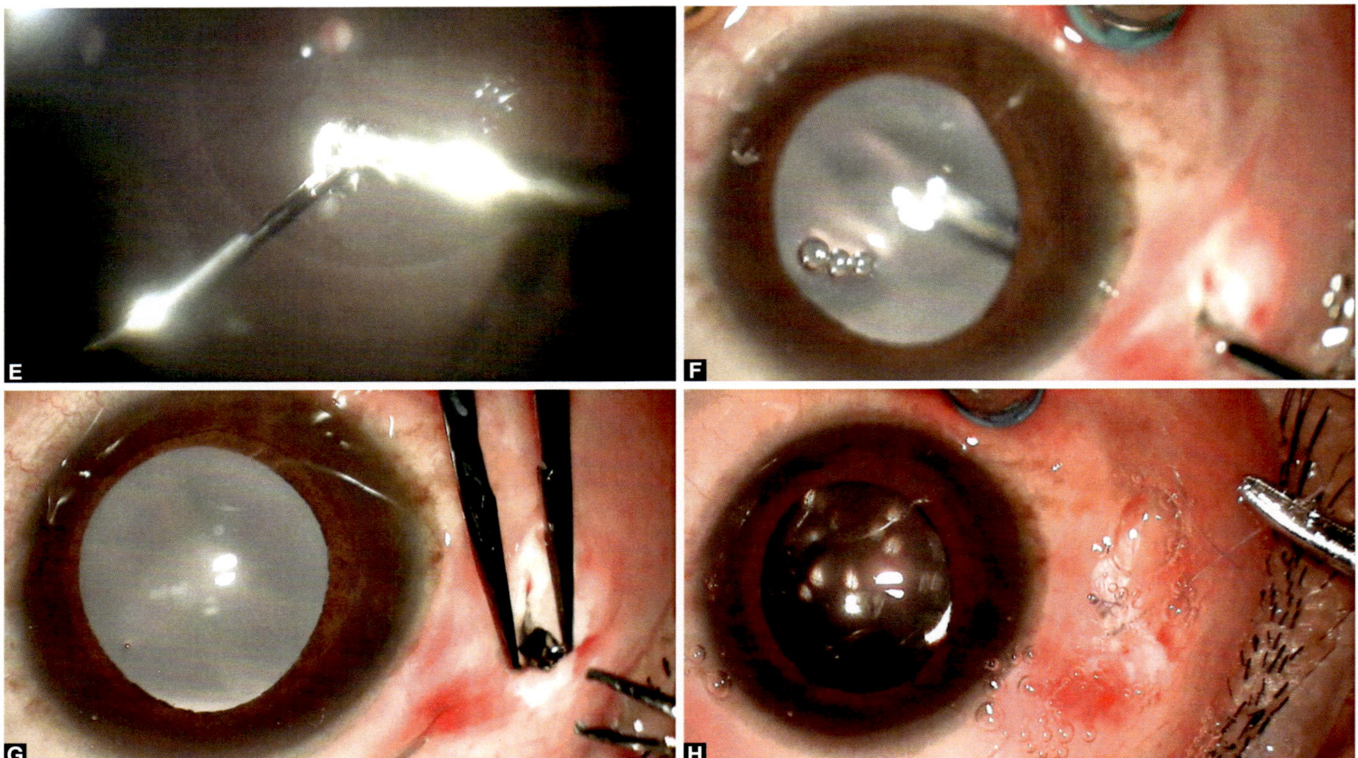

Figs 16.3A to H: Intraoperative steps of surgery for managing intravitreal iron RIOFB with clear lens

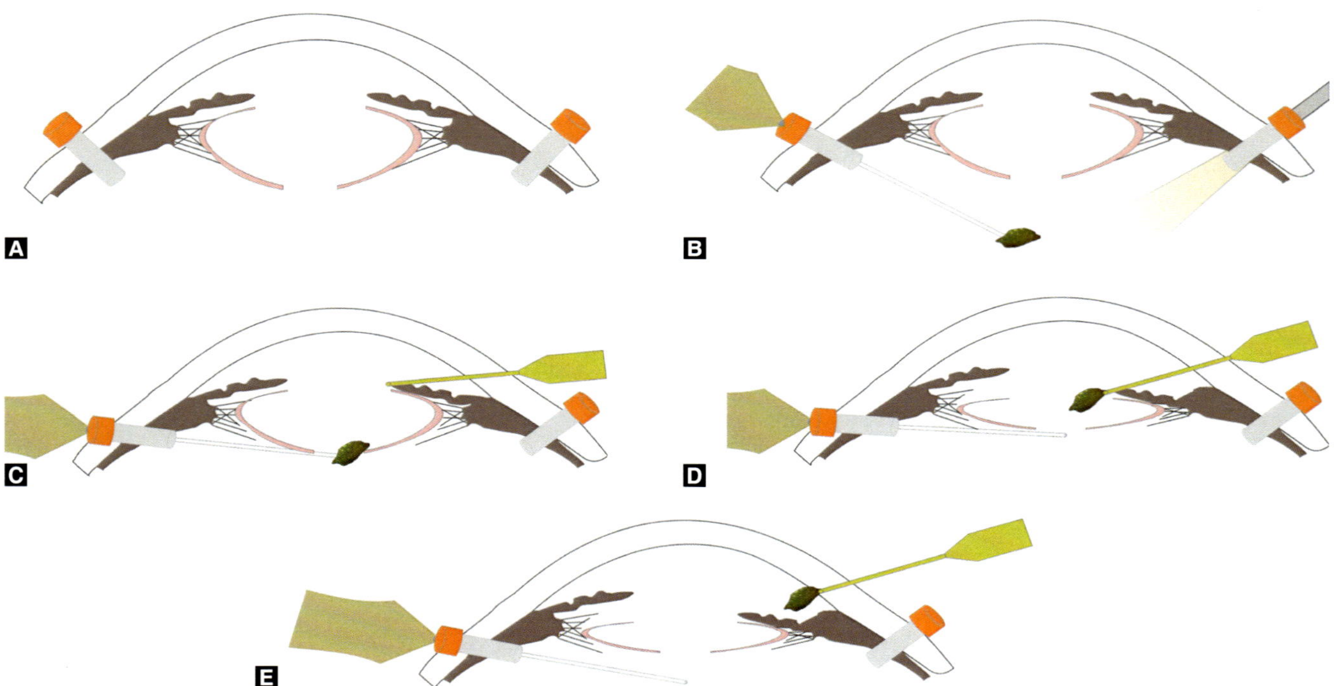

Figs 16.4A to E: Schematic presentation of steps of surgery managing intravitreal iron RIOFB with cataract

- A magnet should be used through the limbal route to release the RIOFB from the cutter port and bring into the anterior chamber (Fig. 16.4D)
- The RIOFB should be removed through the same limbal route (Fig. 16.4E).

Case discussion *(Video 2, Chapter 16)*:

- A post-traumatic case with advanced cataract with radiopaque RIOFB on orbital X-ray
- Lens capsule was found to be yellowish, may be secondary to early siderotic change (Figs 16.5A and B)
- Lens aspiration was done and a small opening at posterior capsule was noted
- IOL was not implanted
- Torpedo light is always helpful to keep both hands free to remove RIOFB
- RIOFB was made free of vitreous
- It was partially embedded within retina
- A 24G needle was bent at it's tip, so that it can be passed through the 23G cannula
- The bent needle was used to dislodge the RIOFB from retina
- Suction of the cutter was used to pick up RIOFB and to bring it just behind the PC opening (Fig. 16.5C)
- Now a magnet was introduced through the PC opening to bring the RIOFB into the anterior chamber (Fig. 16.5D)
- Viscoelastic was used to deepen anterior chamber and to keep posterior capsule posteriorly
- RIOFB was successfully removed through the limbal route (Fig. 16.5E) and it was 2 mm × 1 mm
- Now foldable PCIOL was implanted into the capsular bag (Fig. 16.5F)
- Posterior capsulectomy was made by enlarging the PC opening
- Laser was done around the site of RIOFB (Fig. 16.5G) as well as 360° periphery
- Periphery was checked for any other break

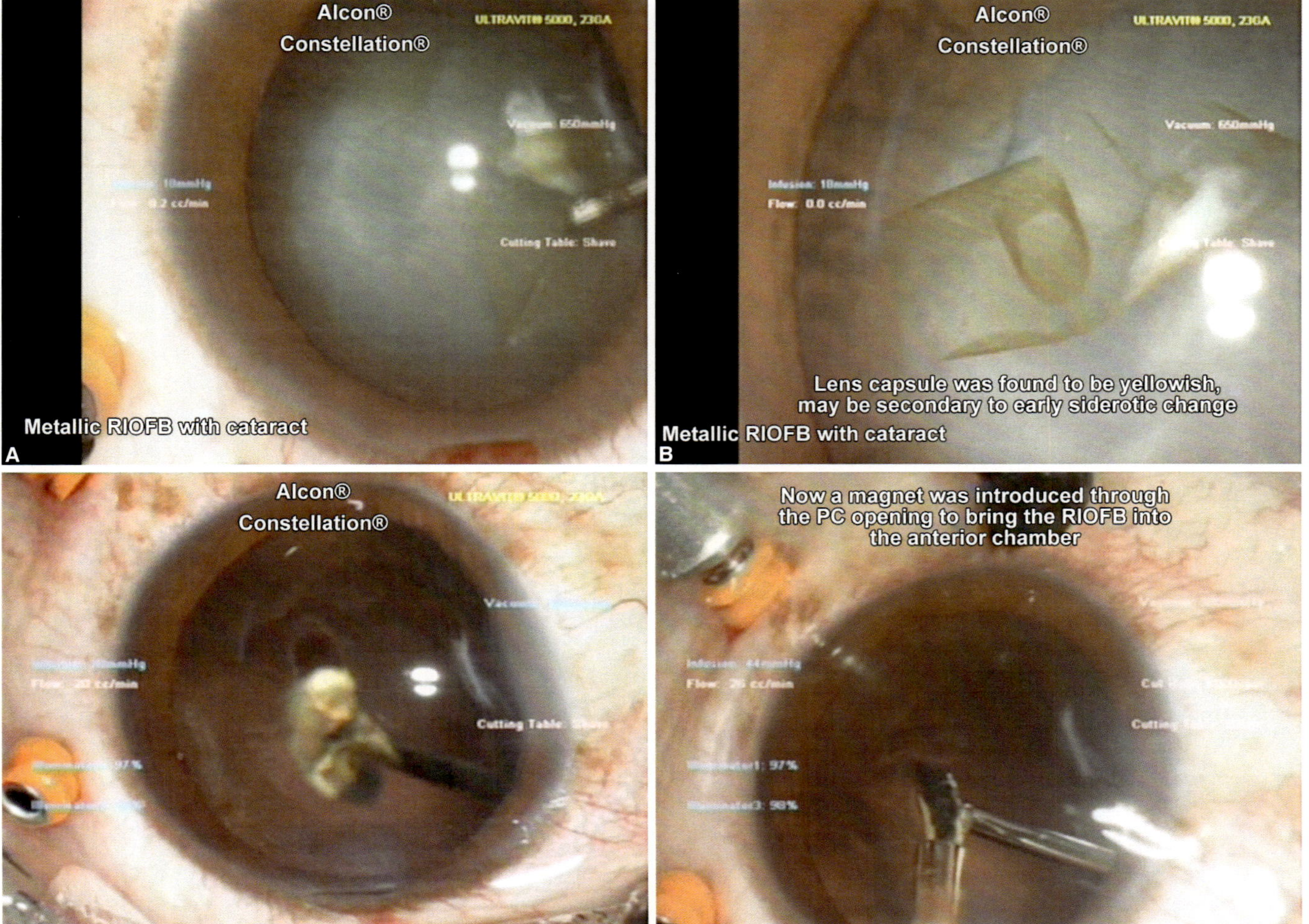

Figs 16.5A to D

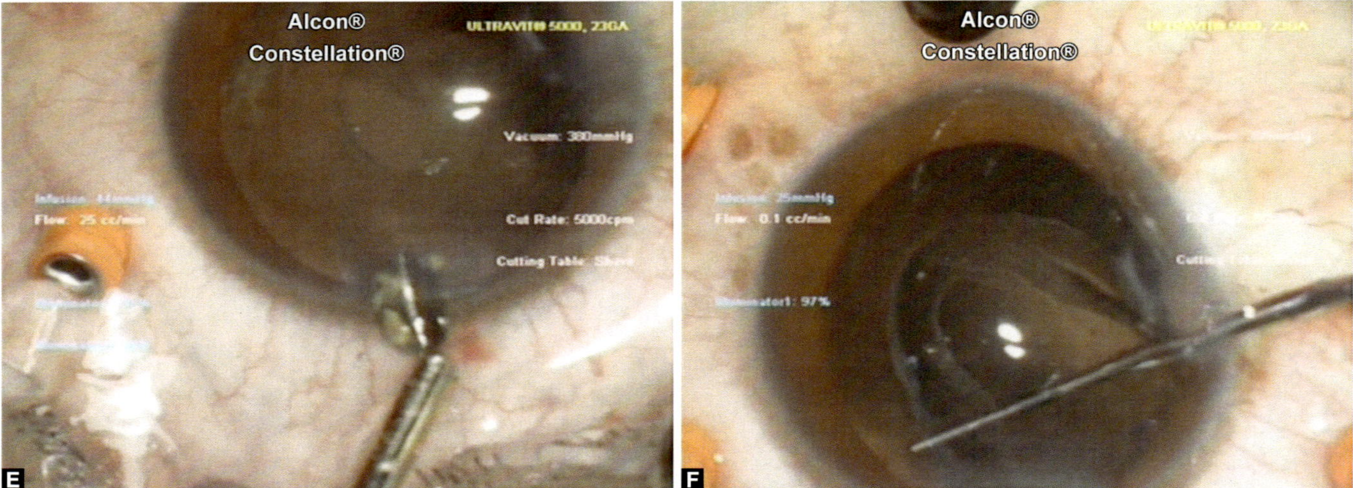

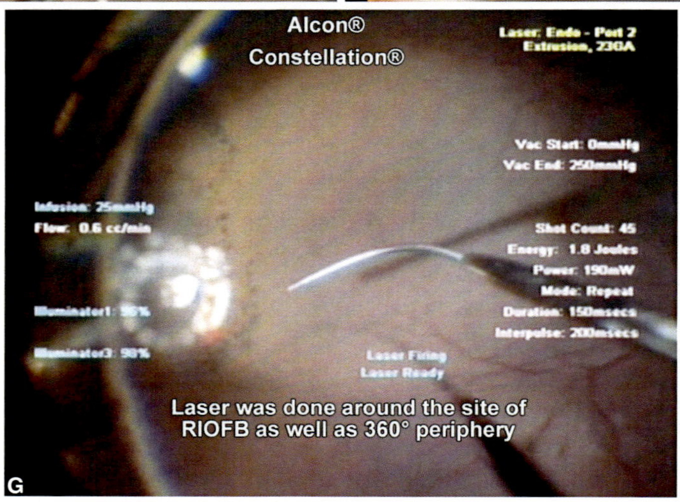

Figs 16.5A to G: Intraoperative steps of surgery managing intravitreal iron RIOFB with cataract

- Fluid-air exchange was done
- All cannulas and torpedo light source were removed
- Intravitreal long-standing gas injection was done at the end of surgery.

3. Metallic RIOFB with endophthalmitis *(Video 3, Chapter 16)*

   Case discussion:
   - A case of RIOFB with self-sealed corneal perforation with cataractous lens with endophthalmitis
   - Lensectomy done (Fig. 16.6A)
   - There was dense vitreous exudates and vitrectomy was started with antibiotics in the infusion bottle (Fig. 16.6B)
   - An encapsulated RIOFB was detected (Fig. 16.6C)
   - It was removed from the capsular coat
   - Now flute needle was held over the RIOFB and with the help of active suction (Fig. 16.6D)
   - RIOFB was bring at aphakic pupillary area (Fig. 16.6E)
   - It was removed through a limbal entry with the help of a magnet
   - It was 3 mm× 5 mm—Base excision was done
   - Fluid air exchange was done (Fig. 16.6F)
   - Laser was done around the site of RIOFB (Fig. 16.6G)
   - Inferior PI and Silicone oil injection was done
   - Cannulas were removed.

4. Nonmetallic RIOFBs

   Case discussion *(Video 4, Chapter 16)*:
   - A case bomb-blast injury with multiple intravitreal nonmetallic RIOFBs
   - RIOFB was picked up with the suction of the cutter (Fig. 16.7A)
   - And removed through the aphakic pupillary area (Fig. 16.7B).

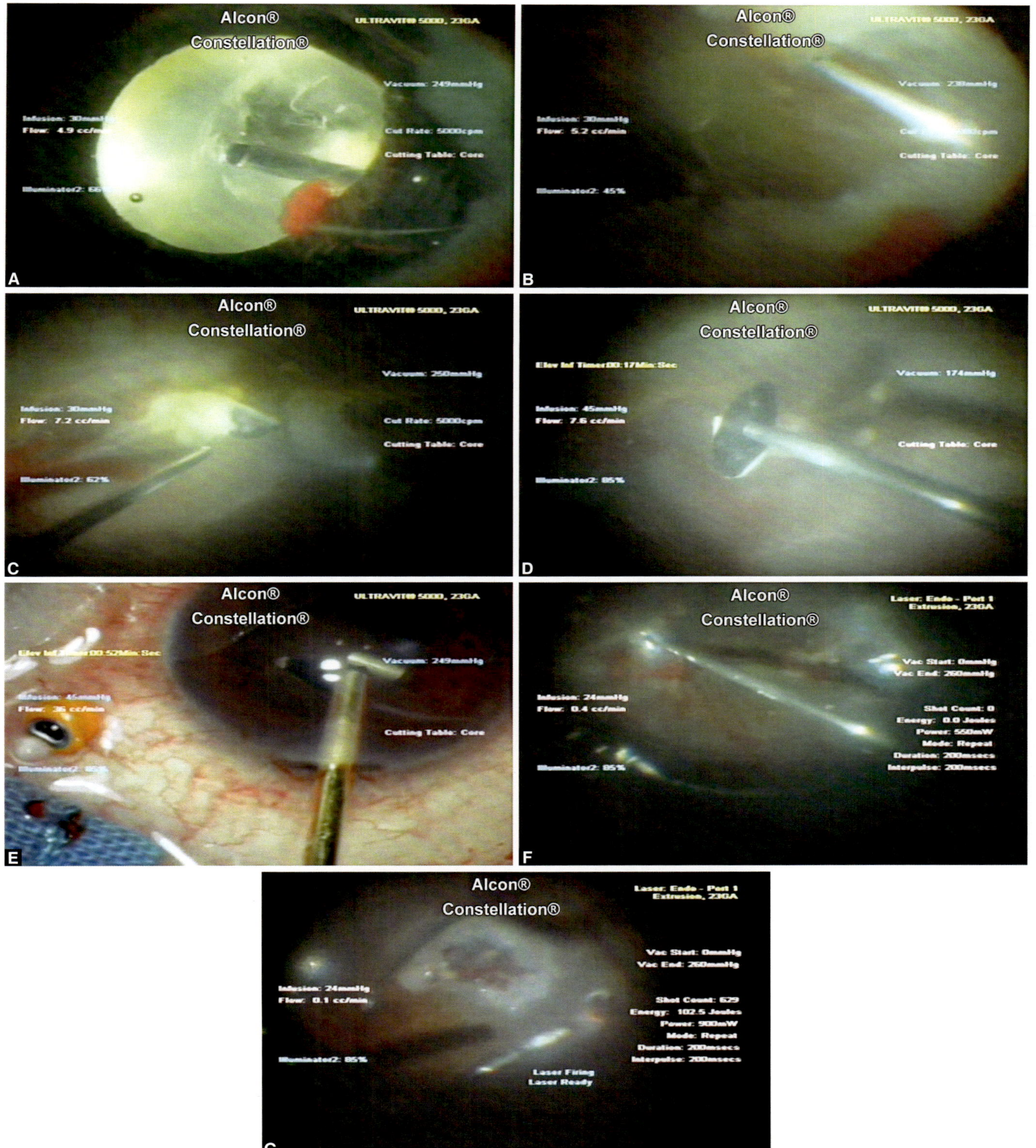

Figs 16.6A to G: Intraoperative steps of surgery managing metallic RIOFB with endophthalmitis

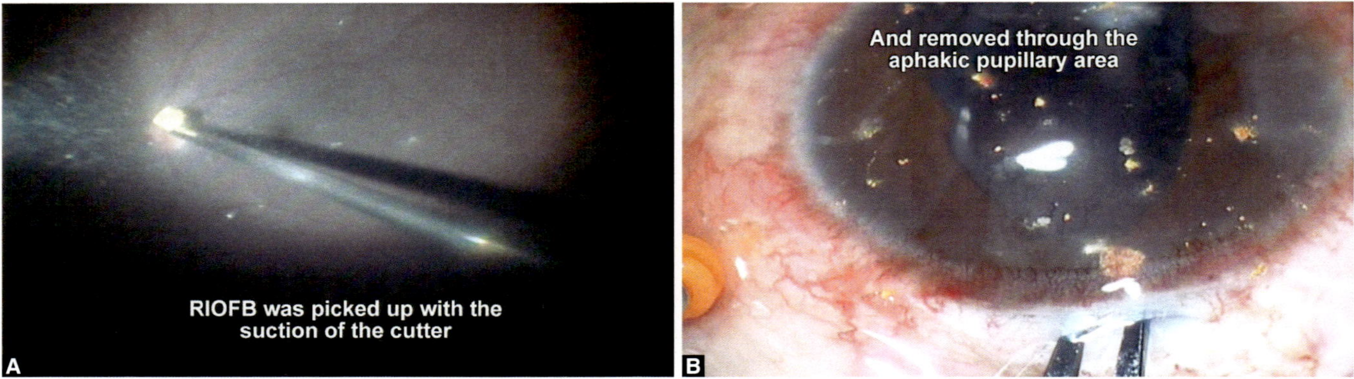

Figs 16.7A and B: Intraoperative steps of surgery managing nonmetallic RIOFBs in a case of bomb blast injury

Kindly scan the QR code below to access the online Video.

CHAPTER 17

Endophthalmitis

Endophthalmitis is a devastating ocular emergency in which there is exudation of purulent materials into the vitreous cavity due to inflammation of internal layers of the eye resulting from bacterial, fungal, parasitic or viral invasion. It is a rare but sight-threatening complication that can occur after ocular surgery or trauma or as a consequence of systemic infection. To optimize visual outcome, early diagnosis and treatment are essential. Leading symptoms and signs of endophthalmitis are:

1. Sudden onset rapid worsening of pain.
2. Poor recovery or rapid diminution of vision.
3. Disproportionate anterior chamber reaction.
4. Pupillary membrane.
5. Hypopyon.
6. Presence of vitritis or vitreous exudates on ultrasonography.

ENDOPHTHALMITIS MANAGEMENT

Endophthalmitis management depends on the etiology.

Exogenous Endophthalmitis

Due to breach in corneoscleral integrity. It can be:

1. *Postoperative Endophthalmitis:* Endophthalmitis after ocular surgery is the most common form of the condition. Cataract surgery is by far the most frequently performed intraocular surgery. Approximately 90% of postoperative endophthalmitis cases develop after this procedure with an incidence following such surgery ranging from 0.08% to 0.7%. It can present as—
   - Acute onset postoperative endophthalmitis (Fig. 17.1A): Most present within 1-2 weeks, usually 5-7 days after the surgery and is most likely to be caused by *Staphylococcal epidermidis* or coagulase negative cocci (rarely fungi). Fulminant variety develop usually within about 4 days after the surgery and is usually caused by gram negative bacteria, streptococci and *Staphylococcus aureus*.
   - Subacute postoperative endophthalmitis: Patients with similar symptoms who presented later than 8 days were defined as having subacute postoperative endophthalmitis.
   - Chronic postoperative endophthalmitis (Fig. 17.1B): usually develop after 4 weeks after the surgery. It may be due to—
     - Delayed entry—e.g. bleb-related endophthalmitis and
     - Delayed onset—The organism involved are fungi, *Propionibacterium acne or S. epidermides.*

       In the EVS, only 69.3% of cases met the criteria for laboratory-confirmed infection. The reasons that more than 30% of cases failed to obtain positive results from culture vary and include low microbial counts, spontaneously sterilizing during the ocular inflammatory response of certain strains (e.g, *Staphylococcus epidermidis*), or even noninfectious inflammations.

       With proper management, chronic postoperative endophthalmitis can be resolved (Fig. 17.1C) after vitrectomy
2. *Post-traumatic Endophthalmitis:* Endophthalmitis is an important complication of open globe injury. About 25% of endophthalmitis cases are a result of ocular trauma and these are more often associated with a poorer visual outcome than otherwise similar globe injuries. The incidence of endophthalmitis in cases of penetrating ocular trauma has been reported to range from 3.3% to 30% and after intraocular foreign body from 1.3% to 61%.

Endogenous Endophthalmitis

Unlike the origin in exogenous endophthalmitis, where the pathogen enters from outside the body into the eye, in endogenous endophthalmitis the infection is secondary to hematogenous spread from a distant infective source within the body. The endogenous form of endophthalmitis accounts for approximately 5% to 10% of endophthalmitis cases.

It occurs when micro-organisms in the bloodstream get into the eye, cross the blood-retina barrier, and infect the ocular tissue. Because of the higher blood flow, choroids and ciliary body are the primary focuses of infection in the eye with secondary involvement of the retina and vitreous.

Causative organisms of endogenous endophthalmitis may be bacteria, as well as fungi (*Candida albicans, Aspergillus*), and rarely parasites.

Risk factors for the development of endogenous endophthalmitis are mainly related to immunosuppression or to procedures that increase the risk for blood-borne infections. Most common factors include—

- Immunosuppressive diseases, such as diabetes mellitus, HIV infection, cancer, renal failure requiring dialysis, cardiac disease, long-term use of broad-spectrum antibiotics, steroids and other immunosuppressive drugs, major surgery, especially intra-abdominal surgery
- Intravenous hyperalimentation, indwelling intravenous catheters, and intravenous drug abuse.

It is important to differentiate postoperative endophthalmitis from toxic anterior shock syndrome (TASS).

TASS

Acute sterile inflammation within 24–48 hours after surgery (Figs 17.1D and E).

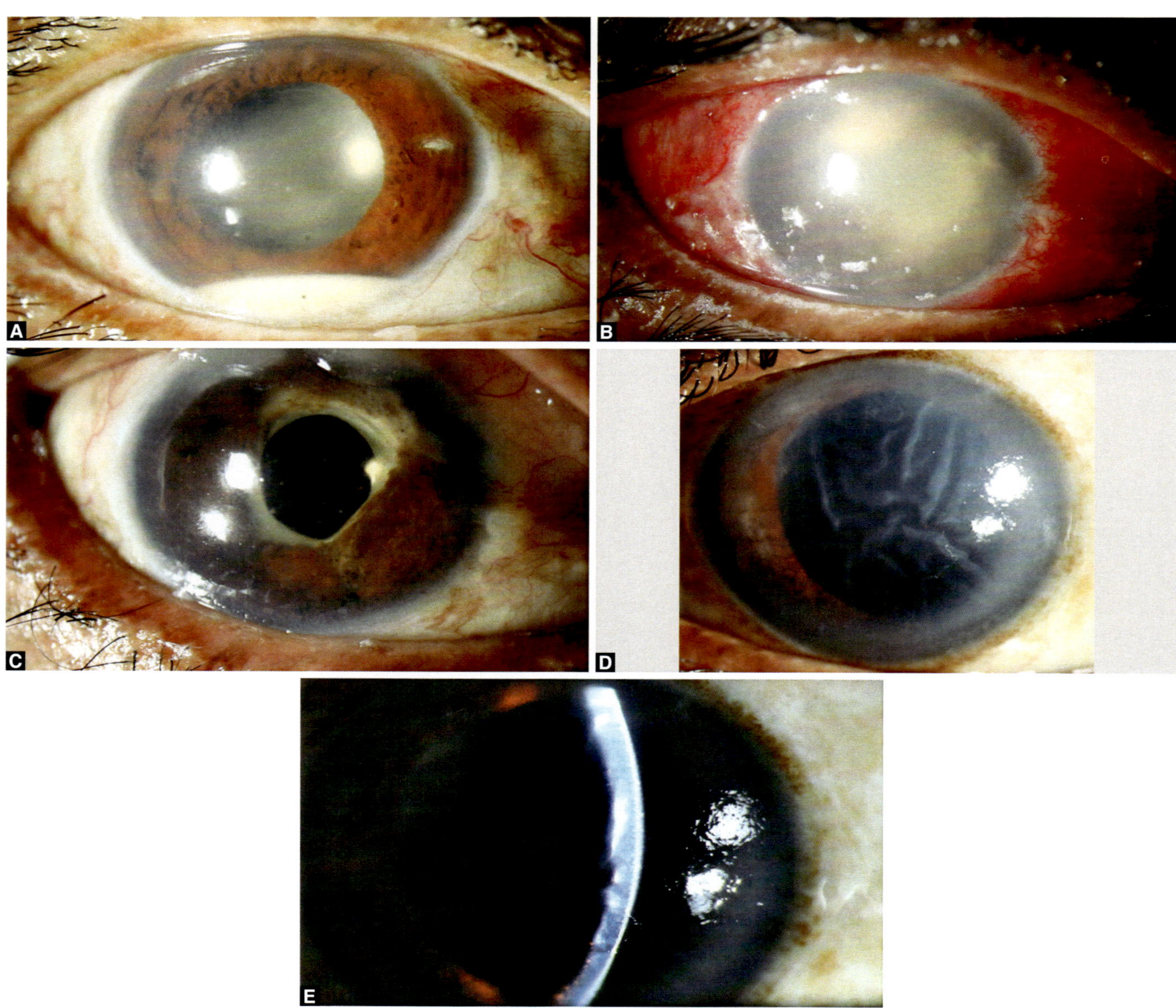

Figs 17.1A to E: (A) Acute postoperative endophthalmitis; (B) Chronic postoperative endophthalmitis; (C) Resolution of chronic postoperative endophthalmitis after vitrectomy; (D and E) Toxic anterior shock syndrome (TASS)

Clinical features

- Diffuse, limbus to limbus corneal edema
- Increased inflammation—Hypopyon
- Fibrin deposition
- Sometimes secondary glaucoma.

Treatment of TASS

- Frequent application of topical steroids and cycloplegics.

Causes

- Toxins from irrigating solution
- Instrument cleaner agents releases heat-stable endotoxins
- Retained viscoelastics.

MANAGEMENT OF POSTOPERATIVE ENDOPHTHALMITIS

Animation *(Video 1, Chapter 17)*

The main difficulty in doing vitrectomy in cases of endophthalmitis (postoperative) is media haziness. Following factors (Fig. 17.2A) hampers media clarity in cases of endophthalmitis:

- Corneal edema
- AC exudation
- Retro-IOL exudation
- Exudates in the vitreous cavity.

Ultrasonography B scan reveals vitreous exudates with low to moderate amplitude spikes (Fig. 17.2B).

Ultrasonography is also important to rule out:

- Retinal detachment
- Choroidal detachment
- Dislocated lens/nucleus
- Parasitic infestation
- RIOFB
- In children

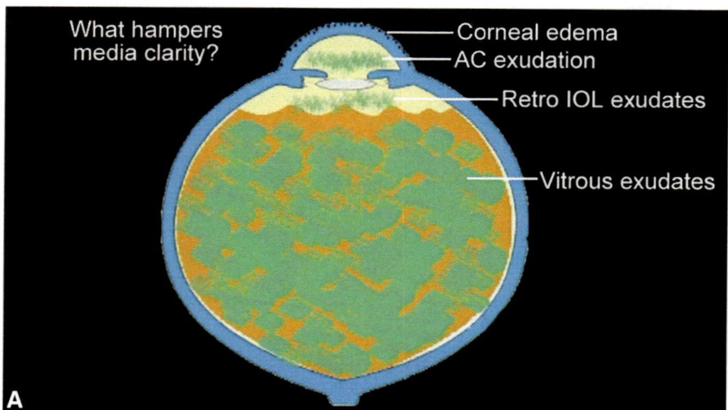

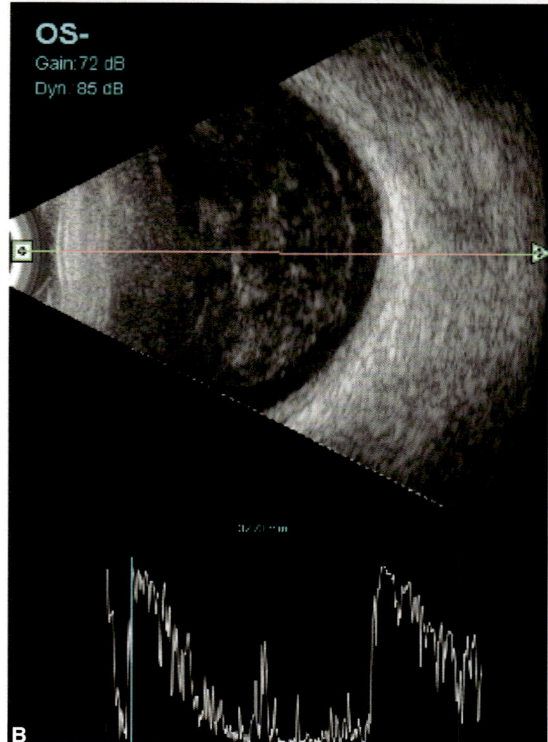

Figs 17.2A and B: (A) Factors responsible for media haziness in postoperative endophthalmitis; (B) Endophthalmitis with echo dense vitreous exudates with low-to-moderate amplitude spikes on A scan

Management

The principal modalities in eradicating the intraocular infections are as follows:

1. Topical antibiotics, steroid and cycloplegics has a supporting and adjunctive role at best and is not the definitive management.
2. Intravitreal antibiotics.
3. Vitrectomy.

Intravitreal injections should be given even in the slightest suspicion of endophthalmitis. One should not forget to take AC tap before intravitreal antibiotic injection (Culture positivity for anterior chamber aspirate is around 25%).

The technique of vitreous biopsy (Fig. 17.3 and Video 2, Chapter 17).

In Case of Propinobacterium acne Endophthalmitis

Propinobacterium acne is an anerobic, gram positive bacillus that is normally present in the conjunctival sac as a commensal. It is now known to be a frequent cause

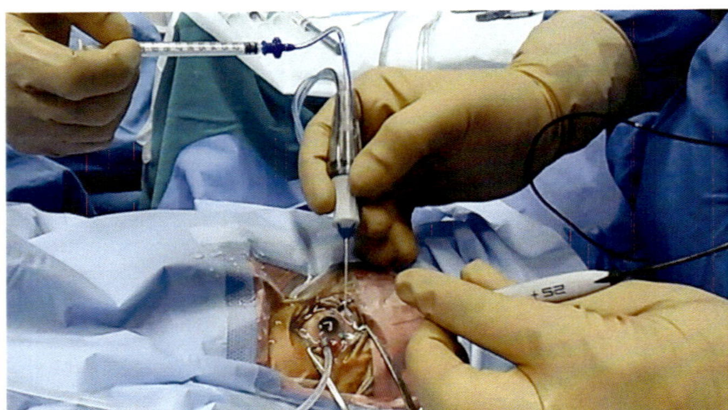

Fig. 17.3: Technique of taking vitreous biopsy by attaching the suction-tubing of the vitrectomy cutter for manual suction with a 1 mL tuberculin syringe.

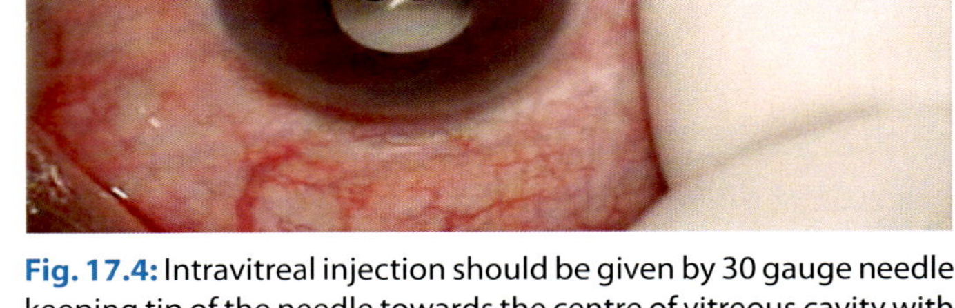

Fig. 17.4: Intravitreal injection should be given by 30 gauge needle keeping tip of the needle towards the centre of vitreous cavity with beveled tip up

of chronic bacterial endophthalmitis. The organism probably act as an adjuvant in stimulating an immune response against soft lens matters remaining after cataract surgery.

Onset—Usually Subacute or Chronic Onset

Presentation—Appears as whitish plaque/fleck like deposits as a sequestrated materials in between capsular bag and optic of IOL. Sometimes, there is history of unexpected inflammation after YAG capsulotomy.

Treatment

- In early stage—in the bag vancomycin injection helps
- In late stage—a large primary posterior capsulectomy (PPC) with vitrectomy with intravitreal vancomycin injection or vitrectomy with removal of IOL along with the capsular bag with intravitreal vancomycin injection.

Intravitreal Antibiotics

Technique (Video 3, Chapter 17)

Intravitreal antibiotics in early/suspected postoperative endophthalmitis

- Before any intravitreal injection ocular surface should be washed thoroughly with 5% povidone iodine followed by saline
- Scleral mark was done 3.5 mm from the limbus
- Intravitreal injection should be given by 30 gauge needle keeping tip of the needle towards the centre of vitreous cavity and beveled tip up (Fig. 17.4)
- Then under direct visualization under microscope, prepared intravitreal antibiotic solutions should be given drop-by-drop
- While removing the needle, a cotton-tip applicator should press the 30 gauge port to prevent vitreous prolapse.

Available Intravitreal Injection Preparations

Antibacterial Drugs

Drugs	*Dose*	*How to make intravitreal dose*	*Organisms against*
Vancomycin	1 mg in 0.1 mL	500 mg in 10 mL sterile solution for injection—take 0.2 mL—make it 1.0 mL—take 0.1 mL	Gram positive bacteria *(Staphylococci, Strepto faecalis, Cl difficile)* and *Neisseria*
Ceftazidime/Cefazoline	2.25 mg/ 0.1 mL	500 mg- add 2.0 mL sterile solution for injection—take 0.1 mL— make it 1.0 mL— take 0.1 mL	Ceftazidime - *Pseudomonas* and Cefazoline - *E coli*, *Klebsiella*

Contd...

Contd...

Drugs	*Dose*	*How to make intravitreal dose*	*Organisms against*
Amikacin	400 microgram/0.1 mL	100 mg in 2 mL— take 0.2 mL—dilute with 2.3 mL sterile solution for injection (10 mg in 2.5 mL)—take 0.1 mL	Aerobic gram negative bacteria with widest spectrum of activity
Gentamycin	200 microgram/0.1 mL	80 mg in 2 mL—take 0.1 mL—add 1.9 mL sterile solution for injection (4 mg in 2 mL)—take 0.1 mL	Aerobic gram negative bacteria
Ciprofloxacin	150 microgram/0.1 mL	200 mg in 100 mL—take 0.15 mL—add 0.05 mL ringer lactate— take 0.1 mL	Aerobic gram negative bacteria (*E. coli*, proteus), also Gram positive ones at higher concentration
Moxifloxacin	200 microgram/0.1 mL	0.05 mL of 0.5% moxifloxacin (preservative free) topical preparation	
Imipenum (250mg)	50–100 µg	250 mg - dilute with 100 mL of distilled water- take 0.2 mL (0.5 mg)-dilute with 0.3 mL sterile water - inject 0.05 mL	Aerobic and anaerobic both gram positive and gram negative bacteria, particularly against *Pseudomonas aeruginosa* and *Enterococcus* species
Piperacillin/ tazobactam (2.25 g)	225 µg	Add 10 mL of distilled water to 2.25 g vial - Take 0.1 mL-Add 0.9 distilled water-take 0.1 mL-Add 0.9 distilled water-take 0.1 mL to get concentration of 225 µg/0.01 mL	Tazobactam expands activity of piperacillin to include beta-lactamase producing strains of S. aureus, H. influenzae, *E. coli*, Bacteroides spp, and other gram-positive and gram-negative aerobic and anaerobic bacteria
Carbenicillin (1 g)	2000 µg	Add 5 mL of distilled water to 1 g vial - Take 0.1 mL solution & add 0.9 distilled water- take 0.05 mL (2000 µg)	Gram-negative coverage specially Pseudomonas aeruginosa
Ticarcillin (with clavulanate (3.1 g)	3000 µg	Add 9.7 mL of distilled water to 3.1 g vial - Take 0.1 mL solution & add 0.9 distilled water - Inject 0.1 mL (3000 µg)	Gram-negative coverage specially Pseudomonas aeruginosa

Antifungal Drugs

Drugs	*Dose*	*How to make intravitreal dose*	*Organisms against*
Amphotericin B	5 microgram/0.1mL	50 mg powder—add 10 mL—take 0.1 mL—add 9.9 mL of 5% dextrose—take 0.1mL	*Candida albicans*, *Aspergillus*
Voriconazole	50–100 microgram/0.1 mL	200 mg powder—add 19 mL of d/w—take 1.0 mL—add 9 mL of d/w—take 0.05 mL/0.1 mL	*Aspergillus* (invasive aspergillosis)—better than Amphotericin B *Candida*—as effective as Amphotericin B

Steroid

Dexamethasone	0.4 mg	8 mg in 2 mL vial—take 0.1 mL directly

Intravitreal Moxifloxacin

Use of fluoroquinolone antibiotics, in particular, the recently developed third- and fourth-generation fluoroquinolones, such as levofloxacin and moxifloxacin, with their enhanced activity against gram-positive pathogens, offer broad-spectrum activity that covers most organisms commonly encountered in bacterial endophthalmitis. After topical administration at two-hourly intervals, moxifloxacin reaches mean aqueous concentrations of 2.3 µg/mL. Systemic moxifloxacin does not exceed anterior chamber concentrations. It reaches intravitreal concentrations 10 times higher than levels achieved by topical use, but to reach *S. aureus* and certain fluoroquinolone-resistant strains, higher concentrations are needed. Recent data from toxicologic testing on ocular tissue indicate that intravitreal moxifloxacin in doses up to 150 µg/mL did not result in significant toxicity on several ocular cell types.
Potential advantages of intravitreal moxifloxacin are:

- It covers both gram-negative and gram-positive pathogens, including those most often implicated in the development of exogenous endophthalmitis
- The administration of only a single substance into the eye.

In Multidrug Resistant Gram-negative Infections

Recently, intravitreal piperacillin-tazobactam have been studied both in animal models and clinically especially in cases of Enterobacter species and multidrug-resistant Pseudomonas endophthalmitis with favorable outcomes. Combination therapy with Piperacillin and tazobactam (225 µgm/0.1 mL) complement in their mechanism of action against beta-lactamaseproducing organisms. Due to the production of high-levels of beta-lactamase, combination therapy with piperacillin and tazobactam is a safe and effective alternative in the management of multidrug-resistant gram-negative infections.

VITRECTOMY SURGERY

Pars plana vitrectomy offers several potential benefits for endophthalmitis treatment. Results from the EVS showed that immediate vitrectomy provides a clear benefit in a well-defined subgroup; patients with light perception only at the time of presentation had a significant, three-fold improved chance of obtaining a visual acuity of 20/40 after vitrectomy. If no result after intravitreal injection—as early as possible.

Advantages of Vitrectomy

- To decrease infective, toxic and inflammatory load
- To provide adequate undiluted specimen for culture studies (Culture positivity for vitreous biopsy is 40%)
- To increase antibiotic concentration and drug diffusion within the eye
- To remove media opacities which enables a rapid recovery.

Technique of Vitreous Biopsy

The safest method to obtain vitreous sample is by vitreous biopsy.

- The short tubing part of the suction line on the vitreous cutter is to be connected with a tuberculin syringe to enable manual suction
- The vitreous cutter is placed in the anterior vitreous and the cutting is actuated without making the preplaced infusion on (when a further vitrectomy has been planned)
- Simultaneously the assistant begins to withdraw the piston of the tuberculin syringe so as to induce suction
- The procedure is to be stopped once 0.2–0.3 mL of the sample has been obtained
- The lost volume of the vitreous can be replaced by injecting intravitreal antibiotic injection if no further vitrectomy has been planned or by opening the preplaced infusion line when a vitrectomy has already been planned
- The undiluted sample of the vitreous biopsy should be sent in a sterile manner to the laboratory.

Types of Vitrectomy

1. Conventional vitrectomy (commonly used for postoperative endophthalmitis)
   - Core vitrectomy means partial vitrectomy, i.e. removal of central 50% of vitreous
   - No intervention made at vitreoretinal interface
   - Peripheral vitreous skirt left untouched.

   Disadvantages:
   - There is a chance of rapid reaccumulation of vitreous exudates
   - Chance of cyclic membrane formation
   - Risk of chronic hypotony.
2. Radical vitrectomy (useful for fulminant cases, especially post-traumatic endophthalmitis)
   - More complete vitrectomy
   - Create PVD, if required
   - Removal of all tractional elements including track of penetrating injury
   - Trim peripheral vitreous skirt close to its insertion at ora
   - Removal of cyclic membrane, if required.

   Disadvantage: Risk of intraoperative retinal break formation and risk of retinal detachment.

Justification of Use of Silicone Oil in Endophthalmitis

1. For long-term intraocular tamponade at the end of vitrectomy.
2. Silicone oil compartmentalize the intraocular cavity into anterior and posterior segment. Anterior segment inflammation will be managed by topical antibiotic steroid and posterior segment inflammation (over retinal surface) will be managed by intravitreal antibiotics.
3. Intravitreal antibiotics will be at high-concentration in the fluid film present in the potential space between silicone oil and retina and these will act directly on inflamed retina for a longer duration, as intravitreal antibiotics in a vitrectomized nonsilicone oil-filled eye will be washed out rapidly after surgery.
4. Antimicrobial activity of SO - high surface tension and low permeability of silicone oil could limit the freedom of movement of the pathogens, concentrating them in the ciliary body or close to the retinal blood vessels where the defence mechanisms could act more effectively. Postoperative endophthalmitis.
5. Space-occupying action of a long-standing tamponade may play an important role in pathogens' and toxins' wash-out.
6. Silicone oil reduces the risk of postoperative retinal detachment, especially in case of undetected retinal breaks.
7. It allows laser photocoagulation.
8. It may also influence intravitreal antibiotic distribution and clearance.
9. Silicone oil prevents postoperative hypotony and ciliary body shock.

Postoperative Endophthalmitis

Case Discussion (Video 4, Chapter 17)

- A case of postoperative endophthalmitis
- The edematous corneal epithelium was removed (Fig. 17.5A)
- The next step is to clear exudates and hypopyon from anterior chamber (Fig. 17.5B)
- Removal of pupillary exudates by cutter (Fig. 17.5C)
- Retro-IOL exudates were removed and posterior capsulectomy was done (Fig. 17.5D)
- Vitrectomy was started to clear the vitreous exudates (Fig. 17.5E)
- The end point of vitrectomy should be the well-visualization of fundus (Fig. 17.5F)
- Intracameral vancomycin and voriconazole (can cause precipitate formation) (Fig. 17.5G)
- Intravitreal injection of antibiotics were given after removal of all cannulas (Fig. 17.5H).

Mixing intravitreal antibiotics which can cause precipitate formation in anterior chamber or vitreous cavity:

- Vancomycin and ceftazidime injection
- Vancomycin and voriconazole injection.

Management of Endogenous Endophthalmitis

In contrast with exogenous endophthalmitis, endogenous endophthalmitis requires systemic antimicrobial therapy. The primary source of infection in endogenous endophthalmitis is outside the eye, but within the body. Systemic antimicrobial therapy, for several weeks to ensure eradication of the infection, is the mainstay of endogenous endophthalmitis treatment. In most cases, treatment is initiated empirically and the infecting organism presumed to be that causing systemic infection.

Although systemic and intravitreal antibiotics may be sufficient in milder forms of infection, vitrectomy seems to be helpful in severe cases of endogenous endophthalmitis because of more virulent organisms, such as endotoxin-producing.

Special Situations

a. Pediatric/unco-operative/mentally retarded patients: The initial assessment can be followed by examination under anesthesia, with AC tap, and intravitreal antibiotics/surgery in the same sitting.
b. Dose adjustment:
   i. Vitrectomized eyes - increased daily frequency of intravitreal injections.
   ii. Silicone oil-filled eyes—half dose injections intravitreally, due to compartmentalization,
   iii. Pediatric age group half volumes injected due to smaller volumes of globe.
c. Other associated factors, like
   i. Corneal involvement—patch grafting in case of tunnel abscess of phaco entry wound or therapeutic penetrating keratoplasty before vitrectomy removes the source of infection as well as improves visualization,
   ii. Before glaucoma surgery, it is essential to manage the area of the filtering bleb or drainage device cautiously.

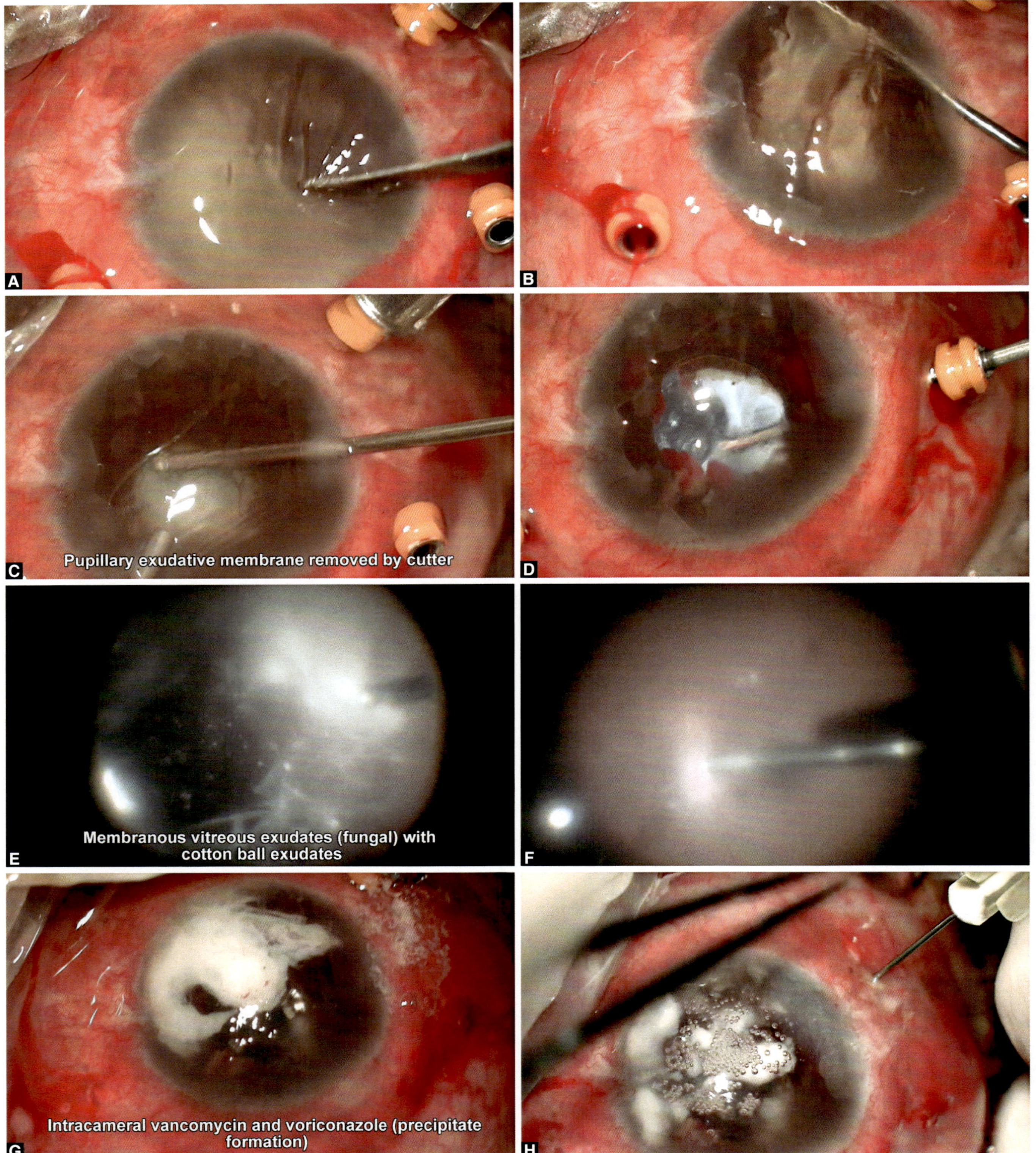

Figs 17.5A to H: Intraoperative steps of surgery managing postoperative endophthalmitis

Kindly scan the QR code below to access the online Video.

CHAPTER 18

Combined Phacoemulsification and Vitreoretinal Interventions

The development and progression of cataracts is an almost invariable consequence of pars plana vitrectomy, with up to 80% of vitrectomy patients developing or having progression of cataracts; thus need subsequent cataract extraction in majority of the eyes.

INDICATIONS FOR COMBINED CATARACT EXTRACTION WITH VITRECTOMY

The indications have expanded to include a variety of vitreoretinal diseases, including diabetic retinopathy, epiretinal membrane, macular hole and retinal detachment, all of which increase in prevalence with advancing age.

Combining two procedures phacoemulsification and vitrectomy into one procedure is known as phacovitrectomy. The reason for increased popularity of this combined procedure are as follows:

1. The prevalence of cataracts also increases with age. So cataract patients are frequently comorbid with these vitreoretinal diseases.
2. Use of intraocular tamponade as an adjunct during vitreoretinal surgery further contributes to the formation and progression of cataracts.

The main advantages of combined phacovitrectomy are:

1. Eliminating a second surgery.
2. Better access to the peripheral retina during phaco and possibly better outcomes.
3. A combined approach minimizes the surgical and economic burden of multiple surgeries.
4. It avoids anesthesias twice and its antecedent risks.
5. Additionally, combination surgery allows for faster patient recovery and earlier visual rehabilitation.

Animation of combined phacoemulsification with VR intervention

- Cataract extraction is required before retinal intervention to improve media clarity and to work with more precision (Fig. 18.1A); as well as for better vitreous base excision (Fig. 18.1B).

Options for Combined Phacoemulsification and Vitreoretinal Surgery

They are as follows *(Video 1, Chapter 18)*:

Option I

First perform phacoemulsification then introduce three ports followed by VR intervention in same sitting.

Option II

Introduce three pars plana ports, then go for phacoemulsification followed by VR intervention.

We generally follow the second option.

General Consideration

1. *Trocar placement*—It is the important first step in combined surgery. By inserting the trocars first, a closed system is maintained; thus making it easier to keep the globe firm during wound construction.

   After the first trocar is placed inferotemporally, the infusion cannula is inserted. Then superior cannulas are placed approximately 160° apart. This provides excellent access to the anterior segment.
2. Some prefer phacoemulsification first, then introduce 3 ports for vitreoretinal intervention.
   Disadvantage of this approach—The globe is difficult to keep firm when inserting the trocars. A long, angled incision is desirable for proper wound construction which is to be aided by flattening the sclera during trocar entry. The pressure on the globe, necessary to flatten the sclera, can cause the corneal incision to leak and destabilize the eye when the trocars are inserted after phacoemulsification.
3. *Timing of IOL implantation*—Foldable IOL is inserted immediately after phacoemulsification, prior to vitrectomy. It improves surgical efficiency.
4. The larger optic size, in conjunction with an appropriately sized anterior capsulorhexis, may help prevent pupillary capture during fluid-air exchange and gas tamponade.

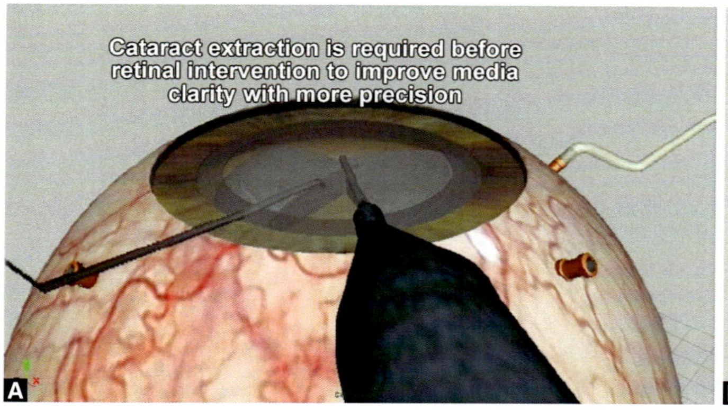

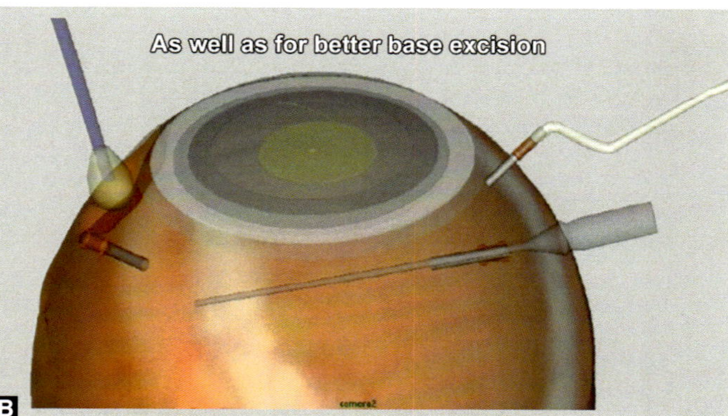

Figs 18.1A and B: (A) Phacoemulsification prior to vitreoretinal intervention; (B) Phacoemulsification facilitates better vitreous base excision

5. Gas tamponade after combined surgery is also associated with myopic refractive error, presumably due to anterior displacement of the IOL.
6. A known complication of cataract surgery is rupture of the posterior capsule, which occurs in 0.82% to 2.1% cases of combined phacoemulsification and vitrectomy. In the event of a posterior-capsule rupture, vitrectomy is performed to remove the anterior hyaloid and to separate the vitreous from the lens materials. Any residual nuclear material is then removed using the 23-gauge vitreous cutter with a low cut rate and high vacuum. The IOL lens can then be implanted into the ciliary sulcus over the anterior capsular rim.
7. Removal of the cataract additionally allows for better access to the vitreous base without the risk of touching the lens. More extensive removal of the anterior vitreous, as required in complex cases of diabetic tractional retinal detachment and in proliferative vitreoretinopathy, becomes easier after cataract extraction.
8. In vitrectomy for macular hole, a more complete vitrectomy allows for a larger gas-fill and a longer duration of tamponade, which may improve the closure rate.

Efficacy and safety of combined surgery for a variety of indications, including macular hole, ERM, proliferative diabetic retinopathy and other complex vitreoretinal diseases have been established.

Case Discussion

Phacoemulsification with Macular Surgery (Video 2, Chapter 18)

Steps of surgery:

- This is a 25G approach for cataract with epimacular membrane
- Phacoemulsification started after introducing 3 pars plana 25G port (Fig. 18.2A)
- Phacoemulsification completed and put foldable PCIOL (Fig. 18.2B)
- 25G Chandelier's illumination source introduced (Fig. 18.2C)
- Vitrectomy started (Fig. 18.2D)
- Triamcinolone injected to identify redial vitreous
- Fluid-air exchange done and trypan blue dye injected under air to stain epimacular membrane(Fig. 18.2E)
- Double dye stained thick epimacular membrane removed with the help of endgripping forceps (Fig. 18.2F)
- BBG dye injected under saline
- Fluid-air exchange done
- Residual ILM removed (Fig. 18.2G)
- Vitreous base checked (Fig. 18.2H)
- Fluid-air exchange done
- All 25G cannulas were removed (Fig. 18.2I).

Phacoemulsification with Diabetic Vitreous Hemorrhage (Video 3, Chapter 18)

Steps of surgery:

- A 25G approach in a case of cataract with diabetic vitreous hemorrhage
- Phacoemulsification started after introducing 3 pars plana 25G ports under no glow situation (Fig. 18.3A)
- Phacoemulsification was completed and put foldable PCIOL (Fig. 18.3B)
- Vitrectomy started (Fig. 18.3C)
- Sub hyaloid blood removed(Fig. 18.3D)
- Thick posterior hyaloids face with bridging TRDs identified and posterior hyaloid face trimmed (Fig. 18.3E)
- Segmentation of membranes done (Fig. 18.3F)
- Bleeders secured with cautery
- Triamcinolone particles injected and TA stained vitreoschisis membranes removed (Fig. 18.3G)
- Laser done and PRP completed (Fig. 18.3H)

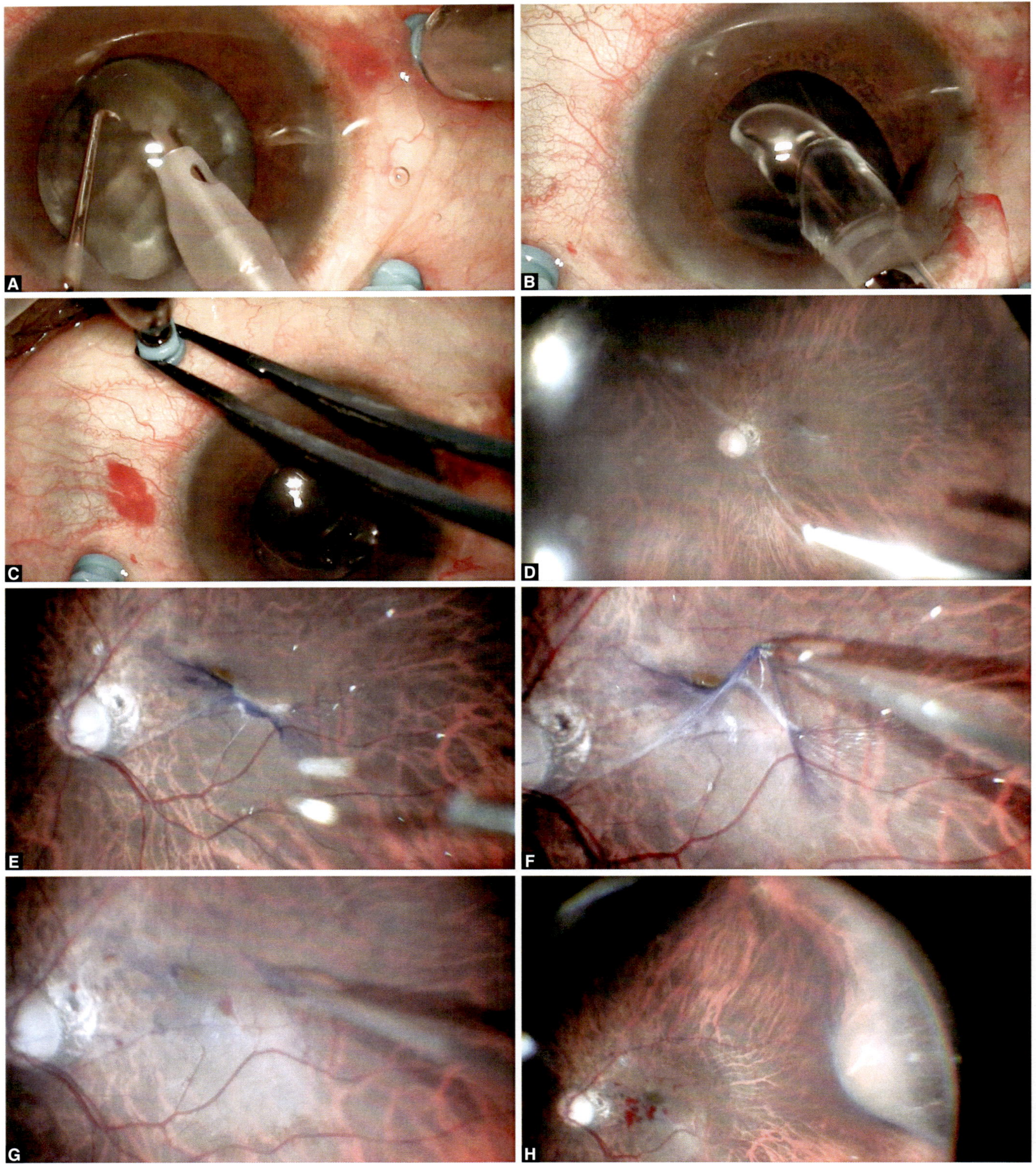

Figs 18.2A to H

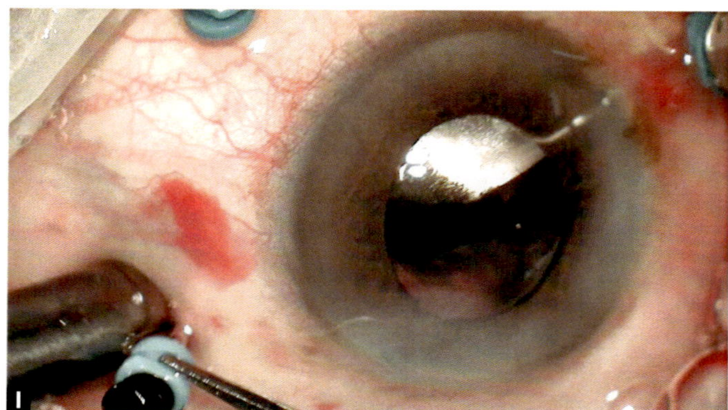

Figs 18.2A to I: Intraoperative steps of surgery managing cataract with epimacular membrane

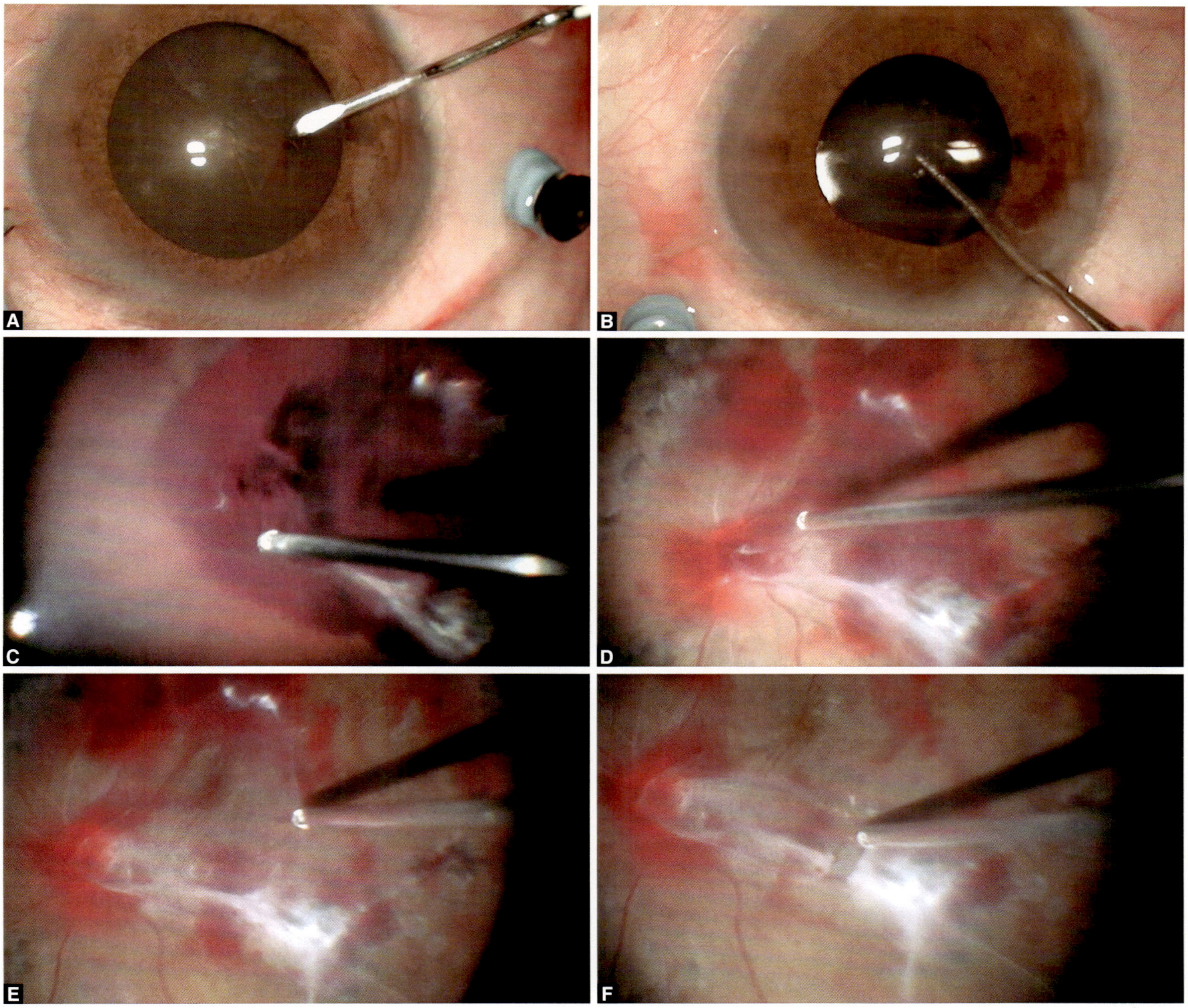

Figs 18.3A to F

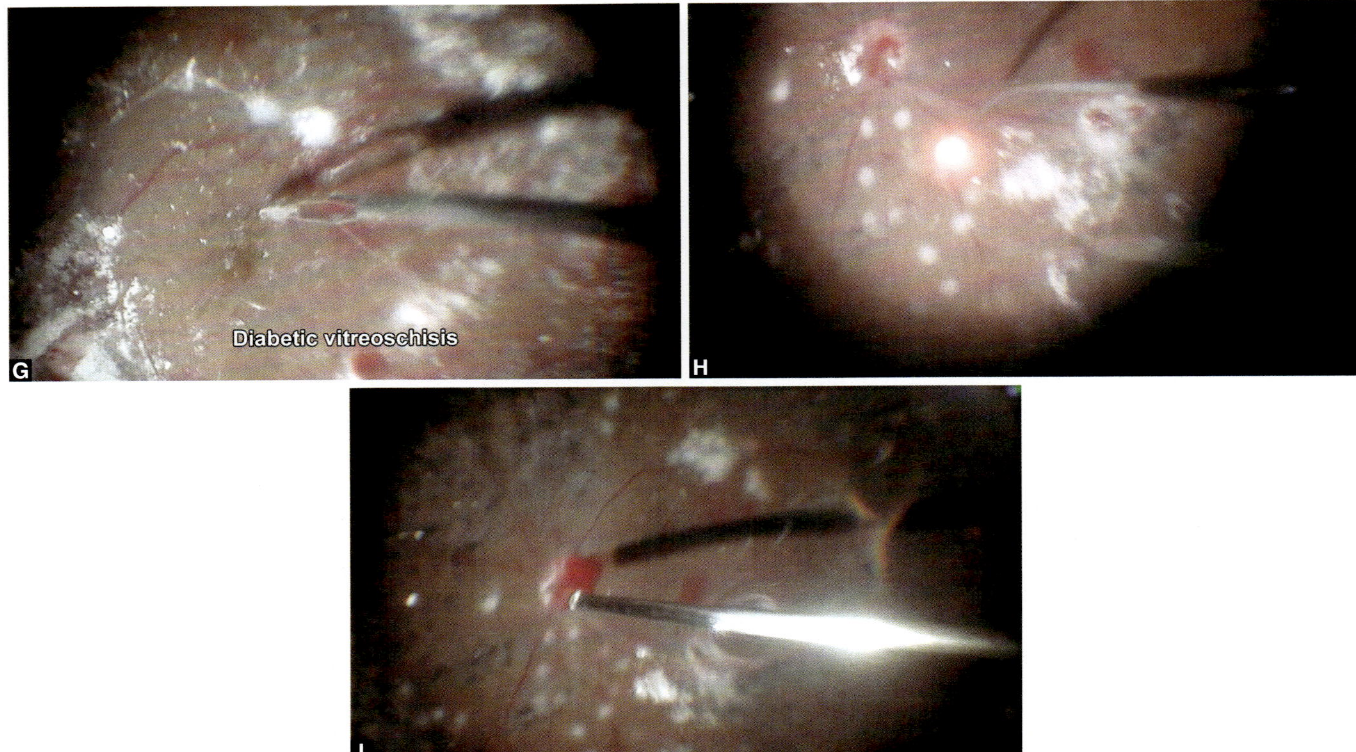

Figs 18.3A to I : Intraoperative steps of surgery managing cataract with diabetic vitreous hemorrhage

- Fluid-air exchange done and long acting C_3F_8 gas injected (Fig. 18.3I).

Phacoemulsification with Retinal Detachment (Video 4, Chapter 18)

Steps of surgery:

- A case of total RD with cataract
- Phacoemulsification started after introducing three pars plana ports (Fig. 18.4A)
- Many times direct chop is preferable (Fig. 18.4B). All lens fragments emulsified under grayish glow and foldable intraocular lens implanted
- 25G chandelier light introduced (Fig. 18.4C)
- Vitrectomy started
- There were multiple horse-shoe tears (Figs 18.4D and E)
- Triamcinolone acetonide injected
- Heavy fluid PFCL injected to stabilize posterior pole (Figs 18.4F and H)
- Vitreous base excision done (Fig. 18.4G)
- Fluid-air exchange started to drain anterior subretinal fluid (Fig. 18.4I)
- Barrage laser done securing all breaks (Fig. 18.4J)
- Silicone oil injected (Fig. 18.4K)

Postoperative problems:

1. Intracapsular IOL implantation in complex pathologies, involving issues such as posterior retinal detachments, uveitis, weak zonules and diabetes, can increase postoperative inflammation and result in posterior synechiae.
2. Decentration and early posterior capsular opacification are also common in phacovitrectomy patients. These often result from pressure from gas (Fig. 18.5) or air tamponade, which can lead to dislocation of the anterior capsule behind conventional IOLs in immediate postoperative period. At the end of surgery, the eye is filled with gas; once the patient gets up 2 to 3 hours after the procedure, the gas bubble creates its own force, which can cause IOL optic to move anterior to anterior

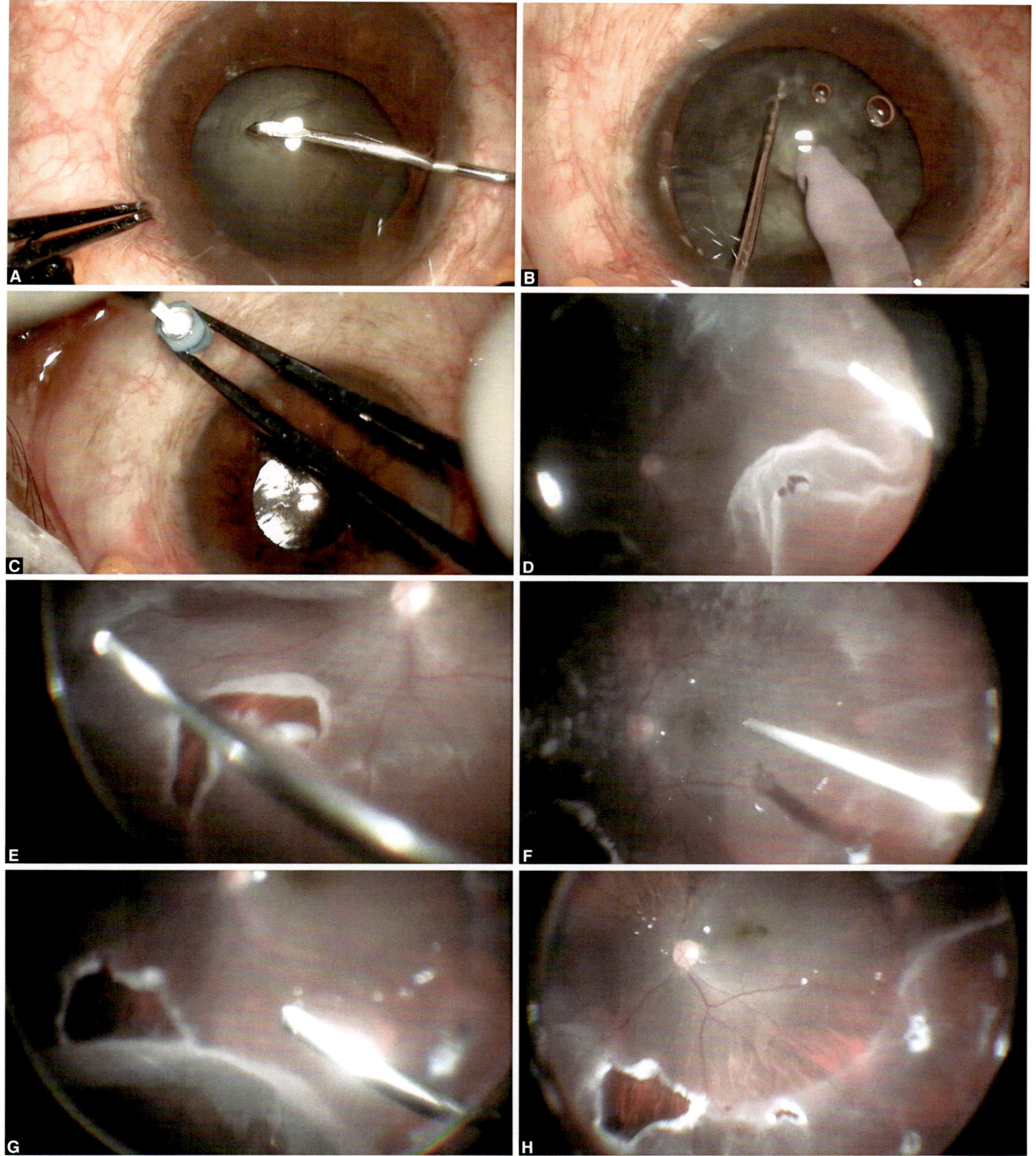

Figs 18.4A to H

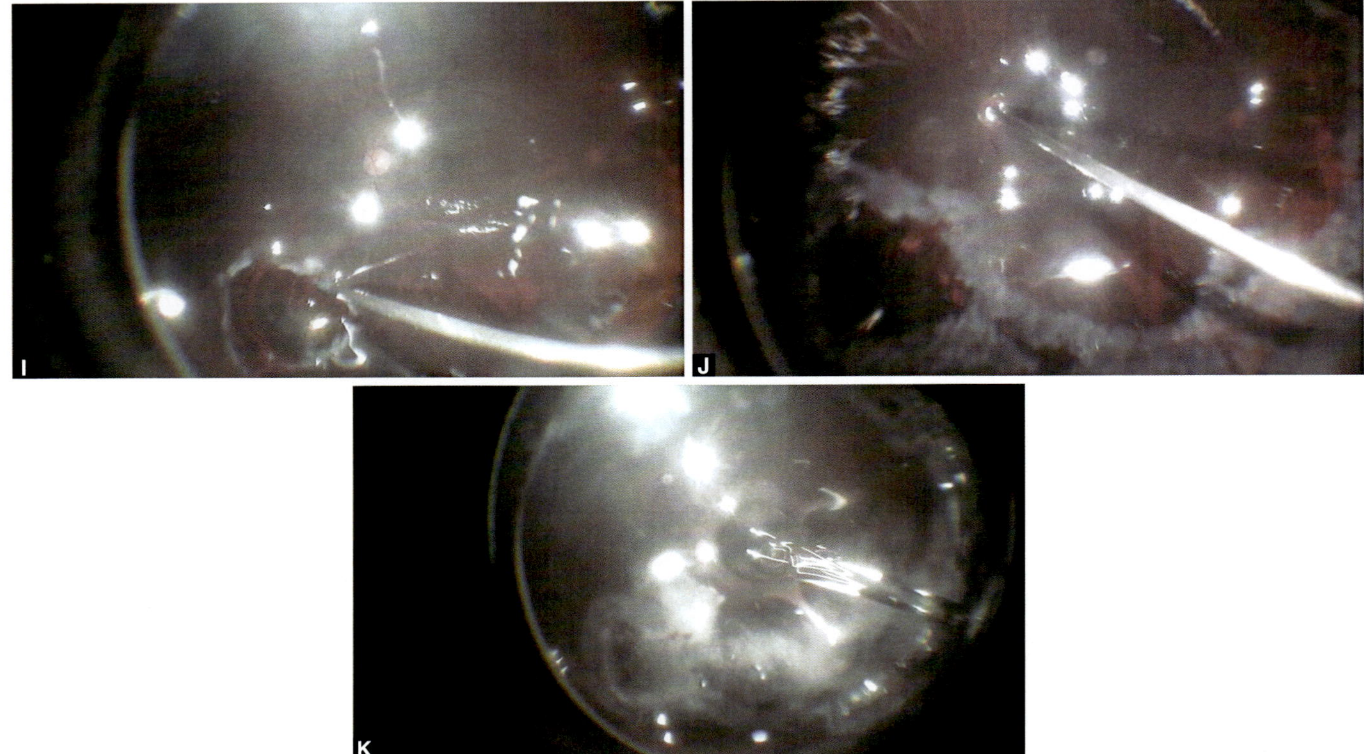

Figs 18.4A to K: Intraoperative steps of surgery managing cataract with total RD

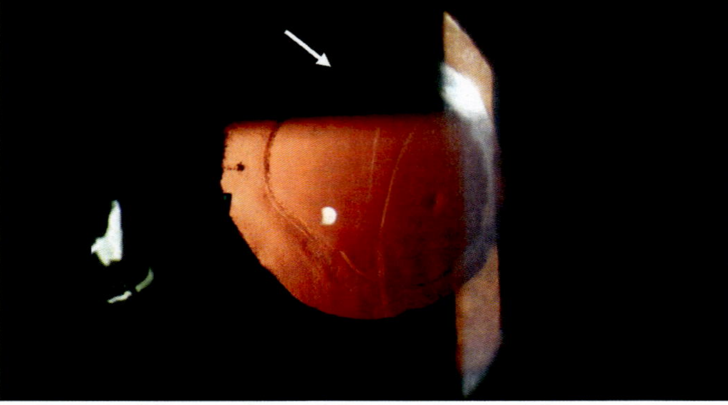

Fig. 18.5: Combined phaco with vitrectomy with retro IOL gas bubble (white arrow)

capsular rim, sometimes resulting in optic capture. This may also result in decentration of IOL as well as early posterior capsular opacification.

3. The inflammatory response may also induce morphologic changes to the ciliary body resulting in shallow anterior chamber and narrowing of the angle that have been observed more frequently after combined surgery compared to vitrectomy alone. Aggressive topical steroid to control postoperative inflammation may minimize these events.
4. Finally, use of an intraocular tamponade cause anterior displacement of the intraocular lens which may induce a myopic shift in the refractive outcome.

Kindly scan the QR code below to access the online Video.

CHAPTER 19

27G Vitrectomy and Recent Updates

INTRODUCTION

- The 27-G surgery was first introduced in 2007, when Oshima et al. introduced a 27-G Chandelier light
- Later Sakaguchi et al. published their experience performing 27-G nonvitrectomy for epiretinal membranes.

Advantages of 27-gauge vitreous surgery are:

- As it is less invasive thus, there is less conjunctival and scleral trauma and less inflammation
- Cause less astigmatism
- There is less postoperative discomfort and early visual recovery
- Smaller wounds are more likely to self-seal and prevent vitreous prolapse and hypotony.
- It reduces the risk of complications like choroidal detachment and endophthalmitis.

Disadvantages are:

- Increased instrument flexibility
- Limited aspiration capacity
- Some tasks difficult or impossible to perform, like removal of foreign body.

Introduction of 27-G vitrectomy system had some concerns like wound leakage, tool fragility and unavailability of corresponding instrumentation in early phase and therefore had very few indications like in myopic eyes with thin sclera, macular diseases, vitreous hemorrhage.

AVAILABLE 27-GAUGE INSTRUMENTS

27-G Vitrectomy Cutter (Fig. 19.1)

- Cut rate—5,000 cpm, now improved to 7,500 cpm.

Faster cut rates allow for safer peripheral vitreous dissection with less likelihood of creating a retinal tear formation at periphery.

Compared with the 25-gauge vitrectomy port, the 27-gauge vitrectomy port is larger (0.079 mm^2 vs 0.066 mm^2) and closer to the cutter tip (0.211 mm vs 0.330 mm). These features aid the surgeon in performing complex maneuvers such as vitrectomy-assisted membrane segmentation and delamination. To address the concern of increased flexibility with 27-gauge instrumentation, Oshima et al. shortened the shaft length of the 27-gauge vitreous cutter from 32 mm to 25 mm, resulting in comparable stiffness to the 25-gauge vitrectomy system.

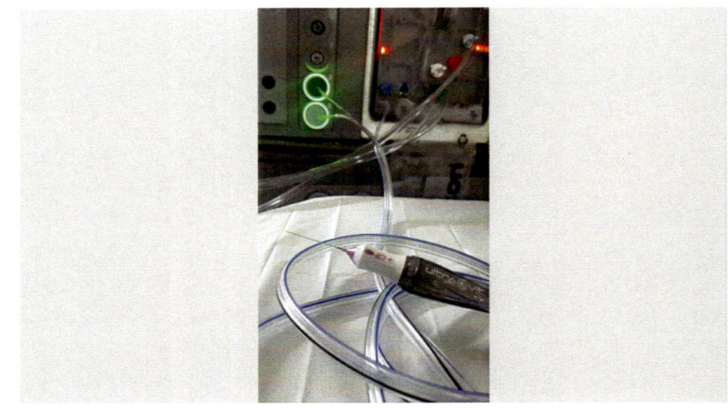

Fig. 19.1: 27-G vitrectomy cutter

Endoilluminator

- Endoillumination efficiency reduces by about 35% when the diameter of the light pipe falls by 20%. Xenon and mercury vapor lamps are powerful enough to provide excellent illumination with 27- and 29-gauge fibers (more than 20 lumens)
- 27-G fibers are available in both focal and wide-angle illumination.

Chandelier Endoilluminator

- The tip is introduced about 3 mm into the vitreous cavity, so the reflected glare from the tip is mostly blocked by the iris during surgery
- The tip of the light fiber is shaped-like a cone for wide-angle illumination

- A polyamide sleeve (arrow) covers the microfiber to prevent thermal burn-induced scleral damage
- Panoramic fundus view under 27-gauge chandelier endoillumination
- Sufficient illumination and wide-angle view of the fundus is obtained without reflecting glare into the surgeon's eyes.

Instruments for epiretinal membrane removal

Shaft of the microforceps—0.40 mm in diameter, is rigid and thin enough for intraocular manipulation. The shape of the grasping end is asymmetric.

Recent Advancement in 27-G Vitrectomy System and Insertion Techniques

- Stiffer instruments
- Wide-angle illuminating light pipe, using xenon/mercury vapor light
- Chandelier endoilluminating optic fibers
- One step vertical non-beveled insertion—trocar cannula, instead of 2 step/angled sclerotomies
- Self-sealing sclerotomies
- Different microarchitecture design of the 27-gauge vitrectomy system with reduced internal diameter results in a decreased flow rate. As compared to 25-G, a 20% reduction in the lumen leads to about 65% reduction in the flow (Poiseuille's law—flow proportional to the fourth power of radius). With a shorter shaft length, 27-G cutters allow approximately 55% less flow rate than 25-G cutters. This decreased flow rate is overcome by using higher aspiration rates and higher infusion rates
- 27-G cutter port is larger and closer to the tip that helps to deal complex maneuvers safely and predictably
- 27-G cutter easily passes between the membrane and the retina
- The duty cycle of 27-G cutter is found to be better than 25-G cutter at 2,500 cpm. The new TDC cutters from DORC (Zuidland, Netherland) go up to 8,000 cpm while maintaining a duty cycle of 92% and a high relatively constant aspiration rate.
- Advanced Ultravit cutter in Constellation system allows 10,000 cpm
- Hypervit dual-blade pneumatic cutter with 20,000 cpm.

Characteristic features of hypervit 27G dual blade vitrectomy probe:

- Continuously open port to improve vitreous flow
- High cut rate (20000 cpm) to reduce pulsatile traction on the retina
- Beveled-tip design to improve access to tissue plane, which improves cutter efficiency
- As the cutter port is very close to the cutter tip (port-surface distance is 0.229 mm), one can reach very close to the retinal surface for membrane dissection. This is particularly important in cases of macular surgeries, which reduces the chances of iatrogenic retinal break formation.

Common Indications for 27-G Vitrectomy

- Macular pathologies, like macular holes, macular epiretinal membrane and puckers, vitreomacular traction, macular edema associated with diabetic retinopathy, retinal vein occlusion, uveitis, persistent cystoids macular edema, subinternal limiting membrane hemorrhage
- Symptomatic extensive vitreous floaters (on patient's choice)—called 'floaters only vitrectomy' (FOV)
- Vitreous hemorrhage and focal tractional retinal detachment
- Simple vitreous hemorrhage
- Vitreous biopsy
- Primary rhegmatogenous retinal detachment
- Moderate PDR with or without focal tractional retinal detachment
- Surgery in myopes with thin sclera.

27-G Vitreous Surgeries

Case-I—Vitreous Hemorrhage (Video 1, Chapter 19)

Case discussion:

- 27-G ports placed (Fig. 19.2A)
- Vitrectomy started to clear vitreous hemorrhage (Fig. 19.2B)
- Preretinal blood removed (Fig. 19.2C)
- Old branch retinal vein occlusion detected along with a large break (Fig. 19.2D)
- Barrage laser around the break as well as scatter laser done (Fig. 19.2E)
- Fluid-air exchange done (Fig. 19.2F)
- Long-acting gas C_3F_8 injected.

Case II—Idiopathic Epimacular Membrane (Video 2, Chapter 19)

Case discussion:

- Three pars plana 27-G ports were introduced along with 27-G twin Chandelier light (Fig. 19.3A)
- Vitrectomy was done
- Epimacular membrane was quite thick (Fig. 19.3B)
- TA-assisted PVD induction was done
- TA-stained epimacular membrane was removed by a 27-G membrane pick forceps (Fig. 19.3C)
- Fluid-air exchange was performed (Fig. 19.3D)

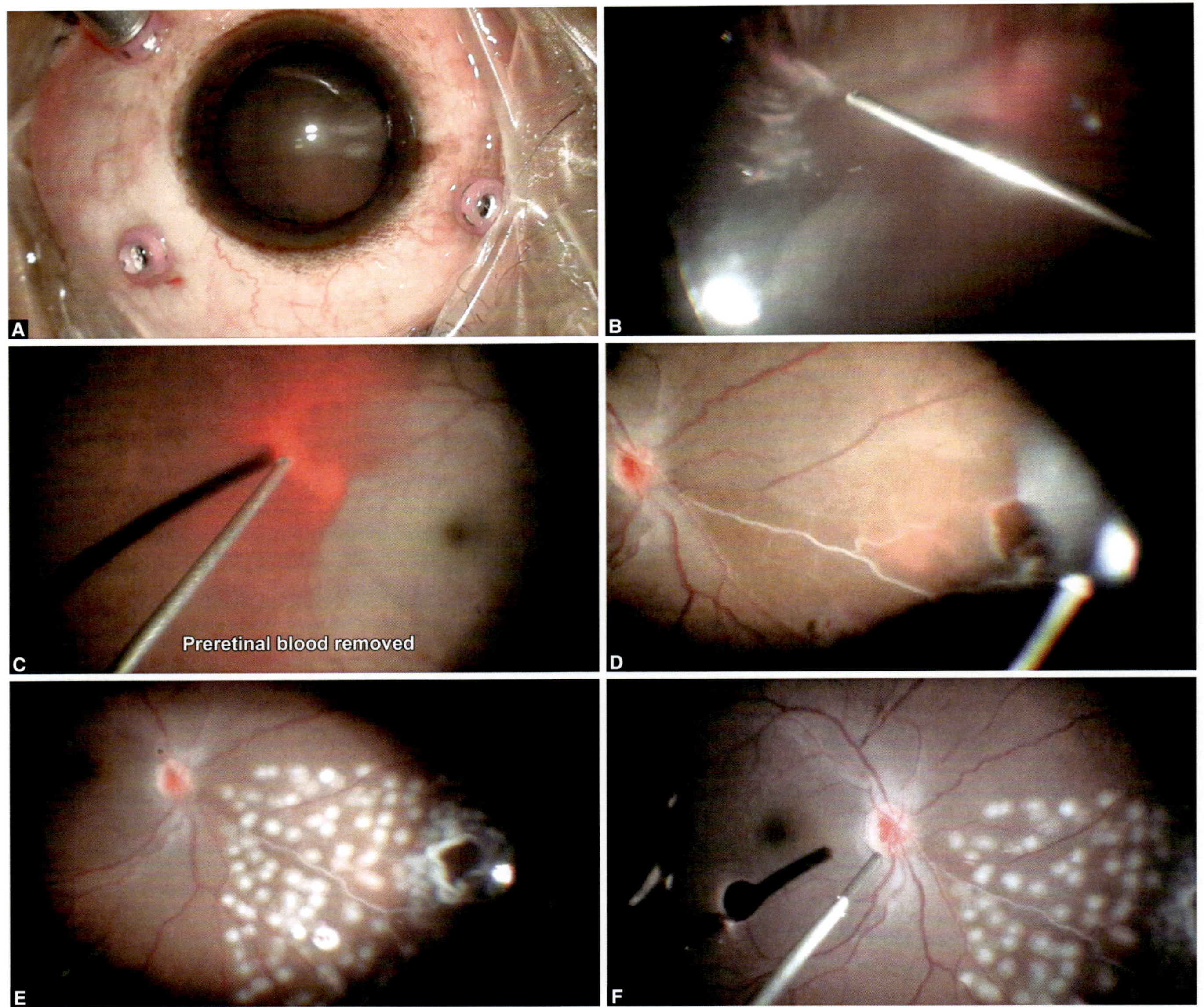

Figs 19.2A to F: Intraoperative steps of 27-G vitrectomy surgery managing vitreous hemorrhage

- 27-G valved cannulas along with twin light sources were removed (Fig. 19.3E).

Case III—Cataract with Full Thickness Macular Hole (Video 3, Chapter 19)

Case discussion:

- Three pars plana 27-G ports were introduced
- Phacoemulsification was completed (Fig. 19.4A) and put foldable posterior chamber intraocular lens (PCIOL)
- 27-G twin Chandelier's light was introduced (Fig. 19.4B)
- Now we started vitrectomy (Fig. 19.4C)
- Triamcinolone was injected—Residual TA particles were removed with the suction of 27-G cutter
- Brilliant Blue G dye was injected in saline (Fig. 19.4D) and waited for 2 to 3 minutes
- We used 27-G membrane scrapper and 27-G membrane pic forceps for ILM peeling
- Excess dye was removed with the suction of a cutter—Dye stained ILM peeling was started creating a flap by 27-G membrane scrapper—ILM peeling was completed in an onion-peel manner by 27-G end gripping forceps (Fig. 19.4E)
- Vitreous base was checked for any break (Fig. 19.4F)
- Fluid-air exchange was done (Fig. 19.4G)
- PI was done with 27-G cutter

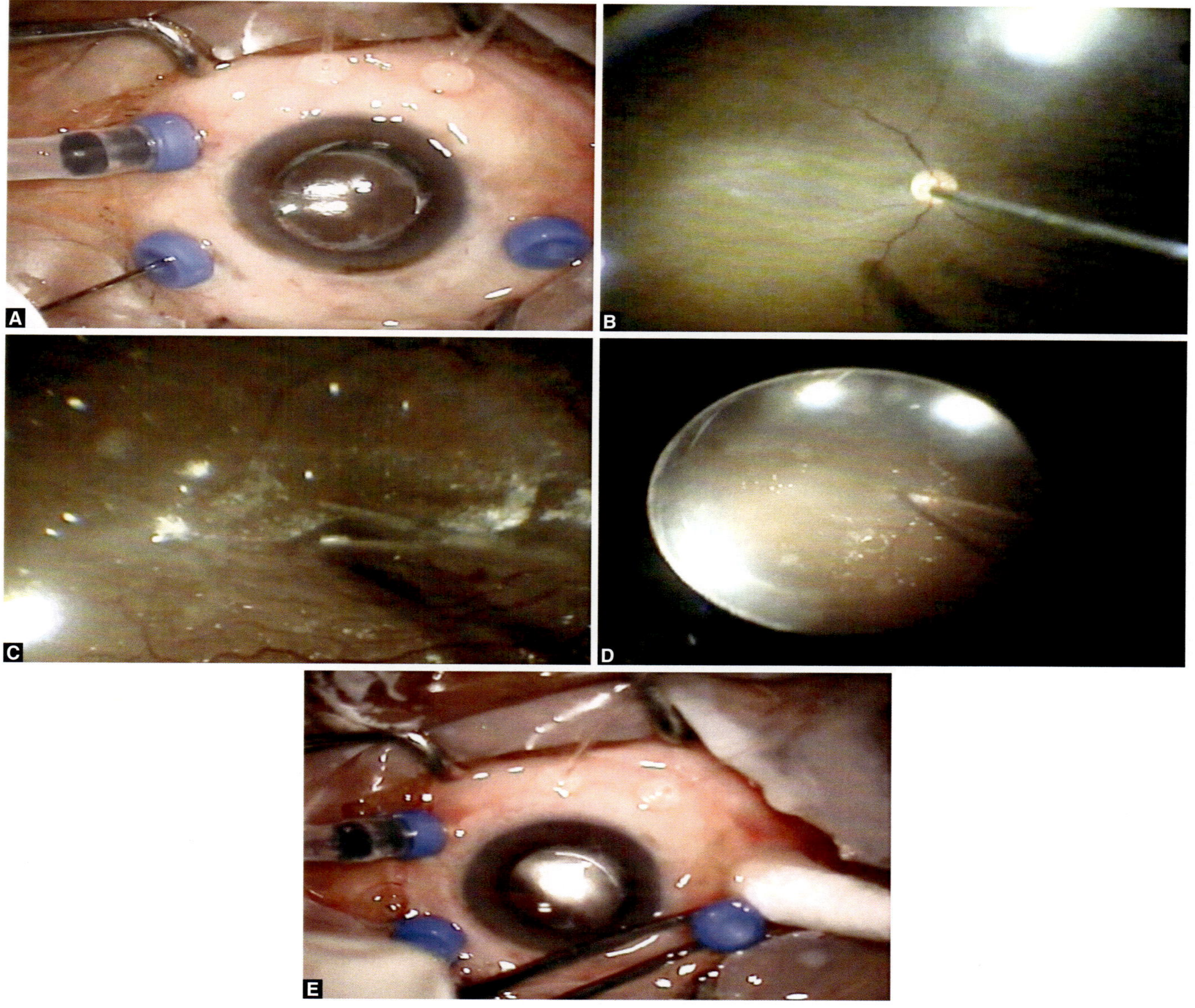

Figs 19.3A to E: Intraoperative steps of 27-G vitrectomy surgery for epimacular membrane

- 27-G valved cannulas along with twin light sources were removed (Fig. 19.4H)
- Long-acting gas was injected at the end of surgery.

Case IV—Retinal Detachment (Video 4, Chapter 19)

Case discussion:

- Three pars plana 27-G ports introduced
- A 25-G valved cannula with trocar-cannula introduce directly to introduce Chandelier light (Fig. 19.5A)
- 27-G vitrectomy started (Fig. 19.5B)
- Vitreous surrounding the inferior horse shoe tears removed and margins trimmed (Fig. 19.5C)
- Triamcinolone particle injected
- PVD was already induced and residual TA particles removed with the suction of cutter (Fig. 19.5D)
- Now heavy liquid PFCL injected to stabilize the posterior pole (Fig. 19.5E)
- Vitreous-based excision started by external scleral depression (Fig. 19.5F)
- Fluid-air exchange started and anterior SRF drained (Fig. 19.5G)
- Laser barrage done around the inferior breaks as well as 360 degres (Fig. 19.5H)
- PFCL removed and silicone oil injected through the 25-G port with endoilluminator in right hand (Fig. 19.5I).

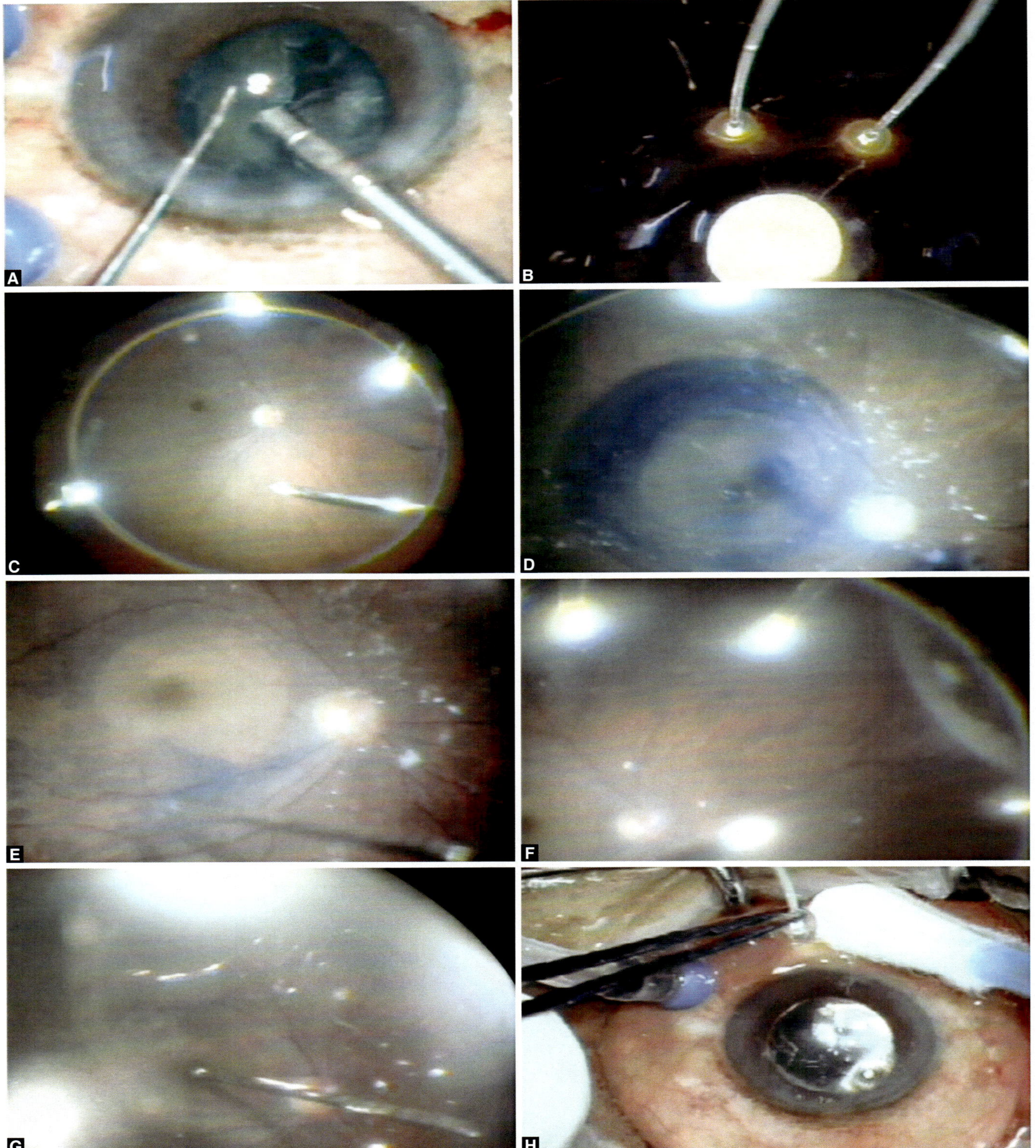

Figs 19.4A to H: Intraoperative steps of 27-G vitrectomy surgery for cataract with full thickness macular hole

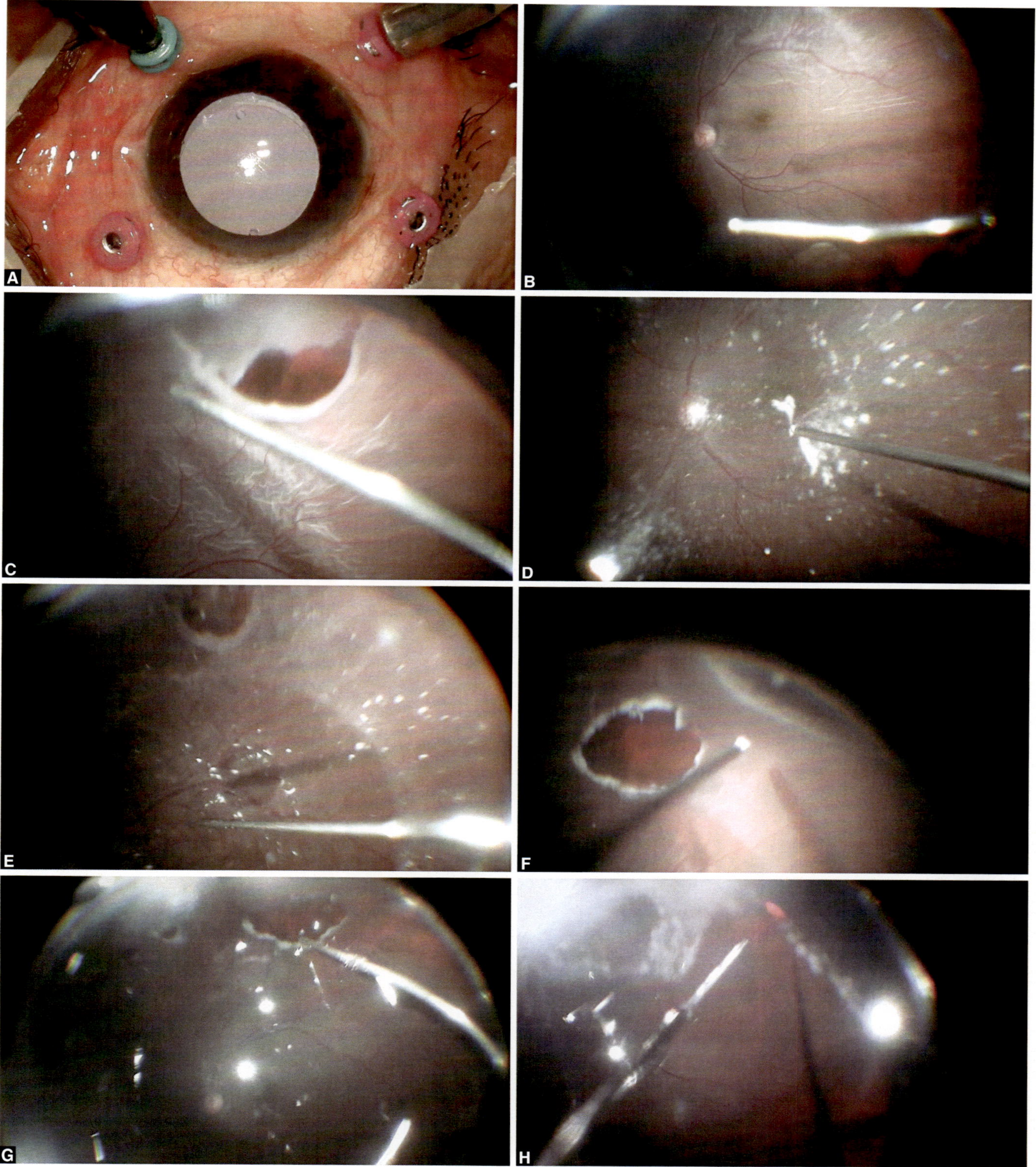

Figs 19.5A to H

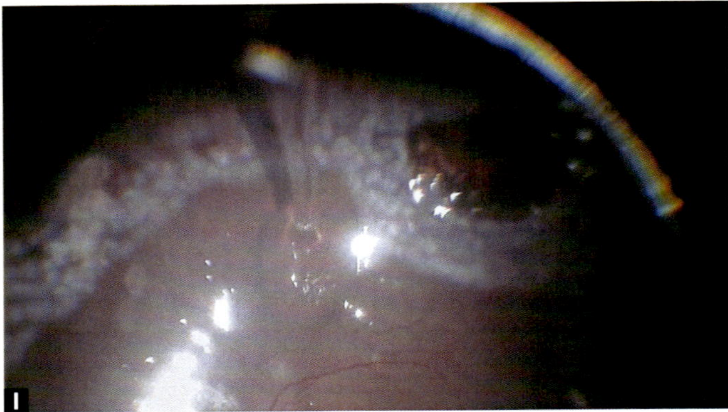

Figs 19.5A to I: Intraoperative steps of 27-G vitrectomy surgery for retinal detachment

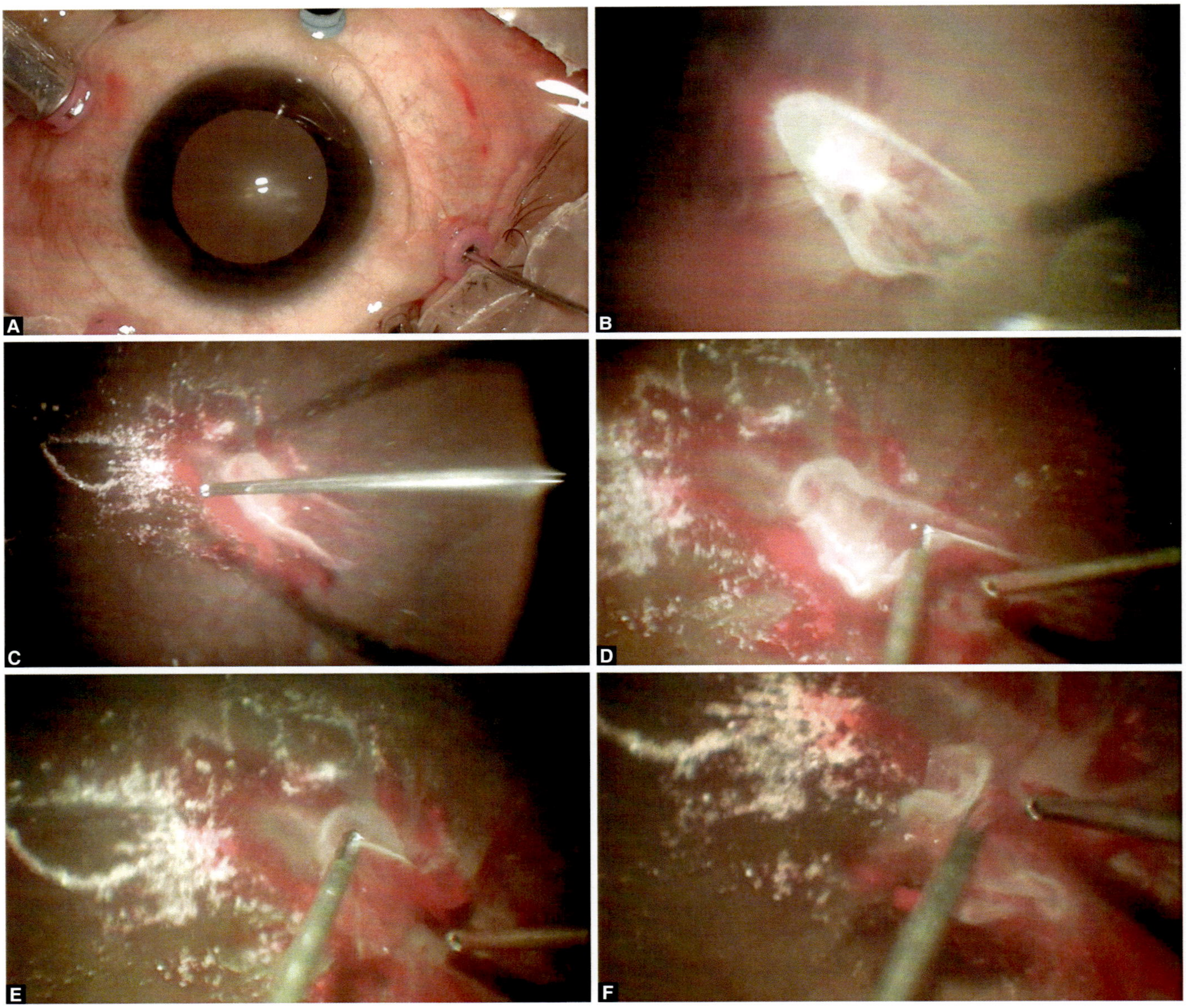

Figs 19.6A to F

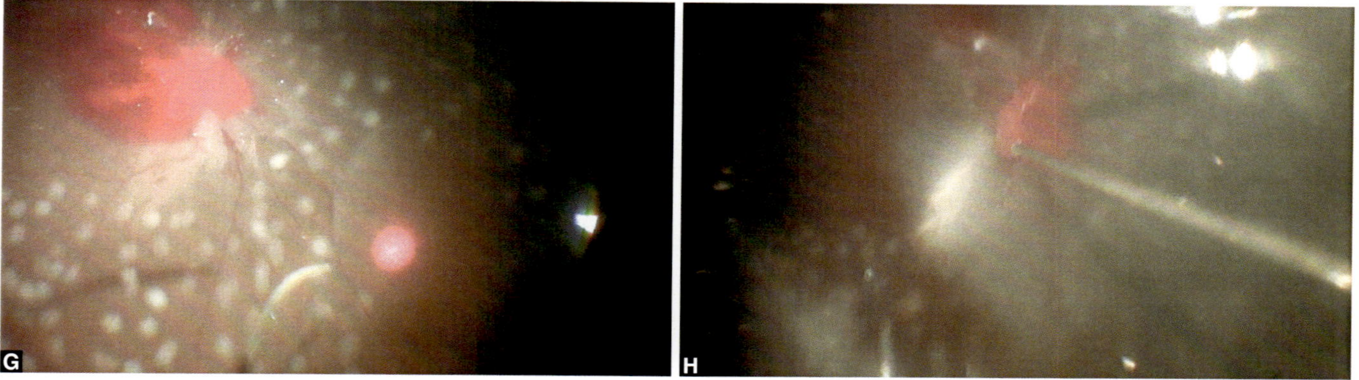

Figs 19.6A to H: Intraoperative steps of 27-G vitrectomy surgery for advanced diabetic TRD

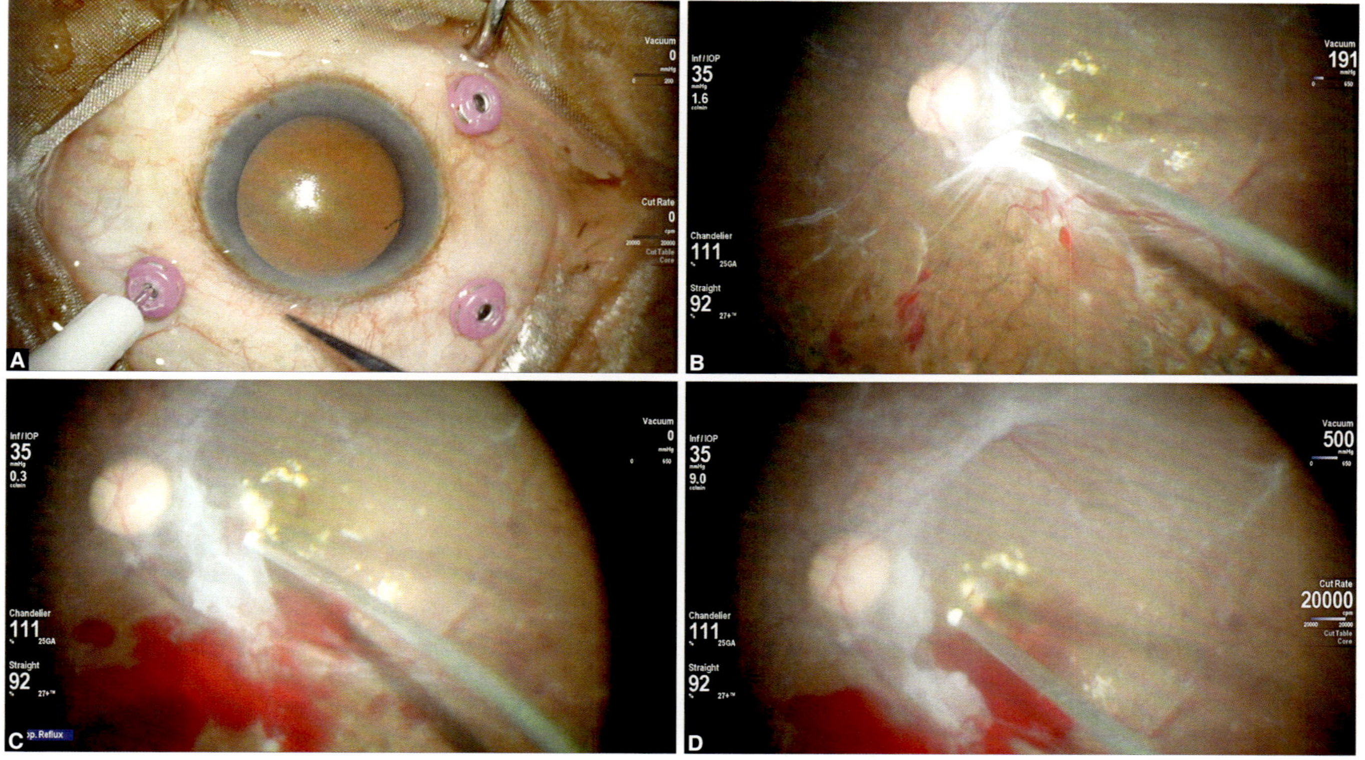

Figs 19.7A to D: Shows intraoperative steps with 27G Hypervit cutter in a case of advanced PDR with florid vascular epiretinal membranes

Case V—Complex Diabetic TRDs (Video 5, Chapter 19)

Case discussion:

- 27-G ports placed
- A 25-G Chandelier light used as fourth port (Fig. 19.6A)
- It was a case of advanced PDR (Fig. 19.6B)
- TA assisted vitrectomy completed (Fig. 19.6C)
- Membrane dissection started bimanually (Fig. 19.6D)
- One edge of membrane held with ILM forceps and segmentation done with cutter (Fig. 19.6E)
- Membrane delamination done (Fig. 19.6F)
- All bleeders cauterized
- Laser done (Fig. 19.6G)
- Fluid-air exchange done (Fig. 19.6H)
- Long-acting gas injected.

Case VI with 27G Hypervit System (Video 6, Section 19)

Case discussion:

- A case of advanced PDR with florid vascular epiretinal membranes
- 27G Hypervit system was used in this case (Fig. 19.7A)

- After vitrectomy, the cutter was used for membrane dissection
- The cutter was used to lift the fibrovascular membrane and to cut all its vascular attachments with the underlying retina (Fig. 19.7B)
- Then the beveled-tip cutter was used to insinuate in between the retina and the membrane and the proportionate reflux mode was activated to separate its vascular attachment with the foveal tip (Fig. 19.7C)
- The membrane was then segmented (Fig. 19.7D)

Kindly scan the QR code below to access the online Video.

CHAPTER 20

Scleral Fixation of IOL With or Without Glue

INTRODUCTION

Options for eyes with weak zonules or a torn capsule are either implanting an anterior chamber (AC) intraocular lens (IOL) or suturing a posterior chamber (PC) IOL into the ciliary sulcus. But in cases of inadequate support of capsular rim, especially inferiorly or in case of complete loss of capsular bag or in case of post-traumatic dislocation crystalline lens, implantation of IOL is a challenging situation. Scleral fixation of IOL with proline suture was a standard technique. But to secure IOLs in these cases in a newer way is "sutureless, fibrin glue–assisted posterior chamber intraocular lens (PCIOL) implantation with intrascleral tunnel fixation." However, "glued IOL" is the shorthand label. The first such implant was performed in 2007 by Professor Amar Agarwal.

Fibrin glue: First developed by Matras et al. in 1972.

Fibrin sealant is now FDA approved for use as a topical hemostat, sealant, adhesive.

Tisseel (Baxter Immuno, Vienna, Austria) was the first FDA approved fibrin sealant. Fibrin glue has two main components that occur naturally in the blood: fibrinogen and thrombin. The additional ingredients are aprotinin and calcium chloride. They are kept separate before use; once they are mixed, the thrombin promotes rapid conversion of fibrinogen to fibrin, producing a local fibrin clot. Macrophages and fibroblasts fully resorb fibrin glue in about two weeks.

I. SCLERAL FIXATION OF IOL WITH GLUE

Technique of Glued IOL

1. Two scleral flaps and sclerotomies, as well as two scleral tunnels or pockets under the flaps, are created exactly 180 degrees from one another, at either 3 and 9 o'clock or 6 and 12 o'clock; a scleral marker is used to ensure precise positioning. Fluid should always be kept in the eye during the surgery, using a trocar cannula or AC maintainer.
2. After performing a partial or full vitrectomy (to prevent retinal traction as the IOL is manipulated), the surgeon uses both hands to place the optic of a three-piece foldable PCIOL into the sulcus. The leading haptic must protrude from the injector while the IOL is being placed.
3. After the IOL optic unfolds within the anterior chamber, the leading haptic is grasped gently at the distal tip and externalized through scleral incisions. A two forceps "handshake" technique is used to reposition the trailing haptic, so it can be passed through the sclerotomy on the other side.
4. Each haptic is tucked securely into a Scharioth scleral tunnel (linear scleral tunnel made parallel to the limbus by a 26G needle).
5. After drying the scleral surface for optimal adhesion, the surgeon places a drop of fibrin glue underneath each scleral flap, over the tunnel entrance. The glue consists of two components that are not mixed until use; these components may be applied through a dual-chamber applicator or placed sequentially with 30-gauge needles and mixed on the ocular surface.
6. Slight pressure is applied to the flap for about 20 seconds to seal securely.

Case Discussion

Basic Steps of Glued IOL

Standard Glued IOL surgery (Video 1, Chapter 20)

- A case of decentered polymethyl methacrylate (PMMA) IOL with large posterior capsular rent (Fig. 20.1A)
- Retro-IOL vitreous removed
- IOL prolapsed in anterior chamber and then removed
- Triamcinolone injected in anterior vitreous to check for vitreous prolapse
- Superior capsular remnant removed
- TA stained prolapsed vitreous removed
- Vitrectomy completed
- Vitreous-based excision done by external scleral depression (Fig. 20.1B)

- Conjunctival flaps made 180 degrees apart along 3 and 9 o'clock (Fig. 20.1C)
- Marking done to make scleral flaps with a scleral marker (Fig. 20.1D)
- 2 mm base/2 mm length scleral flap made 2 mm away from the limbus (Fig. 20.1E)
- Similar scleral flap made in opposite side
- Pars plana separate entry were made at the base of scleral flaps with 23G trocar blade (Fig. 20.1F)
- Now, a 23G end gripping forceps was introduced through left pars plana scleral tunnel (Fig. 20.1G)
- A multipiece IOL introduced through the main scleral tunnel
- Forceps should hold the tip of inferior haptics and it was taken out of sclera tunnel (Fig. 20.1H)
- Superior haptic also introduced and it was made out of scleral tunnel (Fig. 20.1I)
- Linear scleral tunnels were made inferiorly and superiorly at the sides of scleral flaps by a 26G needle parallel to the limbus (Fig. 20.1J)
- Haptic tips had been engaged to the linear scleral tunnel (Scharioth tunnel) in both sides (Fig. 20.1K)
- Now two drops of fibrin glue were applied at the base of scleral flaps (Fig. 20.1L) and they were firmly apposed to the base (Fig. 20.1M)
- Now conjunctival wounds closed similarly with the help of the same glue (Fig. 20.1N).

Dislocated Sutured Scleral Fixated IOL

Case Discussion (Video 2, Chapter 20)

- It was a case of partially dropped scleral fixated rigid IOL with one attachment (Fig. 20.2A)
- Vitreous around the haptic removed
- Pars plana area checked to assess the proline suture fixated haptic with pars plana (Fig. 20.2B)
- Haptic with sutures separated from the pars plana area and removed (Figs 20.2C to E)
- Residual vitrectomy with vitreous base excision done (Fig. 20.2F)
- Standard 2 mm base/2 mm length scleral flaps made 2 mm away from the limbus 180 degrees apart (Fig. 20.2G)
- Pars plana entry with 23G trocar blade done on both sides (Fig. 20.2H)
- Linear scleral tunnels made parallel to the limbus at the sides of scleral flaps and marked with trypan blue dye (Fig. 20.2I).
- Now, a 23 G end-gripping forceps was introduced through left pars plana scleral tunnel
- A multipiece IOL introduced through the main scleral tunnel
- Forceps should hold the tip of inferior haptics and it was taken out of scleral tunnel (Fig. 20.2J)

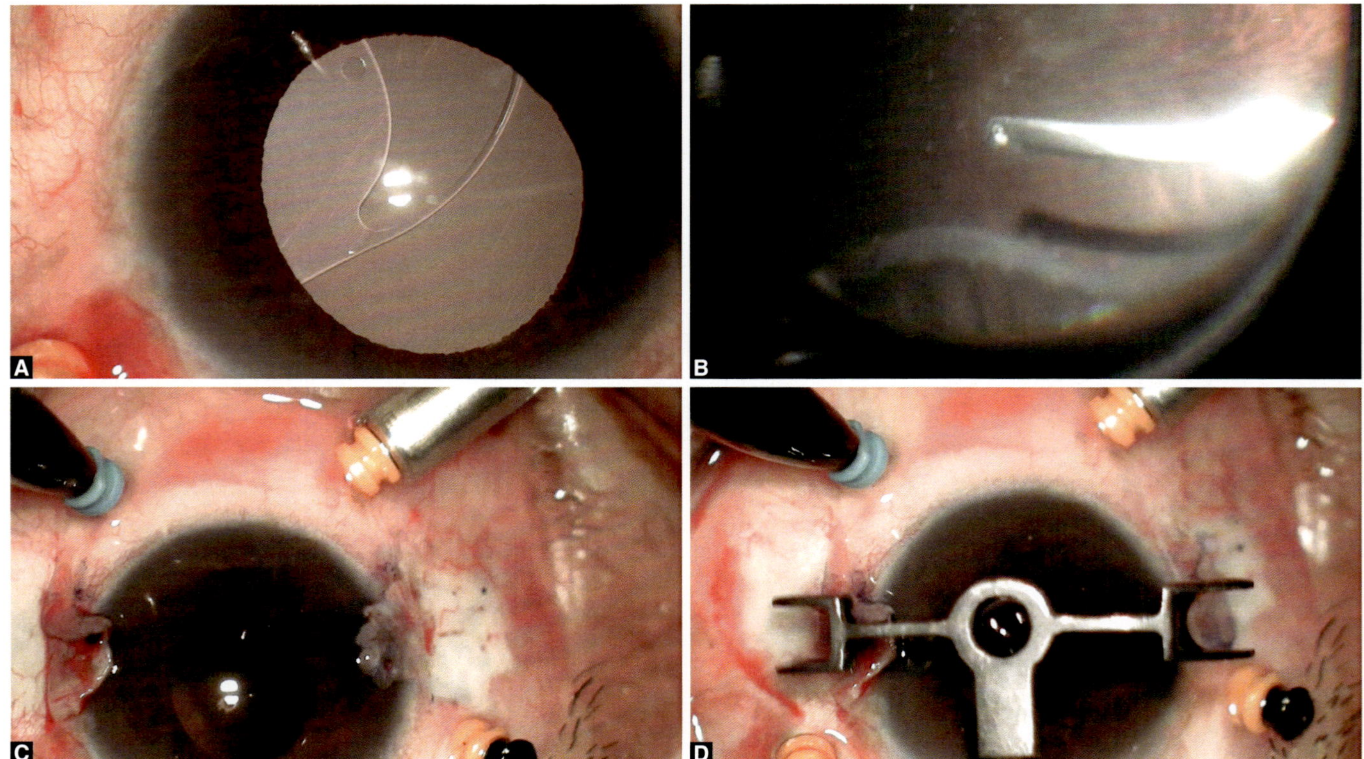

Figs 20.1A to D

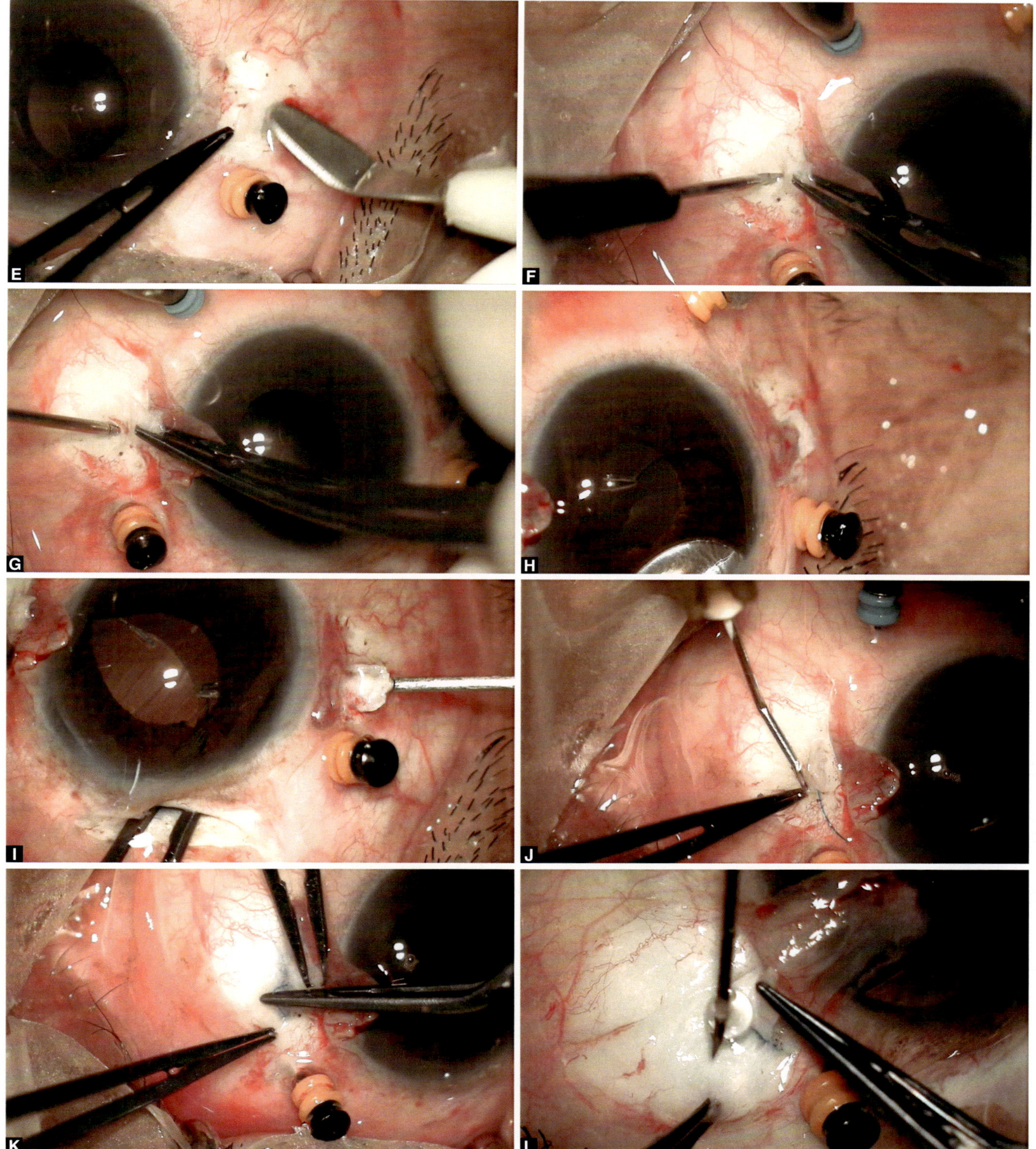

Figs 20.1E to L

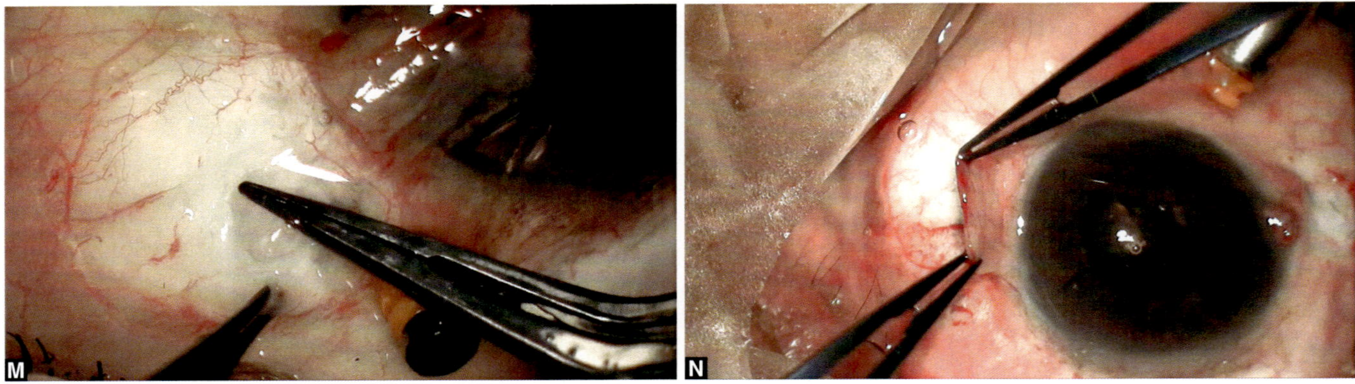

Figs 20.1A to N: Intraoperative steps of standard glued IOL surgery

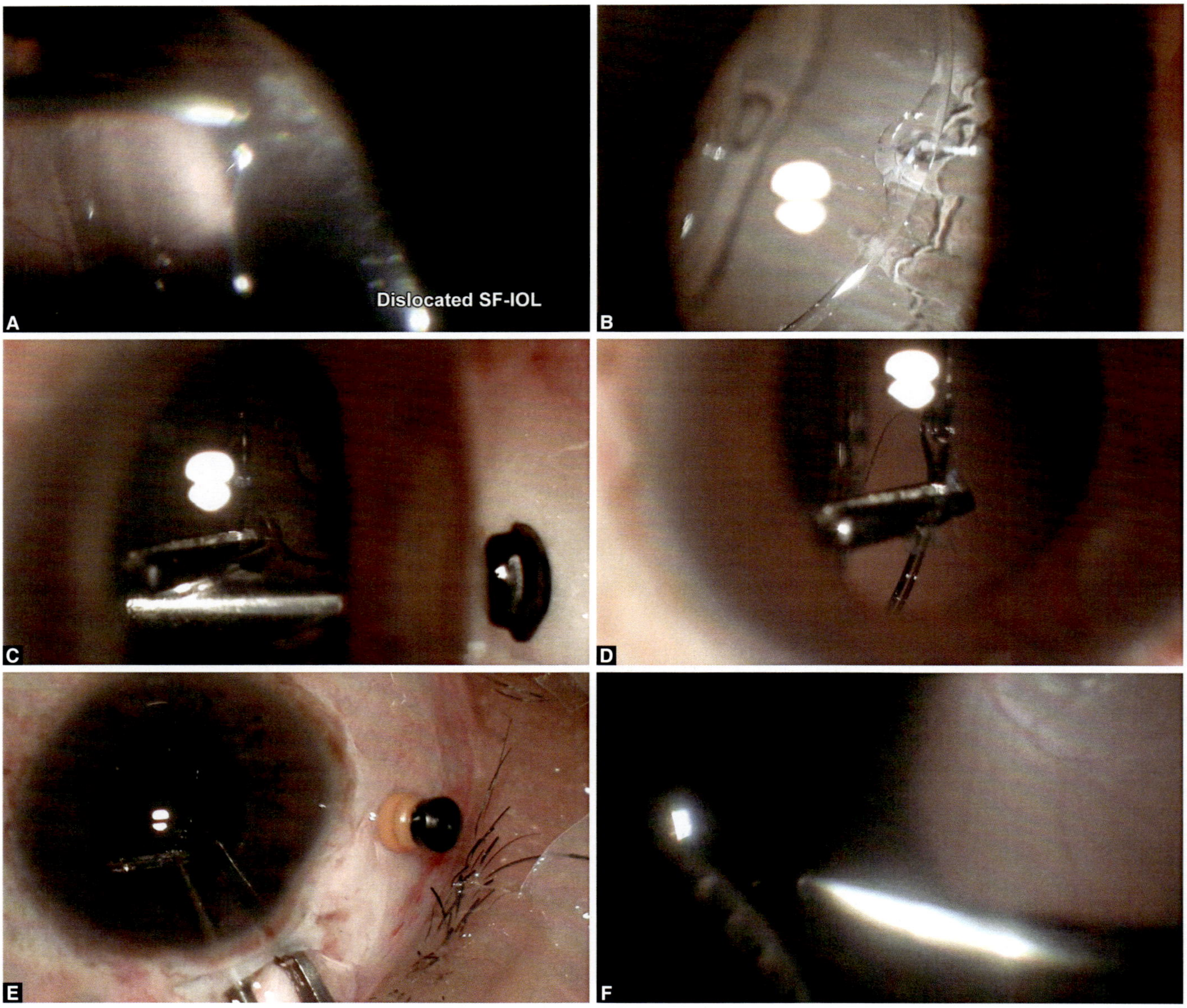

Figs 20.2A to F

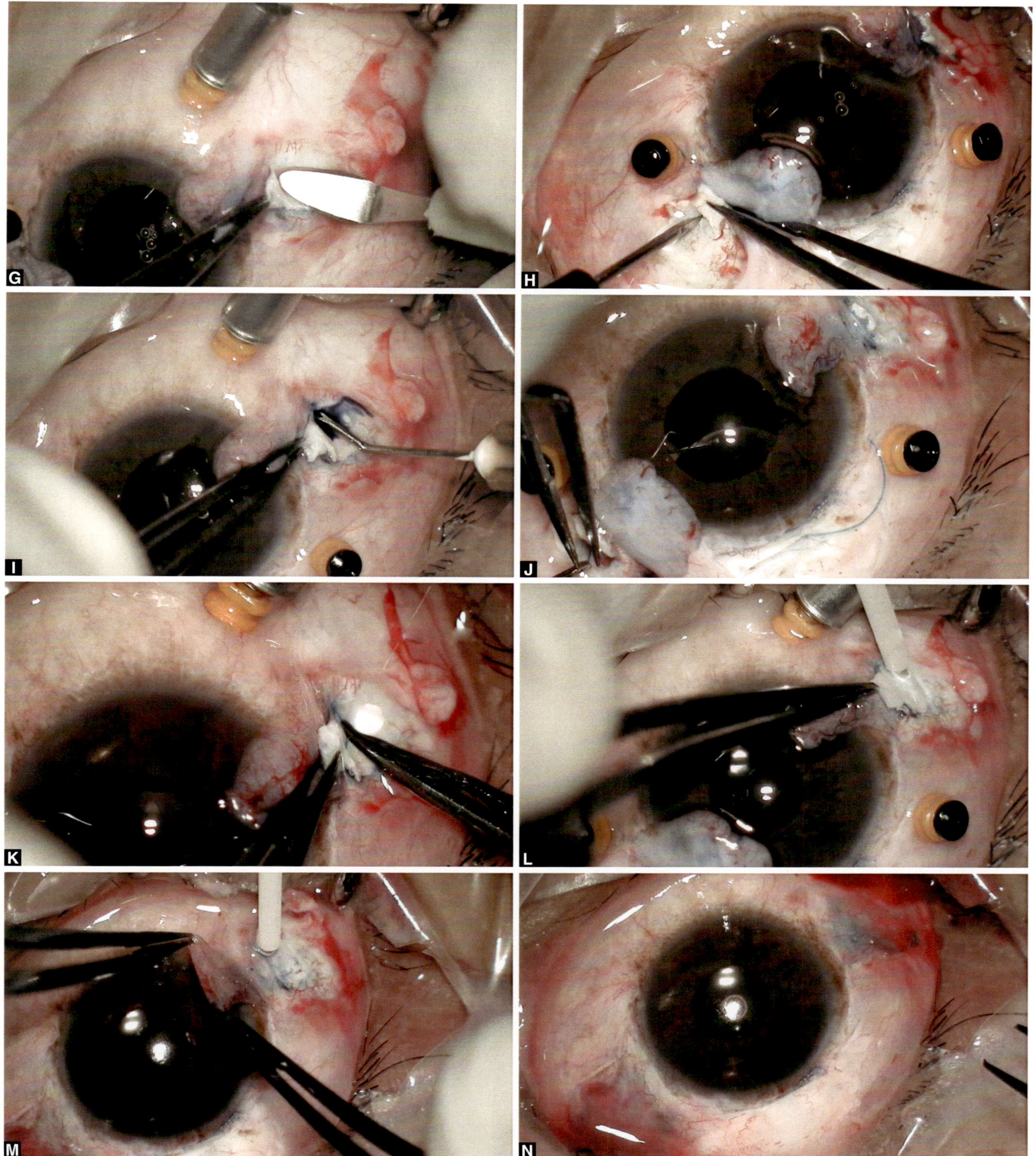

Figs 20.2A to N: Intraoperative steps of glued IOL surgery for dropped scleral fixated rigid IOL

- Superior haptic also introduced and it was made out of scleral tunnel
- Haptic tips had been engaged to the linear scleral tunnel in both sides (Fig. 20.2K)
- Now two drops of fibrin glue were applied at the base of scleral flaps and they were firmly opposed to the base (Fig. 20.2L)
- All cannulas removed
- Now conjunctival wounds closed similarly with the help of the same glue (Figs 20.2M and N).

Endocapsular Dislocation of IOL with CTR

Case Discussion (Video 3, Chapter 20)

- A case of endocapsular dislocation of posterior chamber IOL with capsular tension ring (Fig. 20.3A)
- TA-assisted vitrectomy done
- With the help of passive suction by silicone tip back-flush needle, the whole IOL-CTR complex was bring just behind the pupillary plane (Fig. 20.3B) and prolapsed in anterior chamber (Fig. 20.3C)

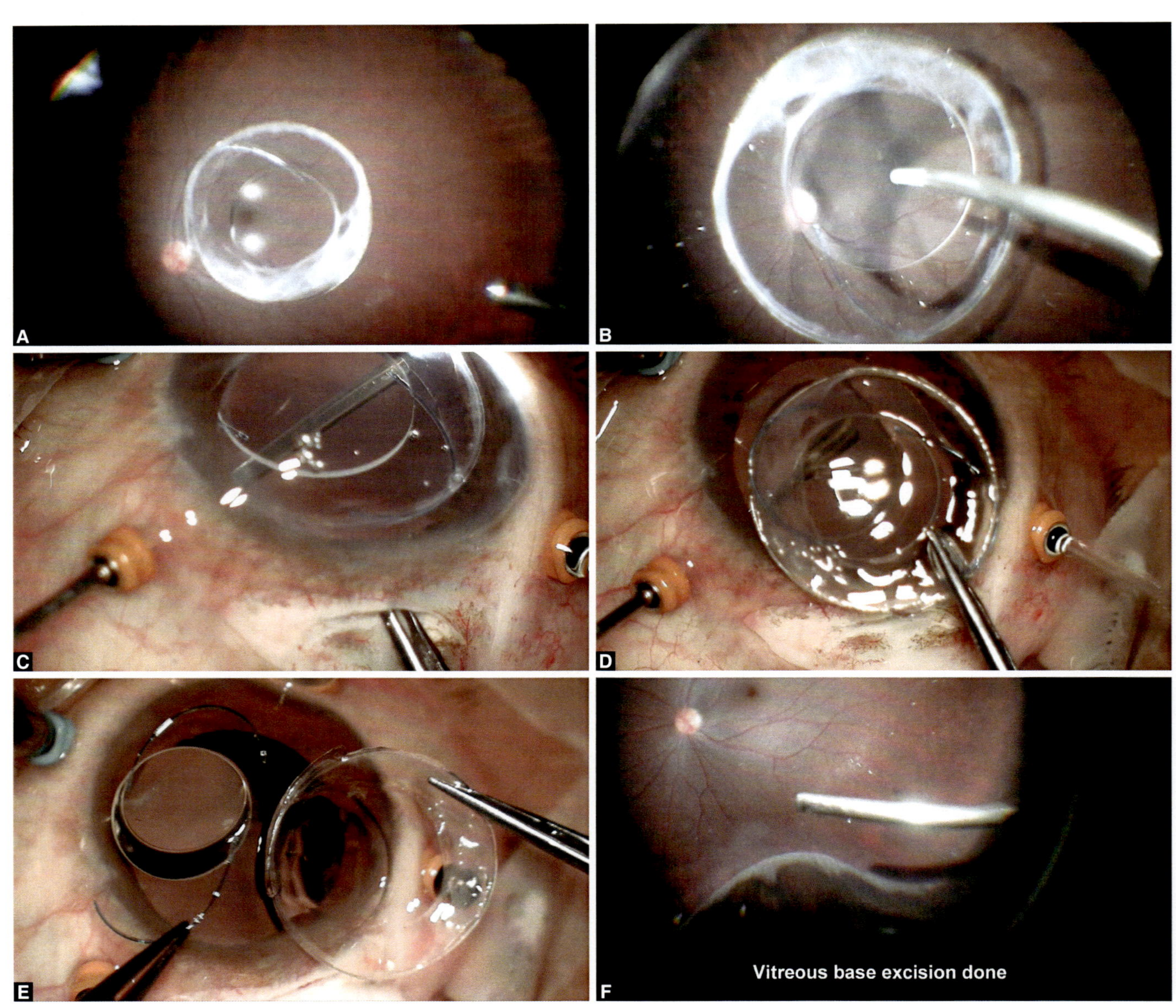

Figs 20.3A to F

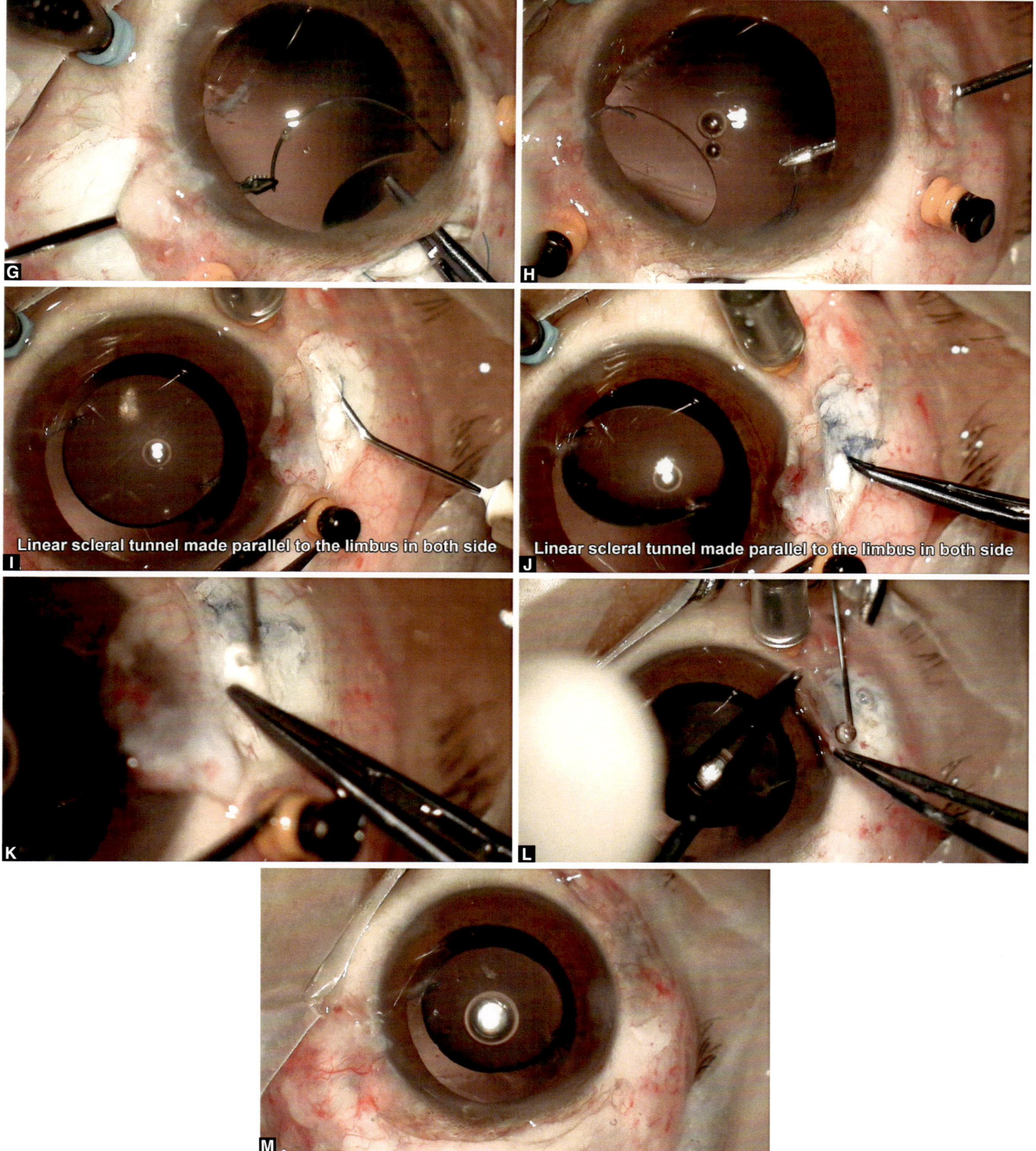

Figs 20.3A to M: Intraoperative steps of glued IOL surgery for endocapsular dislocation of posterior chamber IOL with capsular tension ring

- The IOL-CTR complex removed through the scleral tunnel (Fig. 20.3D)
- Standard glued IOL surgery planned with same multipiece IOL (Fig. 20.3E)
- Vitreous-based excision done (Fig. 20.3F)
- Scleral flaps made horizontally at 3 and 9 o'clock position
- Entry through the base of scleral flap made and inferior haptic brought out first with end grasping forceps (Fig. 20.3G)
- Similarly superior haptic brought through the base of other scleral flap (Fig. 20.3H)
- Linear scleral tunnels made in both sides (Fig. 20.3I) and haptic tips had been engaged into the linear scleral tunnels (Fig. 20.3J)
- Two solutions of glue applied over the bed of scleral flaps on both side (Fig. 20.3K) and scleral flap reapposed
- Conjunctival flap reposition done in a similar way (Figs 20.3L and M).

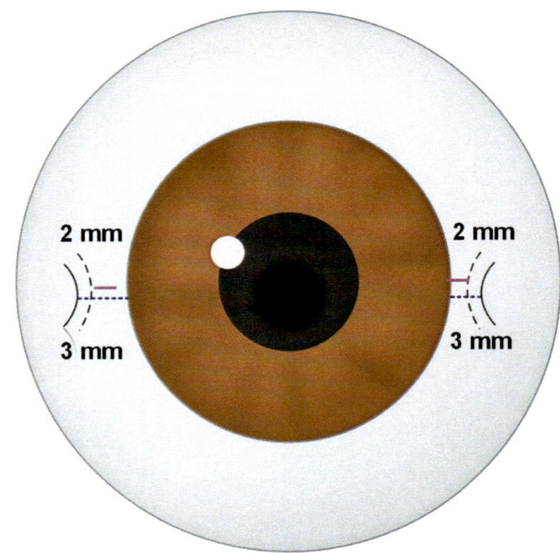

Fig. 20.4: Schematic diagram of self-sealing diagonally opposite scleral pockets for fixing the haptics of SFIOL

II. SCLERAL FIXATION OF IOL WITHOUT GLUE

Scleral fixation of intraocular lenses without suture or glue: Scleral fixation of IOL is the management choice in the absence of posterior capsule support and compromised corneal endothelium. The complete procedure has been highlighted in animated form (Video 4, Chapter 20) and as surgical steps in surgical video (Video 5, Chapter 20):

[Boral SK, Agarwal D. A Simple Modified Way of Glueless, Sutureless Scleral Fixation of an IOL: A Retrospective Case Series. Am J Ophthalmol. 2020;218:P314-319]

- Two diagonally opposite para limbal curved scleral pockets made 3 mm away from the limbus with transscleral 1 mm progression (Fig. 20.4)
- Sutureless vitrectomy (either 23G/25G/27G vitrectomy system) is then performed. Other procedures as required for individual cases (like IOL retrieval, and cataract extraction) were performed. In the case of a subluxated crystalline lens/cataract, a lensectomy was performed with the help of a vitrectomy cutter. In the case of dislocated IOL cases, the same IOL was used for scleral fixation only if it was a multipiece IOL; otherwise, the original IOL was removed and a new multipiece foldable IOL was used for scleral fixation.
- Sclerotomy made by 25G trocar blade at advancing edge of the scleral flap.
- Alcon Acrysof multipiece foldable IOL (Alcon Laboratories, Fort Worth, Texas) was used for scleral fixation.
- Haptics were externalized using 25G serrated end gripping forceps.
- A bent 26G needle, attached to a syringe filled with the trypan blue dye, was used to make a linear scleral tunnel parallel to the limbus underneath the superficial scleral flap of the scleral pockets, and these linear scleral tunnels were stained with this trypan blue dye for better identification to insert haptics. The externalized haptics were subsequently fixed inside these linear scleral tunnels with the help of end-grasping forceps or McPherson tying forceps.
- IOL position was centered
- Haptics did not come back out from the linear scleral tunnel as they were firmly secured inside the tunnel due to the tight distribution of scleral fibers concentric to the limbus. The haptics remained tightly secured inside the linear scleral tunnel underneath the superficial flap of the self-sealed scleral pockets.
- The conjunctival flap was apposed with cautery
- After the surgery, all cannulas were removed
- Sclerotomy sites were checked for wound leakage.

The sutureless glueless technique of SFIOL in Animation (Video 4, Section 20):

- Two diagonally opposite para limbal curved scleral pockets made 3 mm away from the limbus with transscleral 1 mm progression (Fig. 20.5A).
- Sclerotomy made by 25G trocar blade at advancing edge of the scleral flap.
- Haptics were externalized using 25G serrated end gripping forceps (Fig. 20.5B).

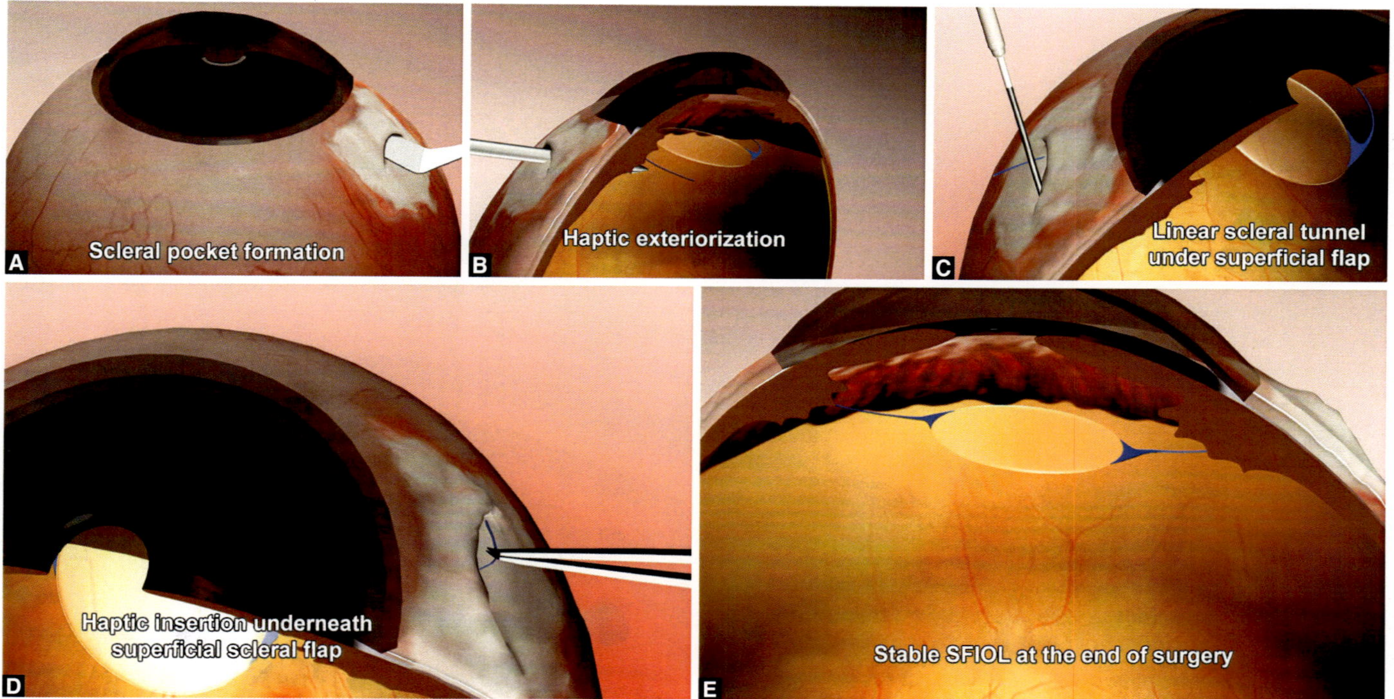

Figs 20.5A to E: Animated form of the sutureless, glueless technique for scleral fixation of IOL

- A bent 26G needle was used to make a linear scleral tunnel parallel to the limbus underneath the superficial scleral flap of the scleral pockets (Fig. 20.5C).
- The externalized haptics were subsequently fixed inside these linear scleral tunnels with the help of end-grasping forceps or McPherson tying forceps (Fig. 20.5D).
- The same procedure was done on the opposite side, centering the IOL position (Fig. 20.5E)

SFIOL in real-life scenarios (Video 5, Chapter 20):

- Two diagonally opposite para limbal curved scleral pockets made 3 mm away from the limbus with transscleral 1 mm progression (Fig. 20.6A)
- 25G vitrectomy performed
- Sclerotomy made by 25G trocar blade at advancing edge of the scleral flap (Fig. 20.6B)
- Alcon Acrysof multipiece foldable IOL (Alcon Laboratories, Fort Worth, Texas) was used for scleral fixation (Fig. 20.6C).
- Haptics were externalized using 25G serrated end gripping forceps (Fig. 20.6D).
- A bent 26G needle, attached to a syringe filled with the trypan blue dye, was used to make a linear scleral tunnel parallel to the limbus underneath the superficial scleral flap of the scleral pockets, and these linear scleral tunnels were stained with this trypan blue dye for better identification to insert haptics (Fig. 20.6E).
- The externalized haptics were subsequently fixed inside these stained linear scleral tunnels with the help of end-grasping forceps or McPherson tying forceps (Fig. 20.6F)
- IOL position was centered (Fig. 20.6G)
- The conjunctival flap was apposed with cautery (Fig. 20.6H)
- These procedures are to be done in cases of dropped IOL, dropped lens matters or nucleus or in cases of subluxated cataracts along with near total vitrectomy with PVD induction and vitreous base excision.
- Postoperatively anterior segment optical coherence tomography (AS-OCT) is done on the Heidelberg SPECTRALIS Spectral-Domain OCT (Heidelberg Engineering, Heidelberg, Germany). AS-OCT showed the haptic positions by a hyper-reflective cross-section of haptics within the sclera. AS-OCT evaluated the optic position for any tilt (Fig. 20.6I).
- Ultrasound Biomicroscopy (UBM B-scan, Appasamy associates/Gantec Corporation, USA) is also performed using immersion technique, with a 50-MHz transducer probe to confirm the absence of optic tilt (Fig. 20.6J).

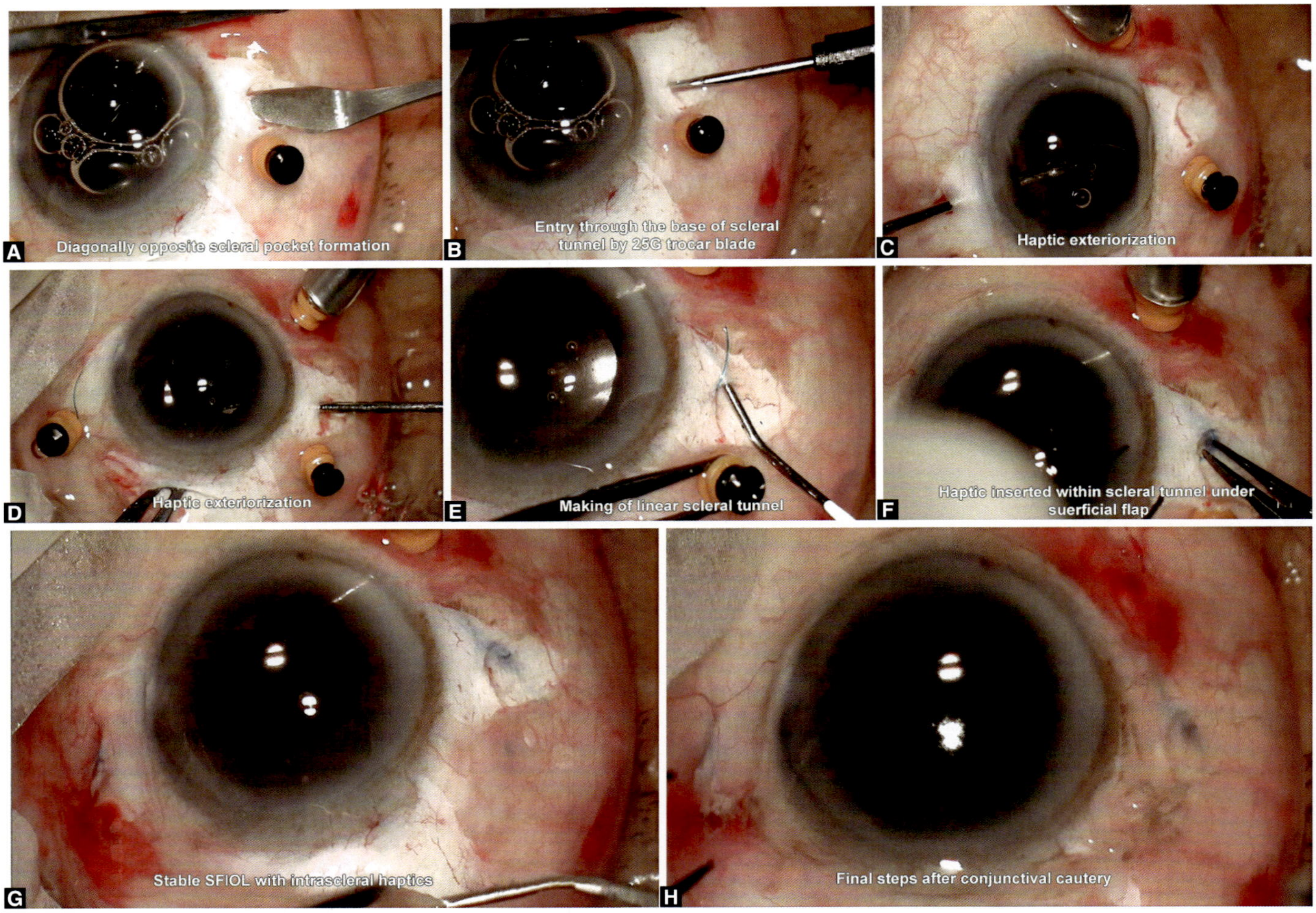

Figs 20.6A to H: Sutureless, glueless technique for scleral fixation of IOL in real-life scenarios

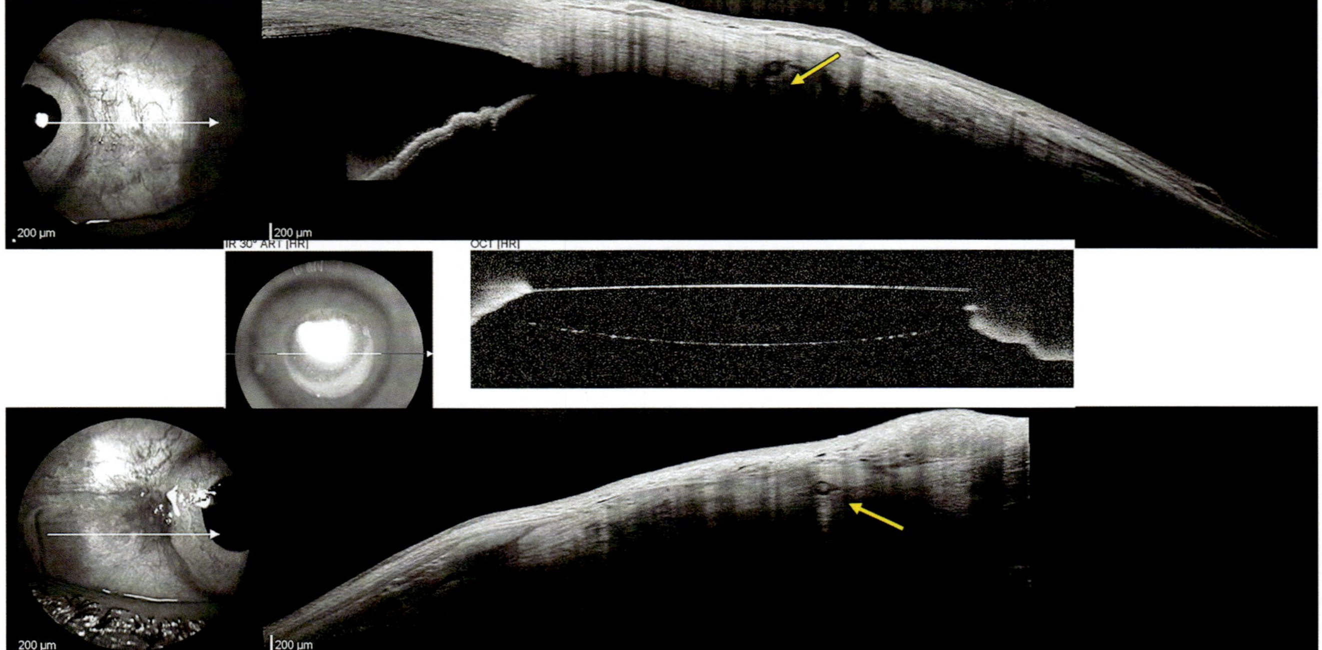

Fig. 20.6I: Postoperative anterior segment optical coherence tomography (AS-OCT) with stable intrascleral haptics of SFIOL (yellow arrows) without any optic tilt

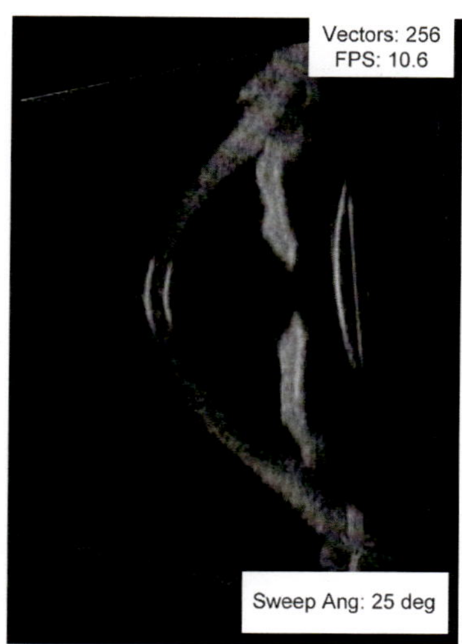

Fig. 20.6J: Postoperative UBM B-scan shows the absence of optic tilt of SFIOL

Advantages of sutureless glueless SFIOL technique:

- Self-sealing scleral pockets usually avoid the need for glue or suture.
- Haptics did not come back out from the linear scleral tunnel as they were firmly secured inside the tunnel due to the tight distribution of scleral fibers concentric to the limbus.
- Haptic insertion on both sides is almost at the same plane which practically minimizes the torque.

This new cost-effective, simple way of scleral fixation of IOL decreases the duration of surgery without any additional complication.

Kindly scan the QR code below to access the online Video.

CHAPTER 21

Intraocular Parasites

INTRAVITREAL *GNATHOSTOMA* WITH RETINAL DETACHMENT

Case Discussion (*Video 1, Chapter 21*)

- A case of progressive tractional retinal detachment involving macula with granuloma formation over optic nerve head
- While doing vitreous base excision, a granuloma detected inferiorly at pars plana
- After removal of adhesion, a worm detected and it started moving actively (Fig. 21.1A)
- A foreign body holding forceps was initially tried to hold the worm, then an end gripping forceps used to separate it from the vitreous base
- But accidentally, it fell down inside. It was removed by forceps from the detached retina
- Optic disk granuloma removed by forceps, followed by intravitreal spatula to separate it from the adjacent macula and disk (Fig. 21.1B)
- Then cutter was used to trim the granuloma
- Retina settled by internal drainage and barrage laser done around the retinotomy, inferior break and 360 degrees periphery
- Silicone oil injection given
- The worm was examined and diagnosed as *Gnathostoma spinigerum* (Figs 21.1C to E).

INTRAVITREAL CYSTICERCOSIS WITH RETINAL DETACHMENT

Case Discussion (*Video 2, Chapter 21*)

- It was a case of intravitreal cysticercosis with retinal detachment
- The cyst was actively motile with a stalk, attached to the detached retina (Fig. 21.2A)
- There was old vitritis
- We trimmed the thick hyaloids face as well as all membrane surrounding the cyst (Figs 21.2B and C)
- Now, the cyst is freely mobile
- A silicone-tipped back-flush needle was held over the cyst wall tried to remove it through the cannula, but failed
- Now a metallic end flute was also tried to remove it similarly, but again failed!
- A 24 G needle was introduced to puncture the cyst wall
- The cyst wall was quite tough to produce a nick
- Now the cyst was in collapsed stage
- The collapsed cyst was now eaten up in-toto by cutter (Fig. 21.2D)
- Now inferior relaxing retinotomy was performed around inferior fixed folds (Fig. 21.2E)
- Lensectomy had to be done for better anterior dissection
- Fluid air exchange was performed to settle retina
- Laser barrage done around the retinotomy, inferior break as well as 360 degrees periphery (Fig. 21.2F)
- And silicone oil injection was given at the end surgery.

INTRAOCULAR TOXOCARIASIS

Characteristic posterior segment findings:

- Mild to moderately elevated granulomatous lesion that can be calcified
- Vitreous membranes extending from granulomatous lesion to posterior pole
- Posterior tractional RD or retinal fold.

Case I (*Video 3, Chapter 21*)

Surgical steps:

- A case of vitritis with mid peripheral retinal granuloma, presumed to be ocular toxocariasis (Fig. 21.3A)
- Vitrectomy done (Fig. 21.3B)
- Vitreous around the granuloma removed (Fig. 21.3C)
- Granuloma very firmly attached to the underlying retina and it was separated bimanually by a forceps and cutter cutting from the base (Fig. 21.3D) of granuloma.
- Granuloma removed by cutter (Fig. 21.3E)

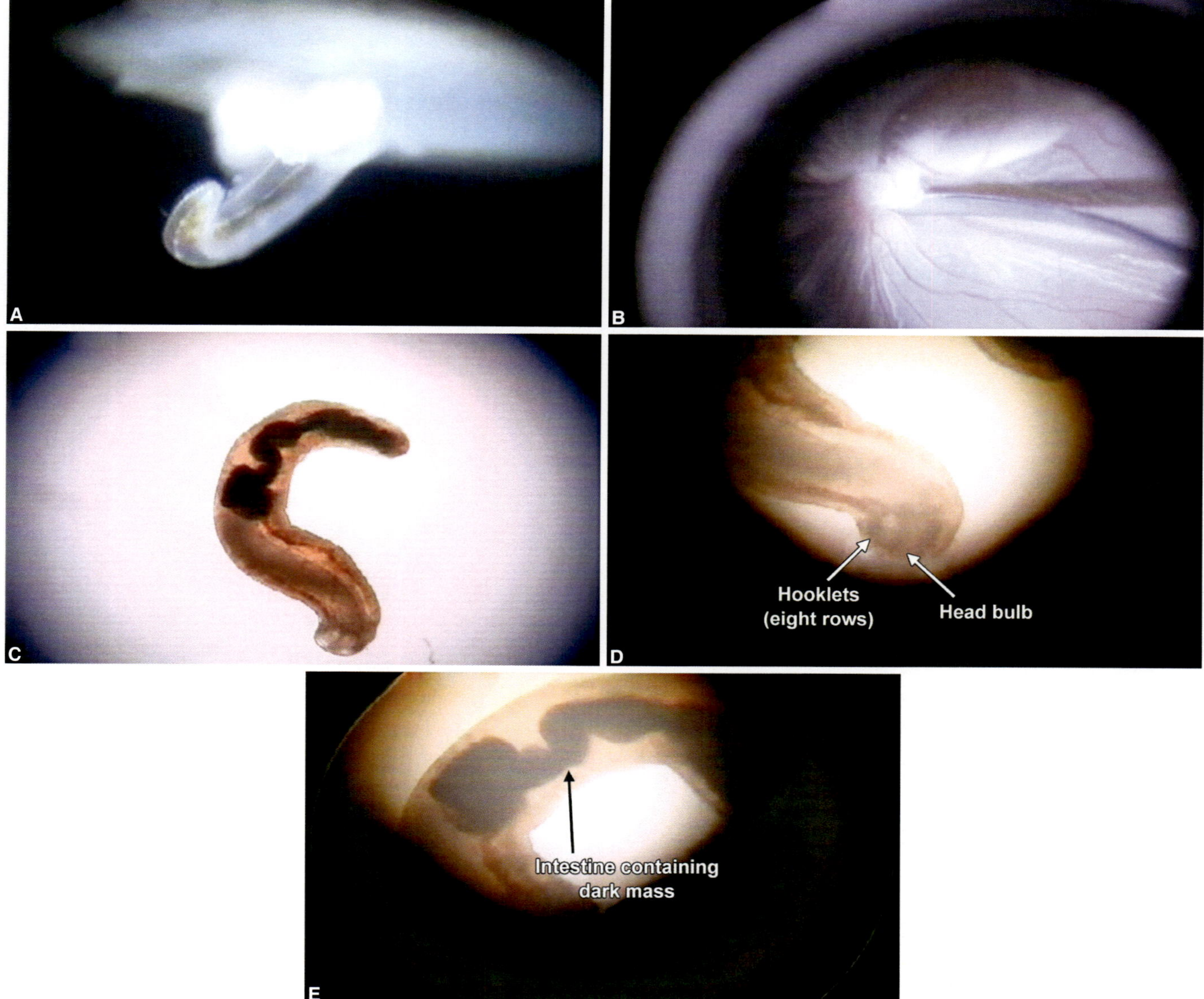

Figs 21.1A to E: Intraoperative steps to manage a case of intravitreal *Gnathostoma spinigerum* with total retinal detachment

- Peripheral vitreous removed
- Triamcinolone stained vitreoschisis membrane removed
- Fluid air exchange done (Fig. 21.3F) and subretinal fluid around the retinal break aspirated
- Laser done around the break (Fig. 21.3G)
- Case ended with SF6 gas injection in iso-expansile concentration (Fig. 21.3H).

Case II *(Video 4, Chapter 21)*

Surgical steps:

- A case of vitritis with inferior vitreous band with inferior peripheral granuloma with macular tractional fold, presumed to be a case of intraocular toxocariasis (Fig. 21.4A)
- Vitrectomy started (Fig. 21.4B)

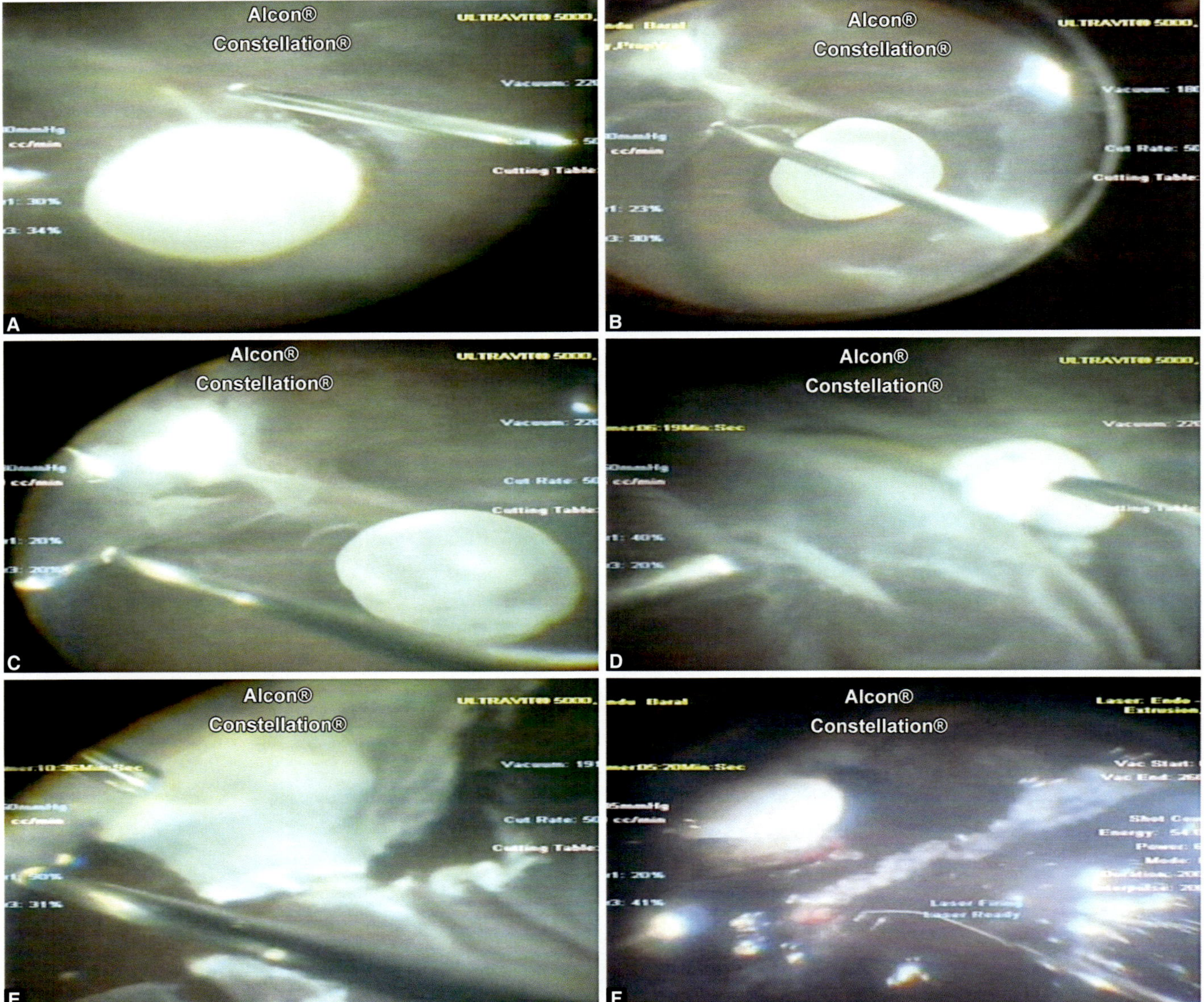

Figs 21.2A to F: Intraoperative steps to manage a case of intravitreal cysticercosis with retinal detachment

- Inferior vitreous band cut (Fig. 21.4C)
- Vitrectomy completed (Fig. 21.4D)
- Triamcinolone acetonide injected
- Vitreous-based excision done (Fig. 21.4E)
- Peripapillary membrane with macular extension removed with end grasping forceps from folded macula (Fig. 21.4F).
- Oozing from the disk secured by keeping the IOP high
- Fluid-air exchange done (Fig. 21.4G)
- Postoperative case with unfolding of macula (Fig. 21.4H).

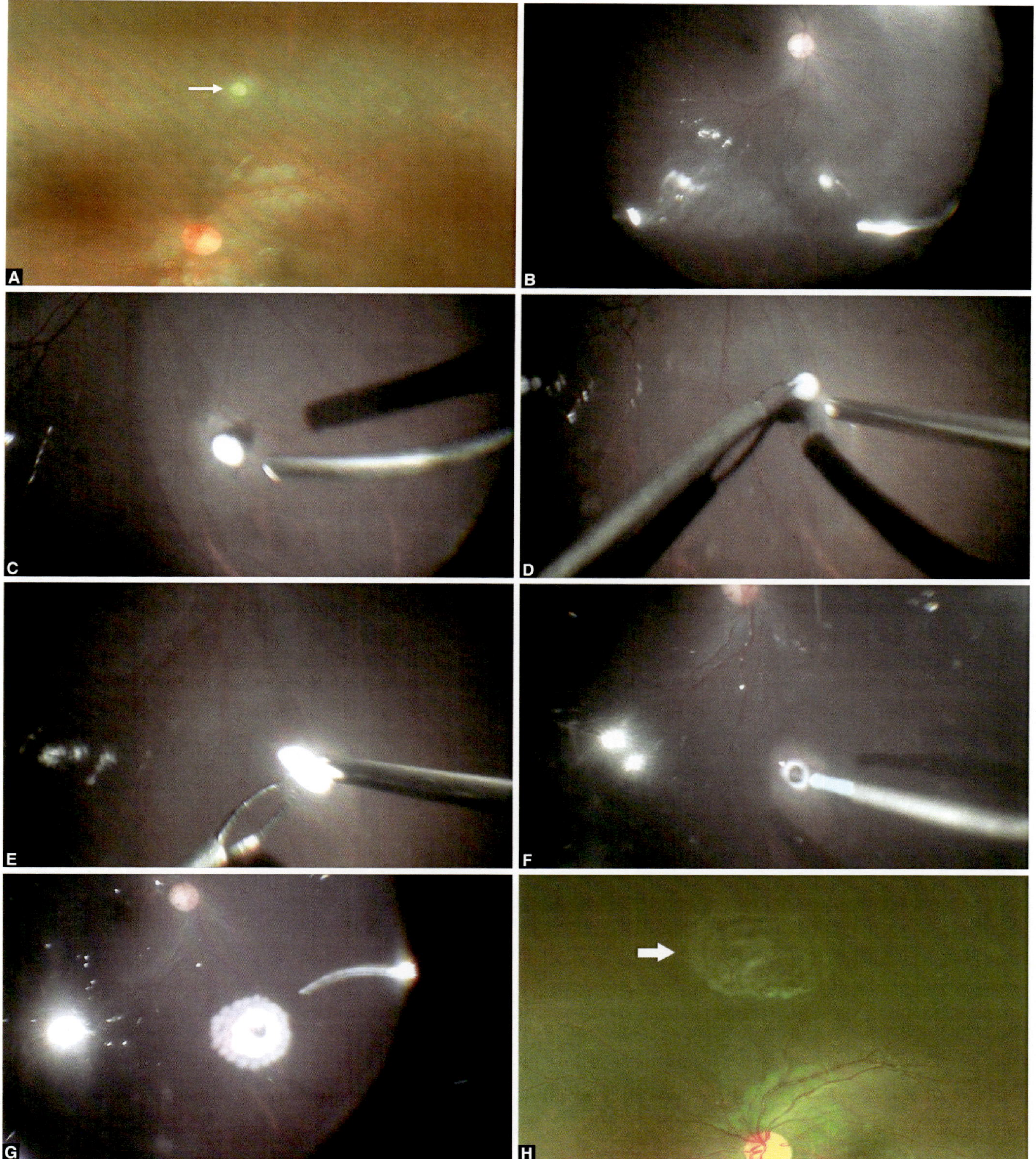

Figs 21.3A to H: (A) Case of vitritis with mid peripheral retinal granuloma (white arrow), presumed to be ocular toxocariasis; (B to G) Intraoperative steps to manage a case of vitritis with mid peripheral retinal granuloma, presumed to be ocular toxocariasis; (H) Postoperative fundus photograph shows laser barraged site of *Toxocara granuloma* (white arrow)

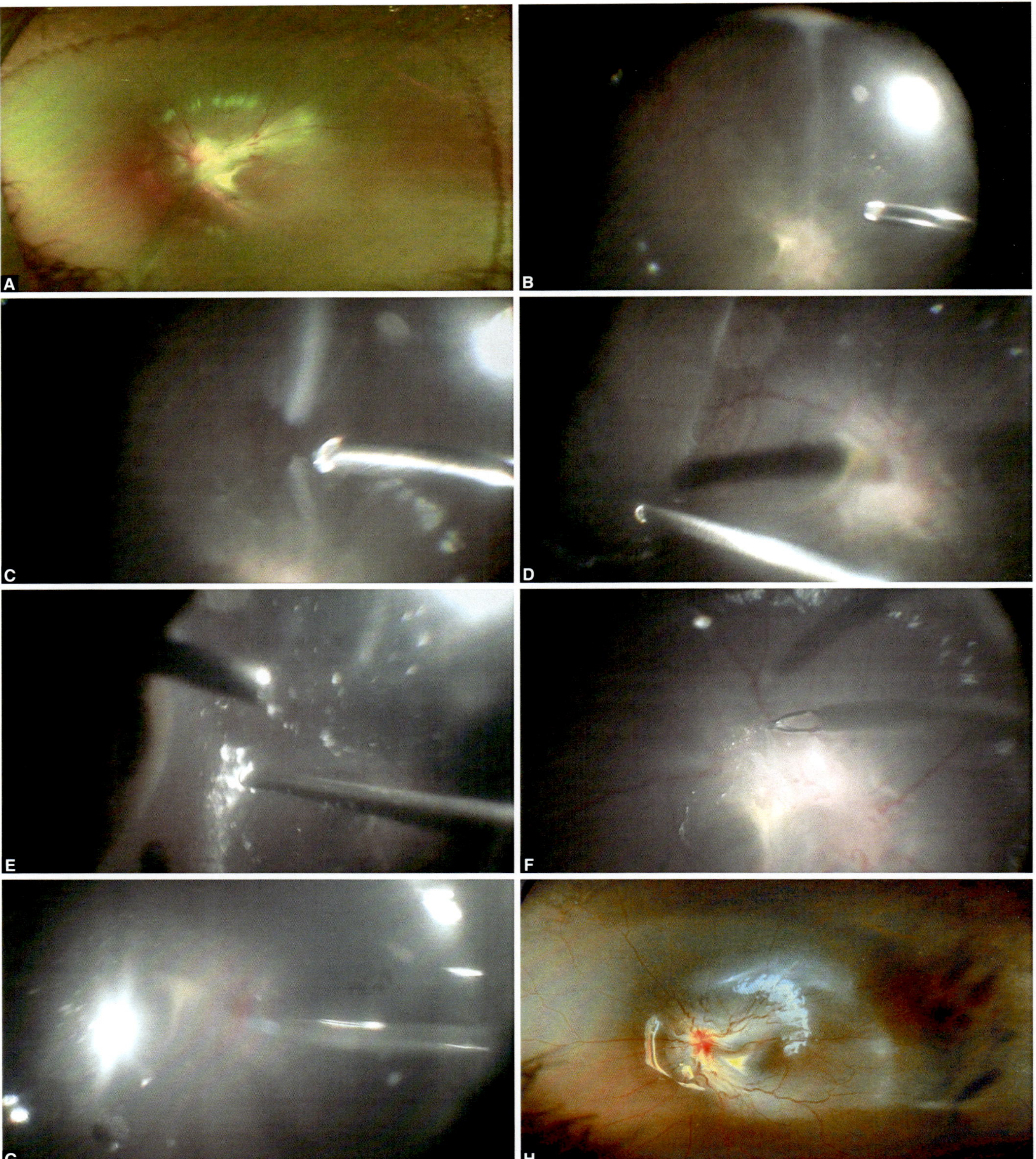

Figs 21.4A to H: (A) Presumed case of intraocular toxocara with vitritis with inferior vitreous band with inferior peripheral granuloma with macular folds; (B to G) Intraoperative steps to manage a case of vitritis with inferior vitreous band with inferior peripheral granuloma with macular tractional fold, presumed to be a case of intraocular toxocariasis; (H) Postoperative case of toxocariasis with unfolding of macula

Kindly scan the QR code below to access the online Video.

CHAPTER 22

Silicone Oil Removal

Removal of silicone oil can be done any time after proper smooth retinal reattachment with stable brownish pigmentary changes of laser or cryoretinopexy. But usually 3 months waiting period after primary intervention is to be followed. Generally, surgeons prefer to remove it in between 3 months and 6 months postoperatively. Delaying oil removal sometimes result in advanced emulsification with it's consequences like secondary glaucoma, epiretinal membrane formation. Moreover, advanced emulsification increase the surgical time to remove silicone oil.

Early removal of silicone oil is necessary—

- When the early emulsification is noted
- Raised IOP due to overfilling of silicone oil
- When significant volume of silicone oil comes into anterior chamber resulting in corneal endothelial changes.

But in the last two situations, removal of whole silicone oil is not necessary. Few drops of silicone oil removal normalize IOP in case of overfilling and in third situation, removal of silicone oil from anterior chamber with approximately same amount of volume replacement intravitreally by injecting silicone oil via pars plana route, taking care of IOP rise, save the cornea.

The incidence of emulsification varies from 5% to 100% and is the result of fragmentation of the oil globule into multiple micelle. It occurs due to:

- Increase in number of low molecular weight silicone oil polymer chains (as impurities)
- Any mixing with biologically active substances like fibrinogen, fibrin, globulin and balanced salt solution.

These particles act as surfactants. Impurities in silicone oil either from the surgical process or during its manufacturing, are extrinsic surfactants and biological elements are intrinsic surfactants. Surface tension is the tendency of a liquid to acquire the least surface area possible, thereby facilitating an inward force at the surface of the liquid. Surfactants promote emulsification by two ways:

1. Surfactants decrease the surface tension and interfacial tension between silicone oil and aqueous, which prevents small droplets of silicone oil from joining the larger bubble.
2. Surfactants also increase the repulsion between the silicone oil bubbles by creating a film around the silicone oil that causes the globules to repel each other.

It has been seen that less viscous silicone oils and silicone oils with lower molecular weight (as the particles can move more freely due to less long-chain branching) emulsify earlier than oils with higher viscosities and higher molecular weight.

Effects of Silicone Oil Emulsification

1. Emulsified silicone oil particles may block trabecular meshwork and cause rise in IOP, that warrants removal of silicone oil.
2. Emulsified silicone oil particles can come into anterior chamber and form inverse hypopyon. These emulsified silicone oils can cause corneal endothelial changes.
3. Epiretinal membrane formation, especially in long-standing silicone oil-filled eyes with advanced emulsification.

Surgical Ways of Silicone Oil Removal

Silicone Oil Removal Passively

Passive removal of silicone oil is always safe, but it takes longer time. Care should be taken to keep tip of the cannula inside as the silicone oil bubbles to facilitate smooth removal of the oil.

Steps of surgery (Video 1, Chapter 22)

- In a case of postvitrectomy emulsification of silicone oil
- Silicone oil removed by two port passively by intravitreal pressure (Fig. 22.1A)
- Retina examined
- Fluid air exchange started keeping tip of back flush needle, then soft tip cannula just at the surface of fluid surface (Fig. 22.1B)
- Partial fluid air exchange done for better closure of scleral tunnel under air.

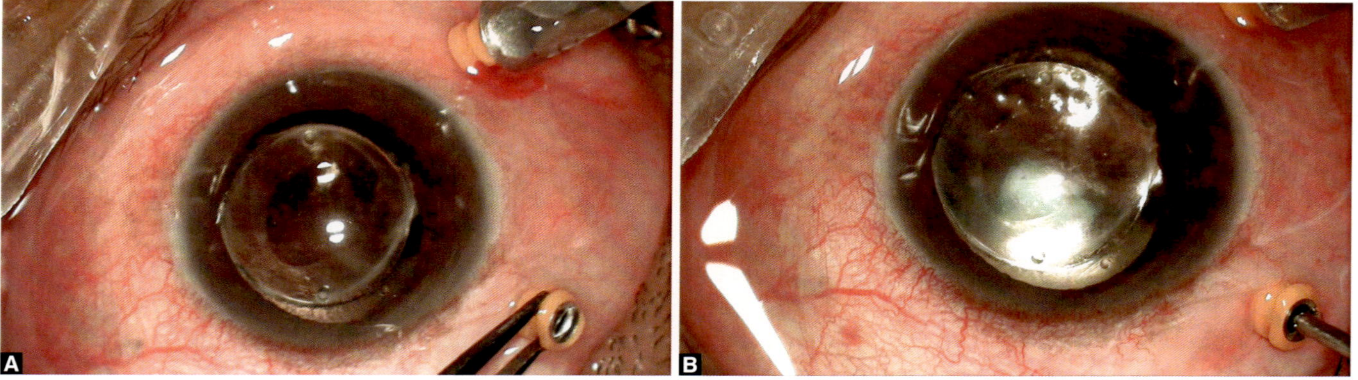

Figs 22.1A and B: Intraoperative steps of surgery to remove silicone oil by two ports passively

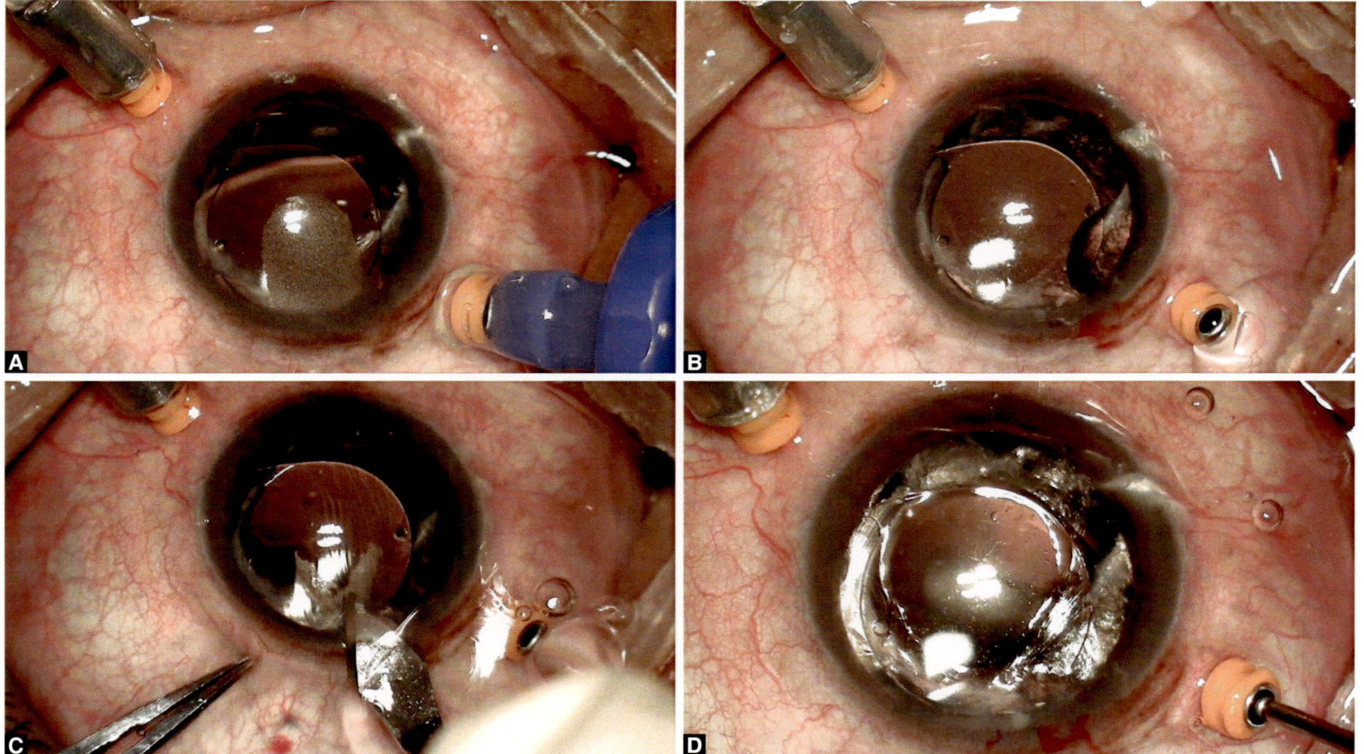

Figs 22.2A to D: Intraoperative steps of surgery to remove silicone oil by active suction

Silicone Oil Removal by Active Suction

Silicone oil removal by active suction VFC (Viscous fluid control) in extraction mode is a rapid way to remove silicone oil, but it may create traction over the uncut peripheral vitreous skirt.

It is better to avoid active suction to remove last globule of silicone oil to prevent sudden collapse of the globe.

Steps of surgery *(Video 2, Chapter 22)*:

- In a case of postvitrectomy emulsification of silicone oil
- Silicone oil removed by two port active suction using VFC (Fig. 22.2A)
- Last bubble of silicone oil removed by passive suction (Fig. 22.2B)
- Emulsified silicone oil particles from anterior chamber removed (Fig. 22.2C)
- Retina examined.
- Fluid air exchange started keeping tip of back flush needle just at the surface of fluid surface (Fig. 22.2D).
- Partial fluid air exchange done for better closure of scleral tunnel under air.

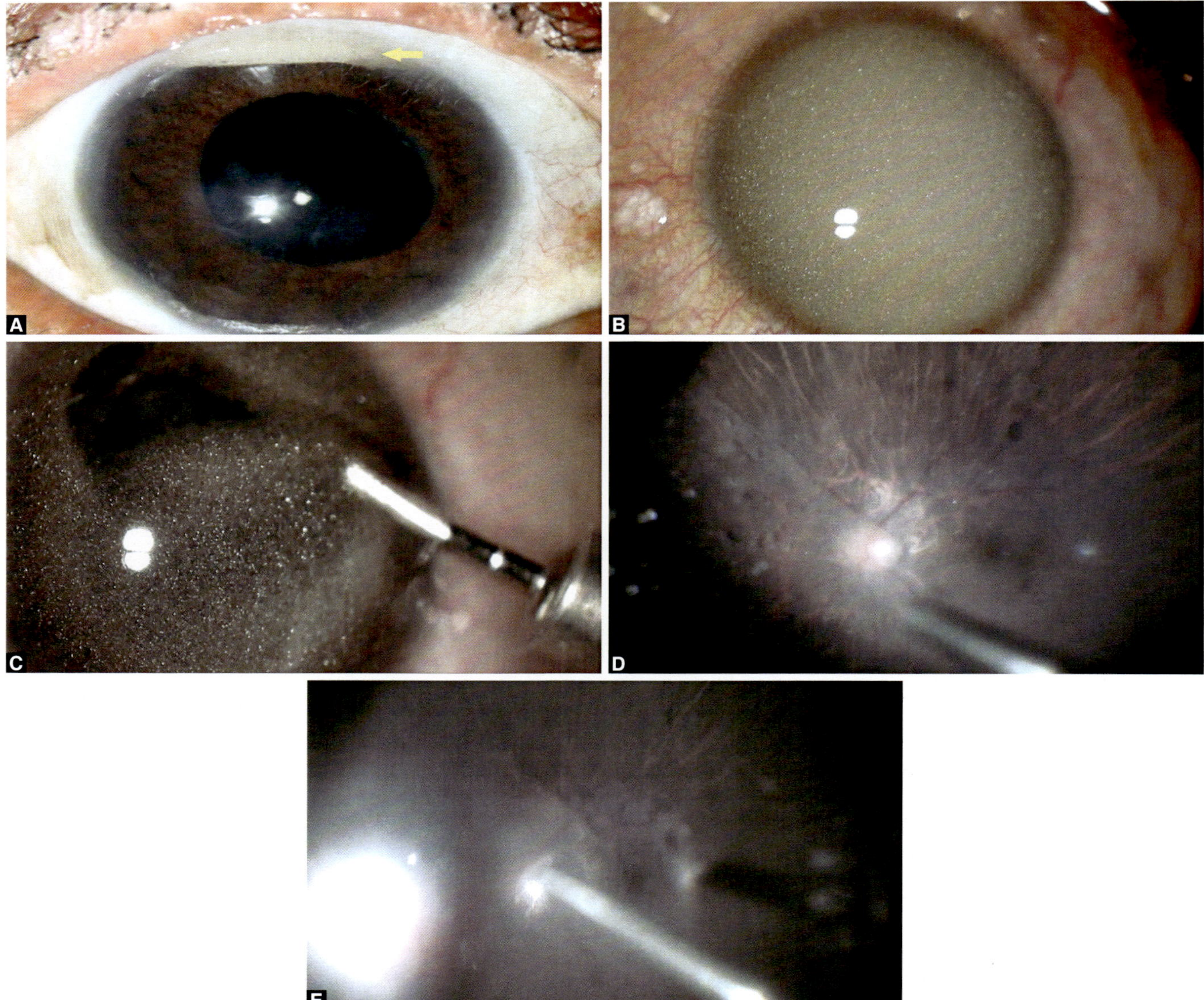

Figs 22.3A to E: (A) Emulsified silicone oil in anterior chamber (yellow arrow); (B to E) Intraoperative steps of surgery to remove totally emulsified silicone oil

Advanced Emulsification of Silicone Oil

Advanced emulsification of silicone oil result in migration of silicone oil particles into the anterior chamber through the zonules. This may partially fill the anterior chamber forming 'inverse hypopyon' or 'hyperoleon' (Fig. 22.3A). Sometimes it may totally fill the anterior chamber obscuring visibility of pupil and iris details.

Steps of surgery *(Video 3, Chapter 22)*:

- In a case of postvitrectomy advanced emulsification of silicone oil with anterior chamber full of emulsified silicone oil (Fig. 22.3B)
- Silicone oil particles removed by introducing metallic end of infusion tip as an anterior chamber maintainer (Fig. 22.3C)
- Infusion cannula placed
- Silicone oil removed using active suction
- Residual silicone oil particles removed by passive suction of back flush needle (Fig. 22.3D)
- Fluid air exchange started keeping tip of back flush needle just at the surface of fluid surface as residual silicone oil particles mostly stay at the surface of saline (Fig. 22.3E)
- Complete fluid air exchange done.

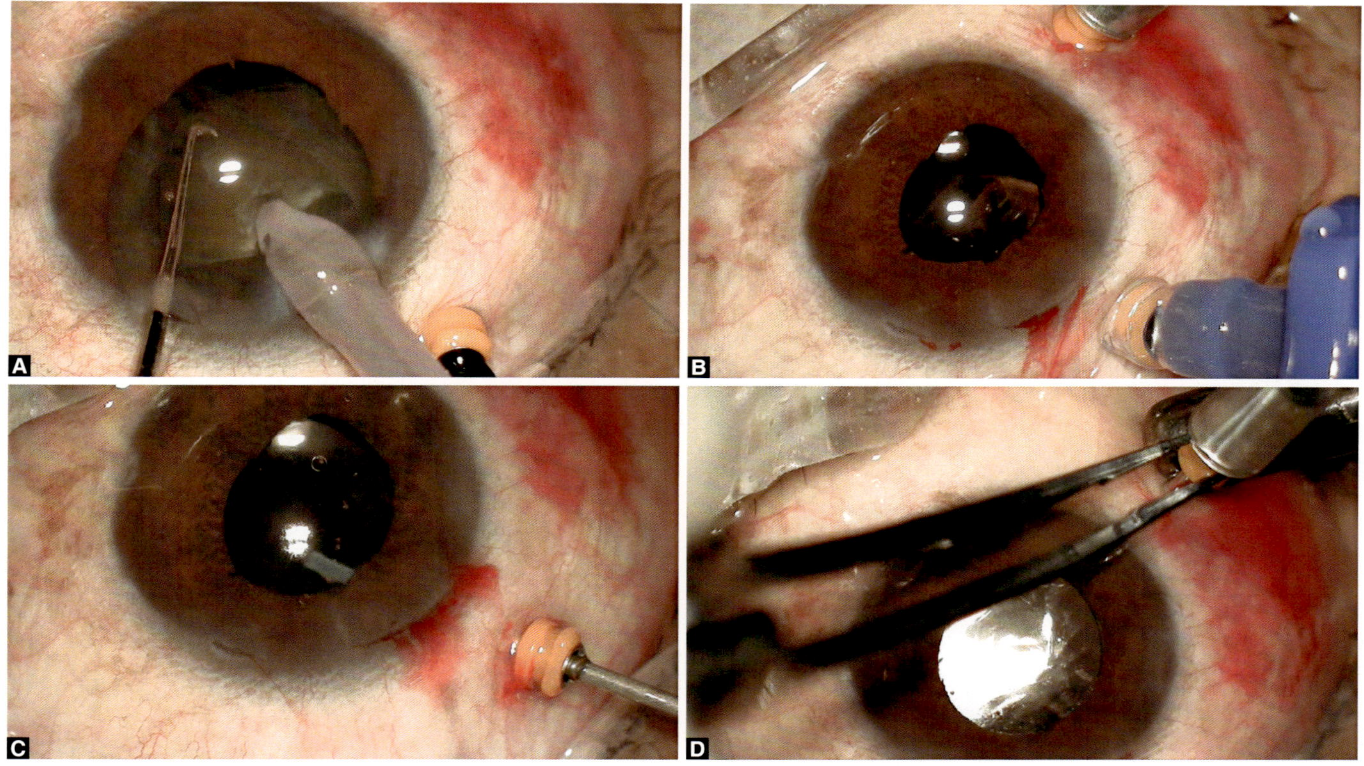

Figs 22.4A to D: Intraoperative steps of combined phacoemulsification and silicone oil removal

Combined Phacoemulsification and Silicone Oil Removal

Postoperative cataract formation in a silicone oil-filled-eye is well-known consequence after vitreoretinal intervention in phakic eyes. Silicone oil removal in these situations should be done along with cataract extraction with IOL implantation.

- Phacoemulsification with foldable IOL implantation is to be completed before removing silicone oil
- Upthrust by silicone oil may result in shallowing of anterior chamber. So, precaution to be taken especially during capsulorrhexis and cortical cleaning
- Sometimes posterior capsular plaques can be removed after silicone oil removal by posterior capsulectomy
- Sometimes dehiscent posterior capsule due to lens touch in previous surgery may result in posterior capsular tear and silicone oil removal through the posterior capsular rent may be possible.

Steps of surgery *(Video 4, Chapter 22)*:

- In a case of postvitrectomy cataract with posterior synechia with emulsification of silicone oil
- Synechia released after introducing two 23G ports
- Capsulorrhexis completed
- Phacoemulsification started
- Direct chop of nuclear fragment is preferable (Fig. 22.4A)
- Cortical aspiration done
- Multipiece foldable IOL placed in the capsular bag
- Silicone oil removed by two port active suction using VFC (Fig. 22.4B)
- Last bubble of silicone oil removed by passive suction
- Retina examined
- Fluid air exchange started keeping tip of back flush needle just at the surface of fluid surface (Fig. 22.4C)
- Partial fluid air exchange done for better closure of scleral tunnel under air (Fig. 22.4D).

Kindly scan the QR code below to access the online Video.

CHAPTER 23

Interface Vitrectomy

CONCEPT AND PRINCIPLE

Interface vitrectomy describes the use of vitreous cutters, scissors, forceps, and other instruments at the interface between silicone oil, air, or perfluorocarbon liquid (PFCL) and residual vitreous, epiretinal membrane, and retina. The term interface was selected to emphasize that the vitreous cutter must be placed outside the air, PFCL, or silicone oil bubble. Vitrectomy, forceps membrane peeling, scissors segmentation/delamination, diathermy, laser, and retinectomy all work well with these agents in the eye. The technique first described by Dr Steve Charles.

Vacuum should not be applied to the vitreous cutter or soft tip cannula within the air, oil, or PFCL bubble to avoid plugging with oil or air lock, and to reduce the risk of loss of oil or PFCL.

Air and silicone oil float in infusion fluid, but PFCL sinks; it is crucial to understand that a fluid layer always exists at the retinal surface and that the retina is more than 90% water as well as immiscible in air, PFCL, or oil.

Interface vitrectomy under air and silicone oil: It can be applied to remove residual vitreous traction and perform retinectomy, epiretinal membrane peeling/segmentation/delamination, subretinal surgery, and bipolar diathermy under air and oil.

AIR-ASSISTED INTERFACE VITRECTOMY

Advantages to Work under Air *(Video 1, Chapter 23)*

- Air widens the field of view and improves visualization (Fig. 23.1A)
- Air stabilizes the retina because of the inherent spring like properties of a compressible gas (called 'spring damping effect')
- Air also reduces unwanted retinal motion (Fig. 23.1B)
- Air confines bleeding to the air-retinal interface and
- Air prevents infusion fluid from flowing into the subretinal space.

INTERFACE VITRECTOMY UNDER PERFLUOROCARBON LIQUIDS

Advantages to Work under PFCL *(Video 2, Chapter 23)*

- The high specific gravity of PFCL (approximately twice of its mass) produces both inertial stabilization and gravitational stabilization (approximately twice of

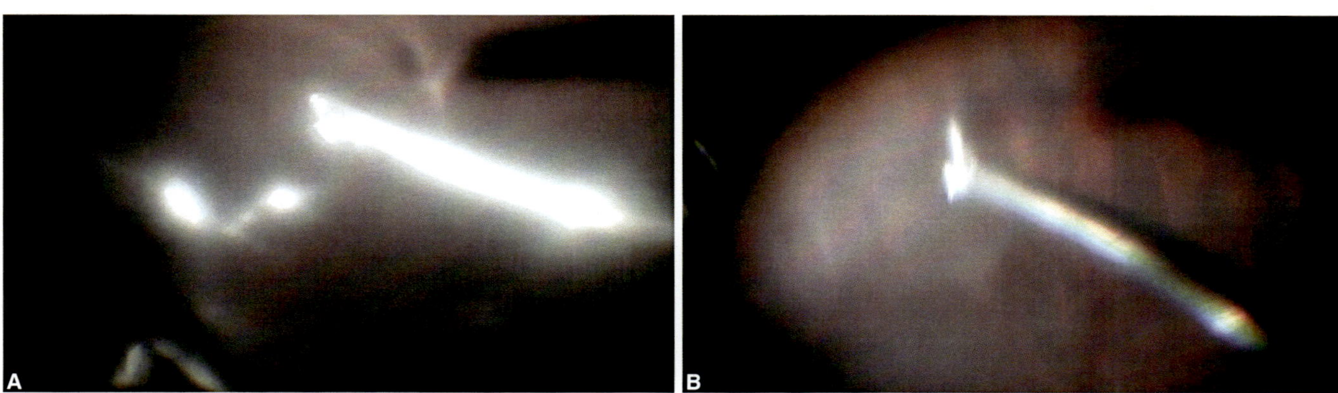

Figs 23.1A and B: Intraoperative steps of air-assisted interface vitrectomy

gravitational force) on the retina to counteract dissection forces ('inertial and gravitational dampening' effect). Thus, blood clots as well as membranes around the PFCL can removed easily by cutter, keeping the cutter port away from PFCL (Fig. 23.2A)
- As subretinal fluid is less dense than PFCL, application of PFCL over posterior pole displace SRF anteriorly to exit subretinal space through retinal breaks or retinotomies
- Laser energy settings must be reduced when treating under PFCL because the subretinal fluid is completely gone (Fig. 23.2B).

SILICONE OIL-ASSISTED INTERFACE VITRECTOMY

Advantages to Work under Silicone Oil

Silicone oil produces viscous dampening, which reduces retinal motion during epiretinal membrane peeling, removal of residual vitreous traction, retinectomy, epiretinal membrane peeling/segmentation/delamination, and subretinal surgery (called 'viscous dampening'). All of these techniques are easily performed just outside the silicone oil bubble, at or near the retinal surface.

Technical steps to identify residual traction by interface vitrectomy:
- Starting internal drainage of subretinal fluid and fluid-air exchange
- Simultaneous reattachment of retina. If subretinal air appears, vacuum should be released as quickly as possible and inspection of the retinal surface initiated to determine the cause of residual traction
- Residual vitreous can be removed using interface vitrectomy technique, and the epiretinal membrane, typically in proliferative vitreoretinopathy (PVR) cases, can be managed with forceps membrane peeling using end-grasping forceps and the internal limiting membrane (ILM) forceps
- If the epiretinal membrane is highly adherent, typically in diabetic traction retinal detachment cases, access segmentation should be followed by inside-out delamination with curved scissors
- If residual vitreous or epiretinal membrane cannot be identified, incremental retinectomy, not "relaxing retinotomy," which leaves tissue anterior to the cut, should be used until the retina gets attached.

Resurgery without Removing Silicone Oil

Reoperation "under" silicone oil in case of recurrent retinal detachment or removal of epiretinal membrane without removing silicone oil.

Silicone oil produces approximately 50% less interfacial surface tension than air or gas interface with infusion fluid or aqueous humor; therefore, the relative force due to interfacial tension and retinal surface contraction can be properly assessed.

Advantages to this approach include:
- Decreased surgical trauma (especially to the lens and cornea)
- Realistic assessment of traction removal, and
- Significantly reduced operating time, cost, and surgical trauma.

Technique (Video 3, Chapter 23)

- Two port system—One for VFC to inject silicone oil and another for cutter, forceps or flute needle is to be used. Chandelier illuminating system is to be used for endoillumination (Figs 23.3A and B). Forceps membrane peeling, cutter delamination, retinectomy, internal drainage of subretinal fluid and endophotocoagulation all can be done well with silicone oil in place
- A vacuum setting of 600–650 mm Hg is required for cutter removal of residual vitreous or cutter delamination.
- Identification of missed break (Fig. 23.3C) and then maximum linear vacuum setting of 600–650 mm Hg

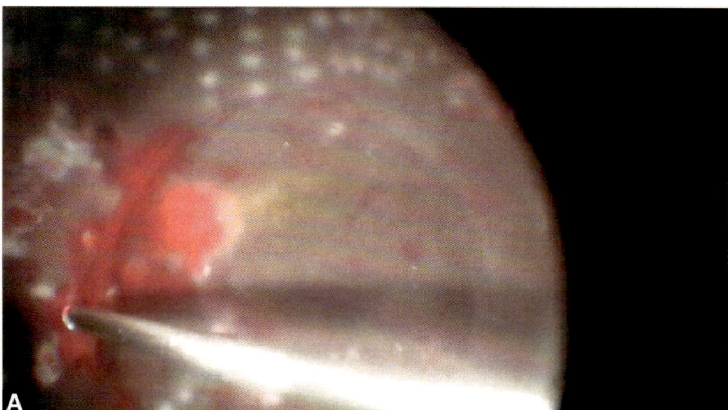

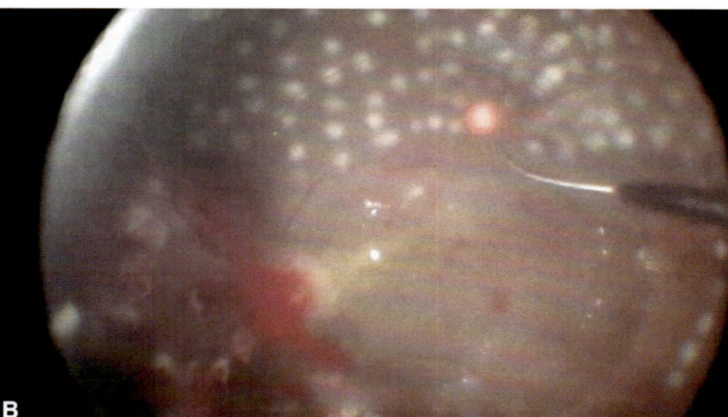

Figs 23.2A and B: Intraoperative steps of PFCL-assisted interface vitrectomy

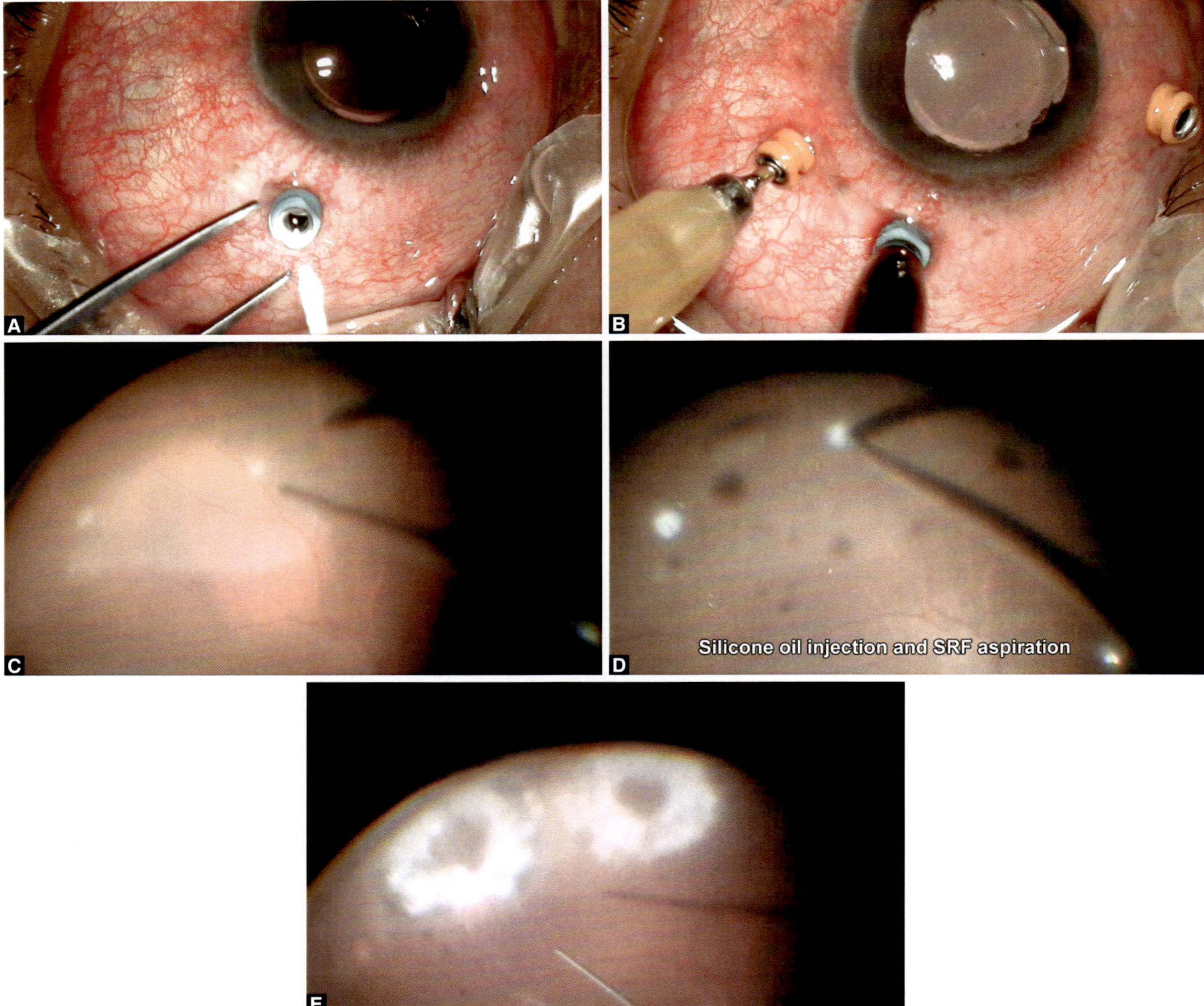

Figs 23.3A to E: Intraoperative steps of interface vitrectomy "under" silicone oil in case of recurrent retinal detachment

is required for internal drainage of subretinal fluid through the break keeping the soft tip cannula out of silicone oil to prevent blockage (Fig. 23.3D). After full internal drainage of residual SRF through the open break, retinal reattachment took place. Now endolaser is possible around the break (Fig. 23.3E). Thus, one can reduce the operative time and cost of surgery

- PVR in diabetic complex RD sometime require retinectomy by cutter (keeping cutter port away from the silicone oil) to remove contracted, stiff retina and epiretinal membrane and subretinal fluid has to be aspirated with the cutter vacuum (maximum around 600 mm Hg). As silicone oil is not conductive, large vessels should be coagulated first with bipolar diathermy with the tip in contact with the vessel.

Kindly scan the QR code below to access the online Video.

CHAPTER 24

Managing Complications of Vitreoretinal Surgeries

PREOPERATIVE COMPLICATIONS

Globe Perforation from Peribulbar/ Retrobulbar Block *(Video 1, Chapter 24)*

Good safe anesthesia is essential for any intraocular surgery.

Conventional method for peribulbar block is injecting the anesthetic solution outside the muscle cone (Fig. 24.1A) and retrobulbar block, inside the muscle cone (Fig. 24.1B). Inferior injection is given at the junction of outer one-third and inner two-third of inferior orbital rim directing the needle towards the apex of orbital muscle cone. Superior injection is given nasally just above the medial cants along the supraorbital bony notch.

Globe perforation occurs from peribulbar or retrobulbar block.

Risk factors:

- High myope with elongated globe
- Thin sclera
- Faulty needle direction
- Uncooperative patients are also to be considered as the etiologies.

Intraocular damage due to:

- Mechanical retinal injury, development of retinal tear and detachment. Intraocular needle entry can cause primary entry break (Fig. 24.1C) and secondary break formation due to further retinal injury (Fig. 24.1D)
- Direct injury to optic nerve
- Sometimes toxic effects of anesthetic agents, administered intraocularly.

Clinically, the situation should be suspected in:

1. Cases with recent history of ophthalmic surgery under local anesthesia.
2. Hypotony.
3. No fundal glow.

On USG: There are vitreous tract formation, vitreous hemorrhage, sometimes retinal incarceration (Fig. 24.1E) and retinal detachment. Retinal incarceration at the entry site or exit sites can cause true foreshortening with tissue loss. In chronic cases, it may also shorten due to fibrous contraction associated with the healing process.

Simple laser barrage around the slit-like superior break sometimes save the eye in single break scenario (Fig. 24.1F).

Perforation with Vitreous Hemorrhage (Video 2, Chapter 24)

Animation: Intraocular entry of needle causes primary entry break and sometimes secondary break due to retinal injury.

Case discussion

- A case of status postcataract surgery with postoperative vitreous hemorrhage
- Primary entry break detected superiorly (Fig. 24.2A) and it was lasered (Fig. 24.2B).

Perforation with Vitreous Hemorrhage with Partial Retinal Detachment (Video 3, Chapter 24)

Case discussion

- A case of postcataract surgery vitreous hemorrhage (Fig. 24.3A) with partial retinal detachment in supero-temporal periphery
- Both primary entry (Fig. 24.3B) and secondary breaks (Fig. 24.3C) detected
- RD settled by FAX and breaks were lasered with long acting C_3F_8 gas injection (Fig. 24.3D).

Perforation with Vitreous Hemorrhage with Total Retinal Detachment (Video 4, Chapter 24)

Globe perforation can lead to retinal detachment (Fig. 24.4A)

Case discussion

- A case of postcataract surgery vitreous hemorrhage with total retinal detachment

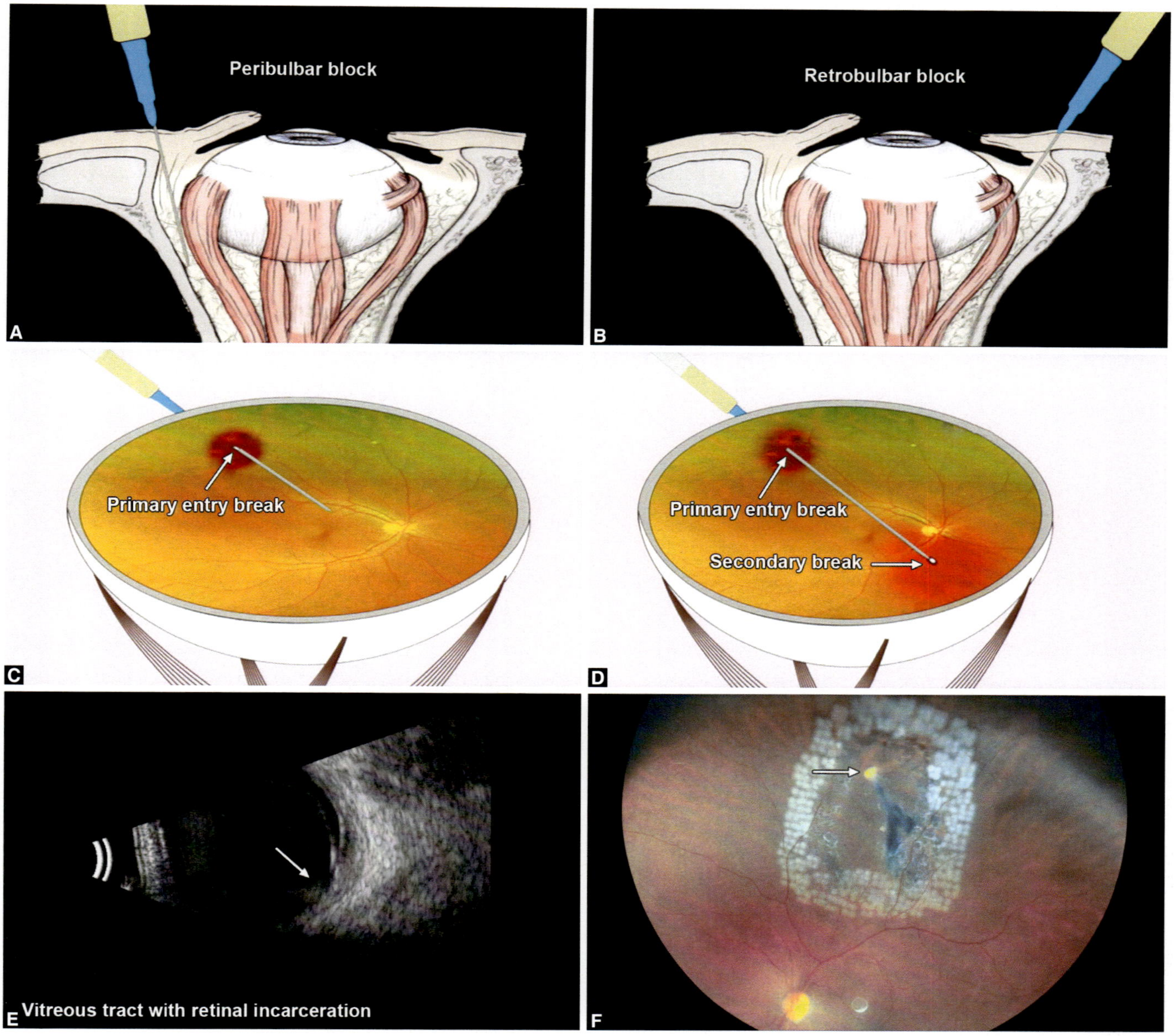

Figs 24.1A to F: (A) Peribulbar anesthesia; (B) Retrobulbar anesthesia; (C and D) Shows intraocular needle entry can cause primary and secondary break; (E) USG shows vitreous tract formation, vitreous hemorrhage and retinal incarceration in a case of globe perforation; (F) Sometimes laser barrage around the visible superior slit-like break saves the vision

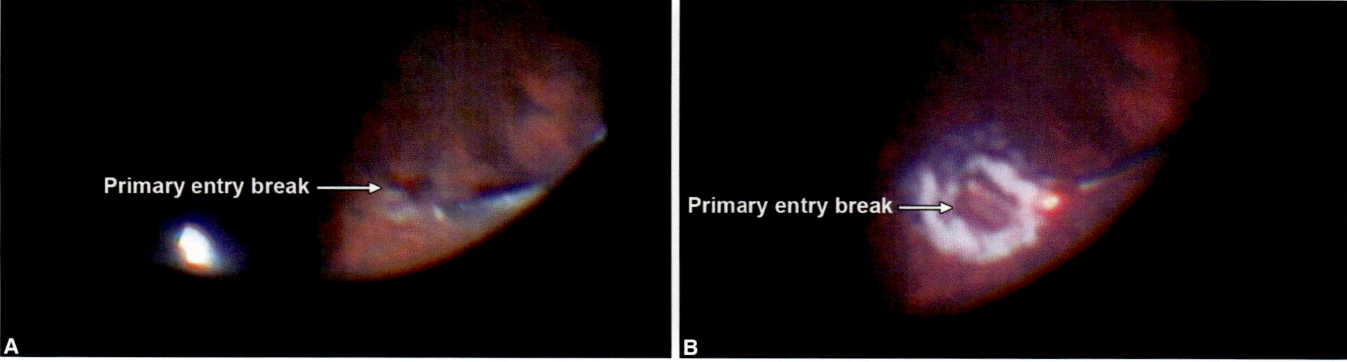

Figs 24.2A and B: Needle entry break in a case of postcataract surgery vitreous hemorrhage

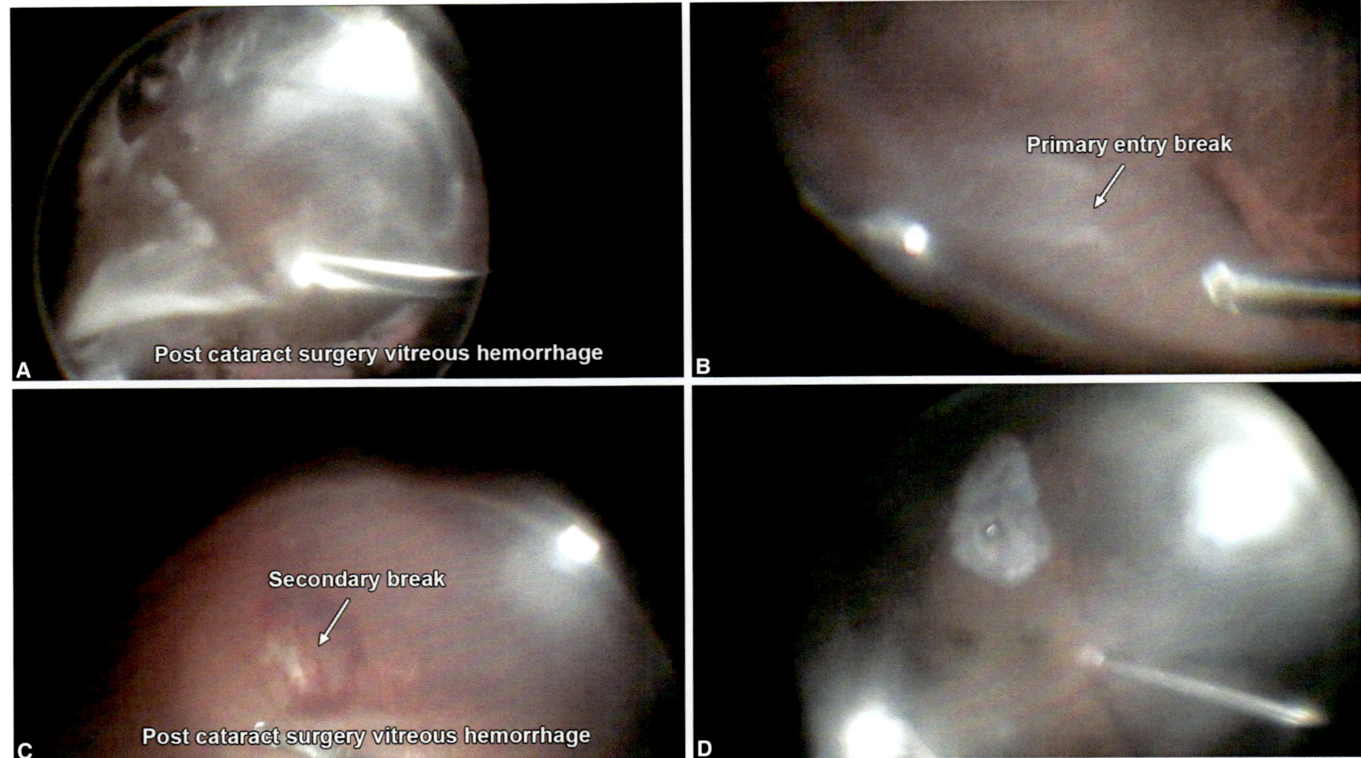

Figs 24.3A to D: Intraoperative steps of surgery managing postcataract surgery vitreous hemorrhage with partial retinal detachment

- Multiple posterior pole secondary breaks, nasal to the optic disc detected (Fig. 24.4B)
- Primary entry was superior, suggesting the needle path (Fig. 24.4C)
- Retina settled with FAX (Fig. 24.4D) and all breaks were lasered (Fig. 24.4E)
- Silicone oil was used as endotamponade (Fig. 24.4F).

Perforation with Macular Break with Retinal Detachment (Video 5, Chapter 24)

- Needle can directly hit macula (Fig. 24.5A) due to globe perforation during periocular anesthesia, carrying very poor visual prognosis.

Case discussion

- A case of postpterygium surgery vitreous hemorrhage with total retinal detachment with secondary slit-like large macular break (Fig. 24.5B)
- Primary slit-like tear detected in superotemporal periphery suggesting wrong site of peribulbar block with globe perforation (Fig. 24.5C)
- PFCL injected (Fig. 24.5D)
- Peripheral vitreous hemorrhage removed (Fig. 24.5E) and vitreous base excision completed (Fig. 24.5F)
- Macular ERM removed (Fig. 24.5G)
- Retina settled by FAX
- All breaks lasered (Fig. 24.5H) and the case ended up with silicone oil tamponade (Fig. 24.5I).

Perforation with Hemorrhagic Retinal Detachment with Retinal Incarceration (Video 6, Chapter 24)

Case discussion

- A case of abandoned cataract surgery with vitreous hemorrhage
- Phacoemulsification completed (Fig. 24.6A) with IOL implantation (Fig. 24.6B)
- Hemorrhagic retinal detachment detected after clearing vitreous hemorrhage
- A large posterior pole secondary breaks, superonasal to the optic disk, extending to macula detected (Fig. 24.6C)
- Subretinal blood removed using back-flush needle (Fig. 24.6D).
- Retina was incarcerated to the RPE-choroid at the break margin (Fig. 24.6E). This incarcerated retinal tags released (Figs 24.6F and G)
- Primary entry break was inferior at 6'O clock (Fig. 24.6H)
- Retina settled with FAX (Fig. 24.6I) and all breaks were lasered (Fig. 24.6J)
- Silicone oil was used as endotamponade.

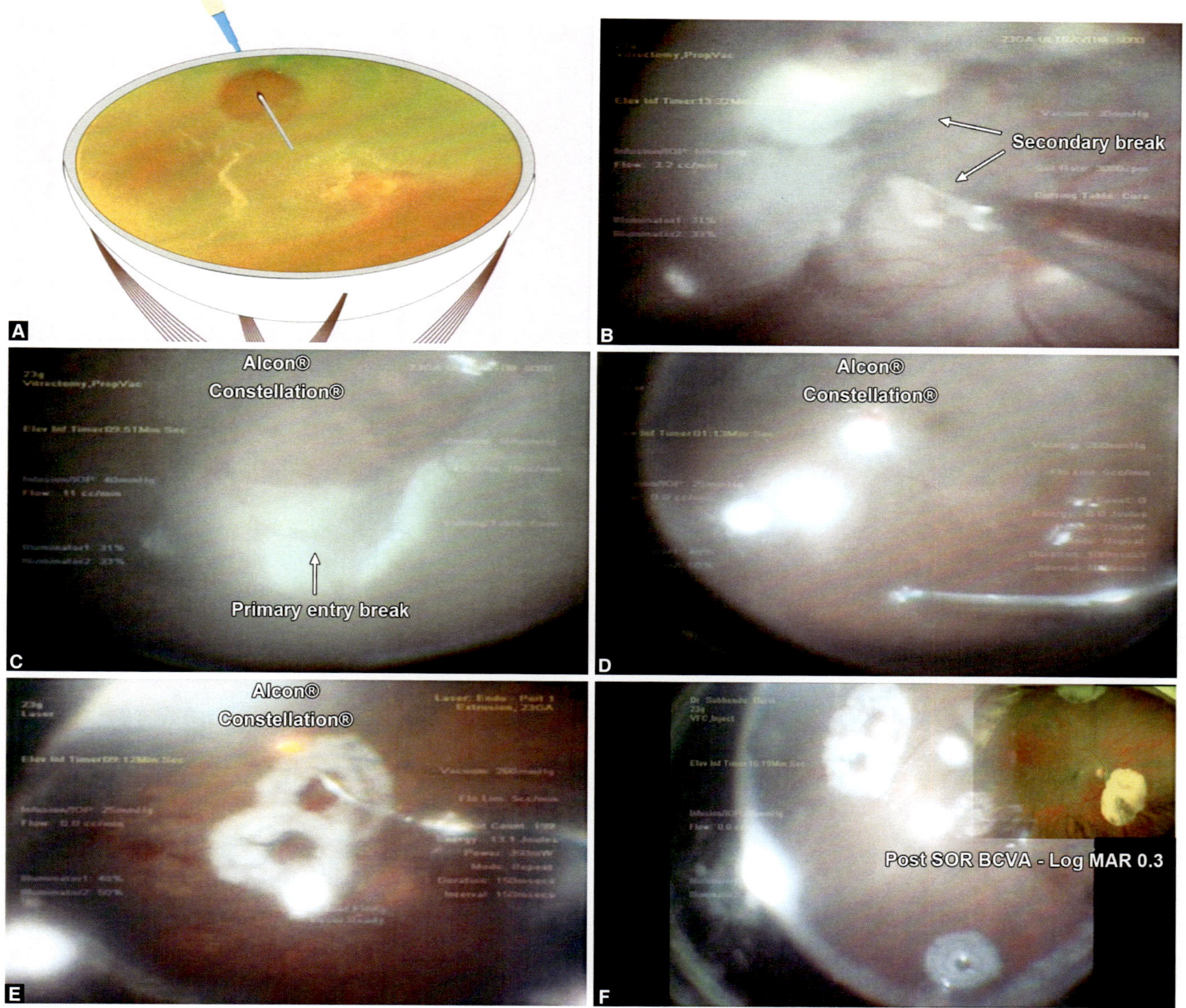

Figs 24.4A to F: Intraoperative steps of surgery managing postcataract surgery vitreous hemorrhage with total retinal detachment

INTRAOPERATIVE COMPLICATIONS

I. Preoperative complications
II. Intraoperative complications

Complications of Scleral Buckling

A. Complications During Tagging Muscles

a. Partial tagging of recti muscles
b. Tagging of oblique muscles
c. Muscle disinsertion and muscle loss
d. Damage to the vortex vein
e. Oculocardiac reflex

B. Complications During Cryoretinopexy

a. Inadequate cryopexy
b. Excessive cryopexy
c. *Scleral rupture:* This may occur in high myopic eyes or eyes with extreme scleral thinning. The surgeon can realize it if there is a sudden gush of subretinal fluid. The surgeon should immediately release the tractional sutures of the muscles and release speculum to avoid further loss of SRF and then should go for repair of scleral rupture. One should pass sutures through relatively healthy areas to repair the scleral rupture.

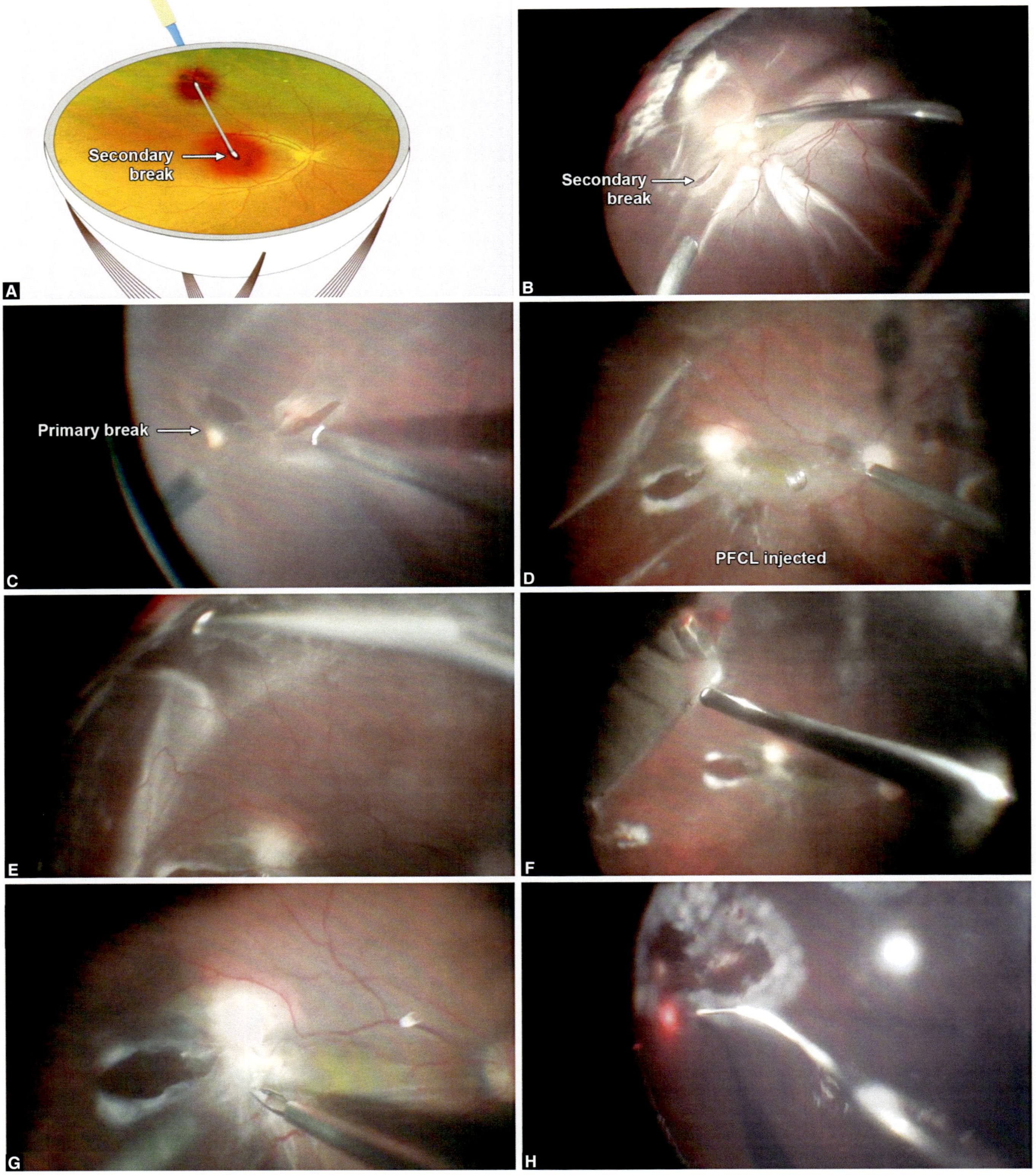

Figs 24.5A to H

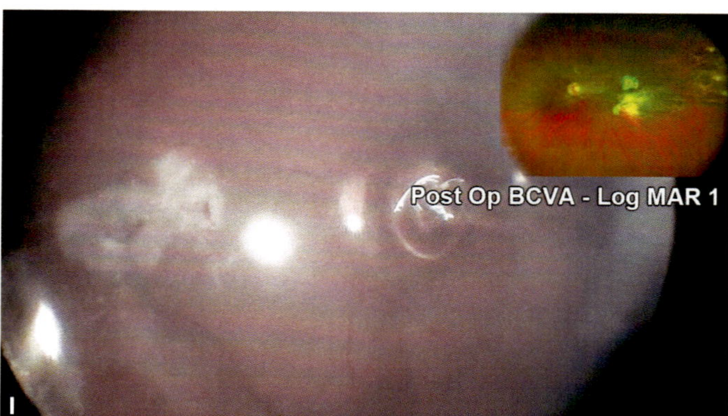

Figs 24.5A to I: Intraoperative steps of surgery managing postpterygium surgery vitreous hemorrhage with total retinal detachment

C. Complications during Drainage of Subretinal Fluid

a. Choroidal hemorrhage and subretinal hemorrhage
   - It occurs in 3–4% of cases with drainage procedures
   - Higher chances in high myopia, glaucoma, patients with diabetes and cardiovascular diseases and sometimes with the preoperative use of warfarin or aspirin.
   - It occurs when a large choroidal vessel is punctured or damaged and if intravascular pressure in the choroidal vessels exceeds the intraocular pressure, especially in cases of profound hypotony, just after drainage of SRF.
   - This complication can be avoided by proper selection of the site of drainage, i.e., just above or below the recti muscles. Prior coagulation of the large choroidal by diathermy or infrared laser lowers the risk of choroidal haemorrhage.

b. Dry tap
   - It means the absence of drainage of SRF through the site of the scleral incision.
   - Improperly chosen site of drainage, i.e., at the area of minimal SRF/no SRF or inadequate full-thickness perforation of sclera-choroid (especially in hypermetropic eyes), can result in a dry tap.
   - Proper site selection is necessary after visualization of subretinal fluid configuration and retinal elevation.
   - If there is 'a dry tap' on the 'first attempt', make sure regarding the depth of the scleral incision and visibility of large choroidal vessels (especially under an operating microscope).
   - If still 'a dry tap' on the 'second attempt' or a dry tap even after the adequate depth of scleral incision, then repeat indirect ophthalmoscopy should be performed to confirm the retina elevation and SRF configuration. In these cases, a second site selection is necessary.

c. Retinal perforation and vitreoretinal incarceration
   - It may occur if drainage is done at the wrong site, where there is minimal or no SRF. Sometimes, vitreoretinal incarceration occurs at the drainage site in 2–3% of cases.
   - If the depth assessment during needle drainage is not adequate, it may lead to retinal perforation. However, large-sized scleral incisions and increased pressure over the globe at the beginning of SRF drainage are two main factors responsible for vitreoretinal prolapse and incarceration. Increased pressure over the globe occurs when the surgeon tries to induce fast drainage in the presence of a large scleral incision.
   - Maintaining a relatively constant IOP is very important during drainage. Globe indentation at the ora serrata in the meridian of the drainage site helps elevate the retina over the site and allows free movement of SRF to the sclerotomy site.
   - If there is a high risk of vitreoretinal incarceration, it is better to close the sclerotomy by suturing or placing a buckle over the drainage site. The vitrectomy cutter should make the scleral drainage site free from any vitreous fibers.
   - If there is already considerable vitreoretinal incarceration, it is better to reposition the herniated tissue, then suture the sclerotomy site, do the I/O, and check for any evidence of a break or any residual incarceration at the drainage site. Gentle cryotherapy and buckle placement over the drainage site is a good option in the majority and rarely is further vitrectomy needed to settle the retina.

d. Suprachoroidal hemorrhage occurs rarely after drainage of subretinal fluid due to precipitation of extreme hypotony after the drainage procedure. Sometimes, an infusion cannula can be placed before starting drainage of SRF to combat severe hypotony if it sets in.

D. Complications During Gas Injection

a. *Fish-egg air/gas bubble:* Single bubble formation after intravitreal air or gas injection is desirable by a smart, gentle push, but sometimes multiple gases or air bubbles may mimic the appearance of fish eggs. The risk factors for this "fish egg air/gas bubbles are:
   i. If the needle is not inserted at the highest point of the eye
   ii. If very slowly or very rapidly injected

   This phenomenon is not welcomed because
   i. It may hamper further visibility for retinopexy and
   ii. A very small air/gas bubble, smaller than the retinal break, can pass into the subretinal space and may complicate the prognosis by delaying the reattachment.

b. *Gas in the canal of Petit:* In young patients with thicker anterior hyaloids, air/gas may be injected between the anterior hyaloid space and crystalline lens, called the Canal of Petit. The gas collects in a ring shape behind the periphery of the crystalline lens, creating an appearance known as the "sausage" or "doughnut" sign. This will never happen if the tip of the needle is well inside the vitreous cavity.

   A small amount of trapped gas inside the Canal of Petit will be absorbed spontaneously, but a larger amount needs overnight face-down positioning or to be

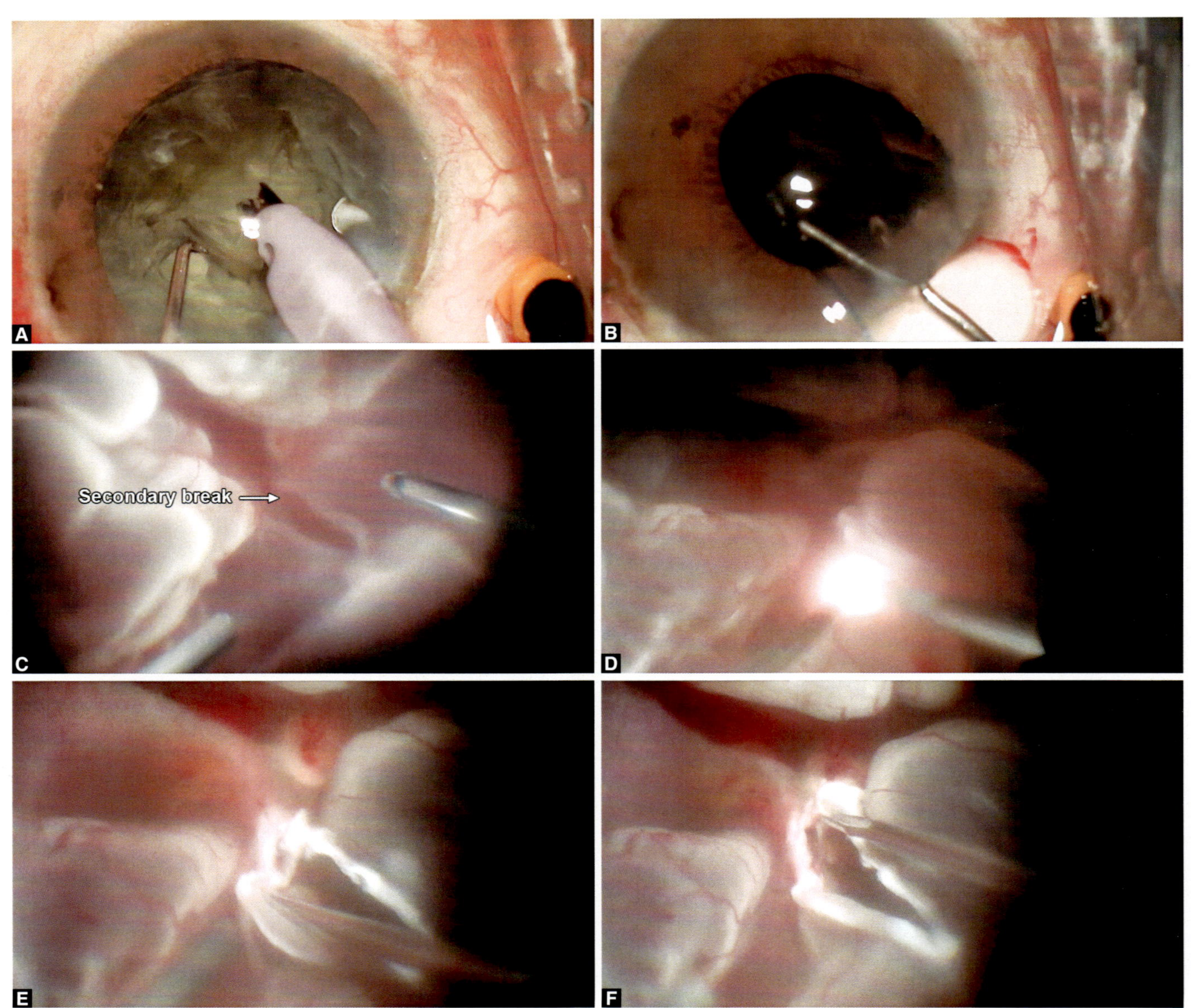

Figs 24.6A to F

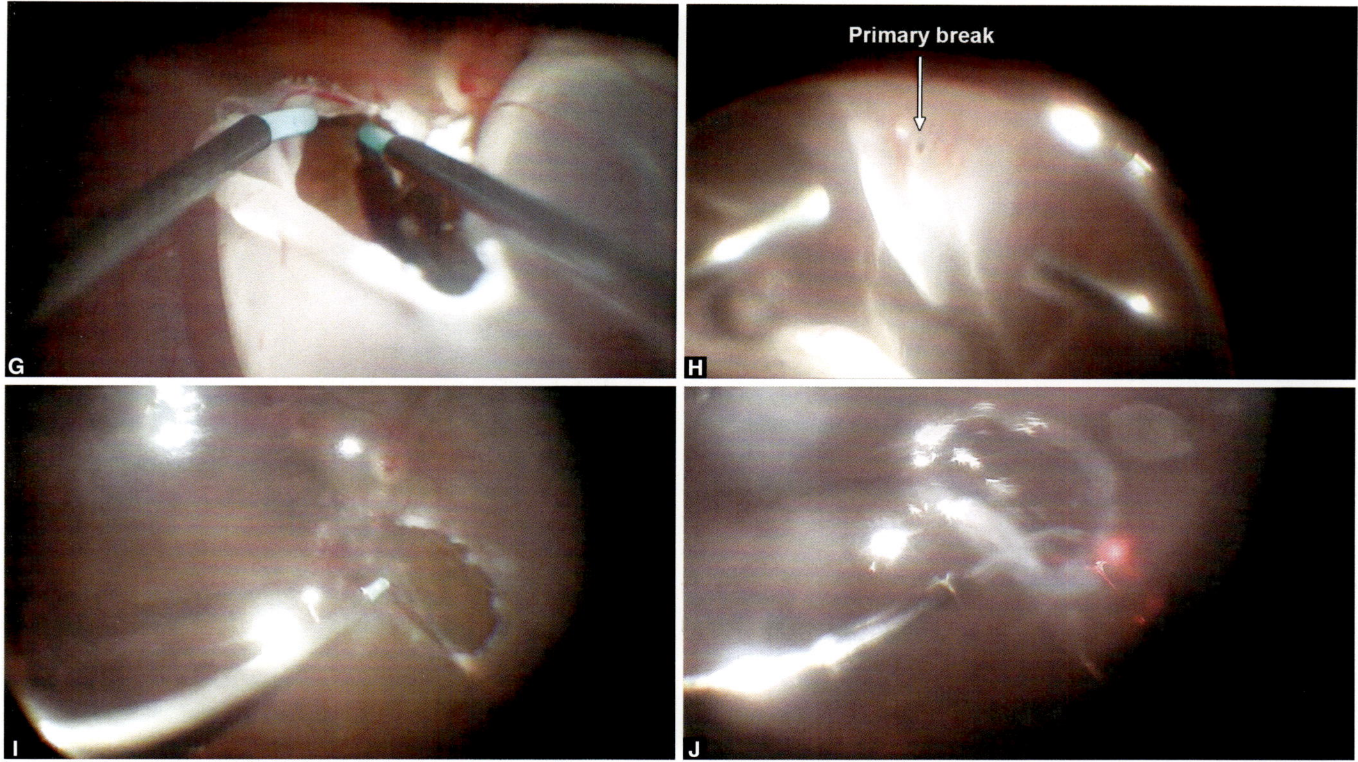

Figs 24.6A to J: Intraoperative steps of surgery managing abandoned cataract surgery with vitreous hemorrhage with hemorrhagic retinal detachment

drained by tuberculin syringe and 30G needle via pars plana route.

c. Subretinal air/gas may occur due to direct injection of air/gas into the subretinal space or entry of a small bubble through the retinal break in case of "multiple small gas bubbles" formation. Sometimes, unrelieved traction can lead to the passage of small gas bubbles into the subretinal space. Many times, it decreases the success rate.

E. Complications of Buckling

a. No break detected
b. Inability to close retinal break on the buckle-radial implant

F. Buckle-related Complications

a. *Buckle exposure:* It can present with or without infection. Without infection, an exposed buckle may be present for a long time without producing any symptoms (Fig. 24.7).
b. Buckle intrusion
c. Anterior migration of buckle
d. Buckle infection—it may present as:
   i *Acute buckle infection:* Where eyes will be congested and there will be exudates or active discharge over the exposed buckle.
   ii. *Chronic buckle infection:* Where eyes will be congested and there will be exudates or active discharge over the exposed buckle.

Management of buckle infection: An infected buckle should always be removed. This should be done under topical antibiotic coverage (preferably a combination of antibiotic drops covering both gram-positive and gram-negative organisms).

Steps of buckle removal:
1. Conjunctival opening
2. Removal of the buckle with buckle sutures
3. Localization of encirclage bands
4. Cutting of band
5. Removal of encirclage band along with all sutures by firm but gentle traction.

Organisms responsible for buckle infection: Mostly *Staph epidermis* and *Staph aureus.*

Complications during buckle removal:

i. Occurrence of retinal detachment
ii. Globe rupture
iii. Vitreous hemorrhage
iv. Infection, i.e., endophthalmitis and
v. Phthisis bulbi.

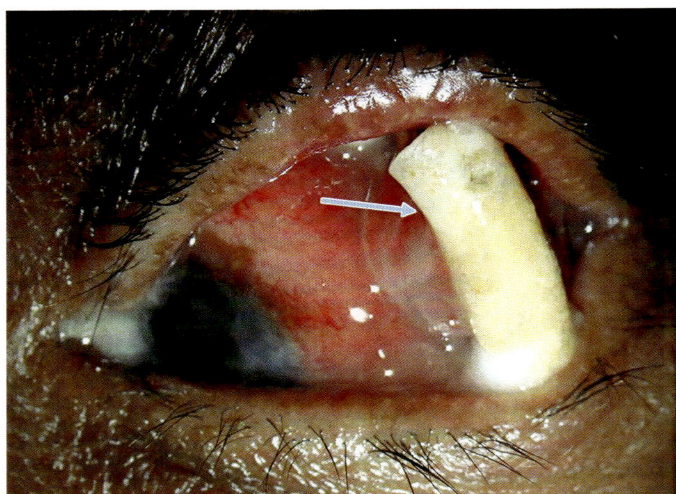

Fig. 24.7: Postoperative exposed infected sponge buckle (blue arrow)

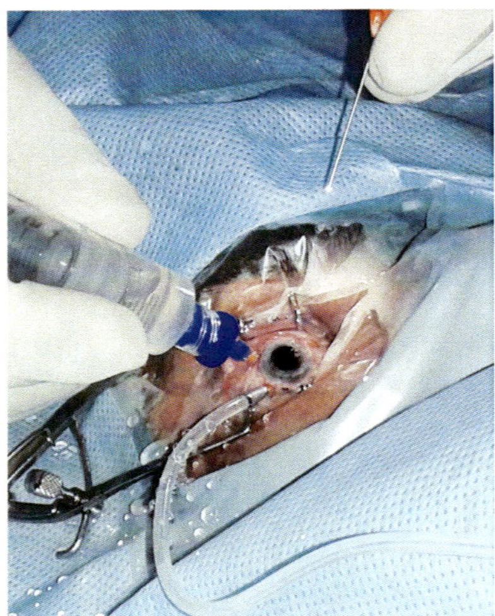

Fig. 24.8: Surgery in a small globe with small palpebral apparture

Problems in Initiating Surgery

Deep Set and Small Eyes (Fig. 24.8)

Causes: Abnormally deep set eyes-skull malformation, congenital (Trisomy 9 Mosaicism), post-trauma with orbital fat atrophy.

Small palpebral fissure: Blepharophimosis, Edward's syndrome, eyes with epicanthic fold, post-trauma scarring.

Small eyes: Congenital (Patau syndrome), microphthalmos, high hypermetropia, nanophthalmos.

Difficulties:

- Difficulty in sclerotomy placement
- Entry site retinal tear at periphery due to narrow pars plana
- Risk of lens touch
- Fogging of wide-angle viewing system (WAVS) due to higher humidity around the ocular surface
- Difficulty in contact lens placement
- Standard-sized instruments too large for smaller eyes
- Risk of choroidal detachment in microphthalmic eyes
- Pooling of fluid
- Difficulty in angulation of instruments.

  Management:

  1. Often temporal approach
  2. Careful position of patient's head
  3. *Cathotomy:* if necessary,
     Cathotomy for small palpebral fissure *(Video 7, Chapter 24)*:
     - In case of eyes with small palpebral fissure, a straight artery forceps is to be held at lateral canthus at the junction of two limbs of 'Y' and the lateral canthus is to be crushed with the artery forceps along the straight limb of 'Y' up to the bony margin of orbit for one to two minutes (Fig. 24.9A). Then the crushed straight limb of the lateral canthus is to be cut with a scissor with small snips (Fig. 24.9B). This will widen the palpebral aperture to introduce trocar-cannula complex easily.
  4. Tractional sutures.

Scarred and Adherent Conjunctiva

Making of sclerotome ports are difficult as shifting conjunctiva to make sclerotomies are difficult (Fig. 24.9C). One has to choose different places to get movable, loose conjunctiva and to avoid previous sites of sclerotomies.

Slippage of Infusion Cannula *(Video 8, Chapter 24)*

Case Discussion

- Soft part of infusion cannula came out during vitreous base excision in a case of retinal detachment (Fig. 24.10A)
- Metallic end of infusion cannula along with cannula was removed
- A new infusion cannula was fitted in the superonasal cannula to build up the intravitreal tone (Fig. 24.10B)
- Now a trocar-cannula was introduced in the same scleral tunnel and trocar blade was removed
- Infusion cannula was removed from the superonasal cannula and fitted to the inferotemporal cannula again.

Suprachoroidal Infusion *(Video 9, Chapter 24)*

Case Discussion

- It was also a case of Giant Retinal Tear with choroidal detachment

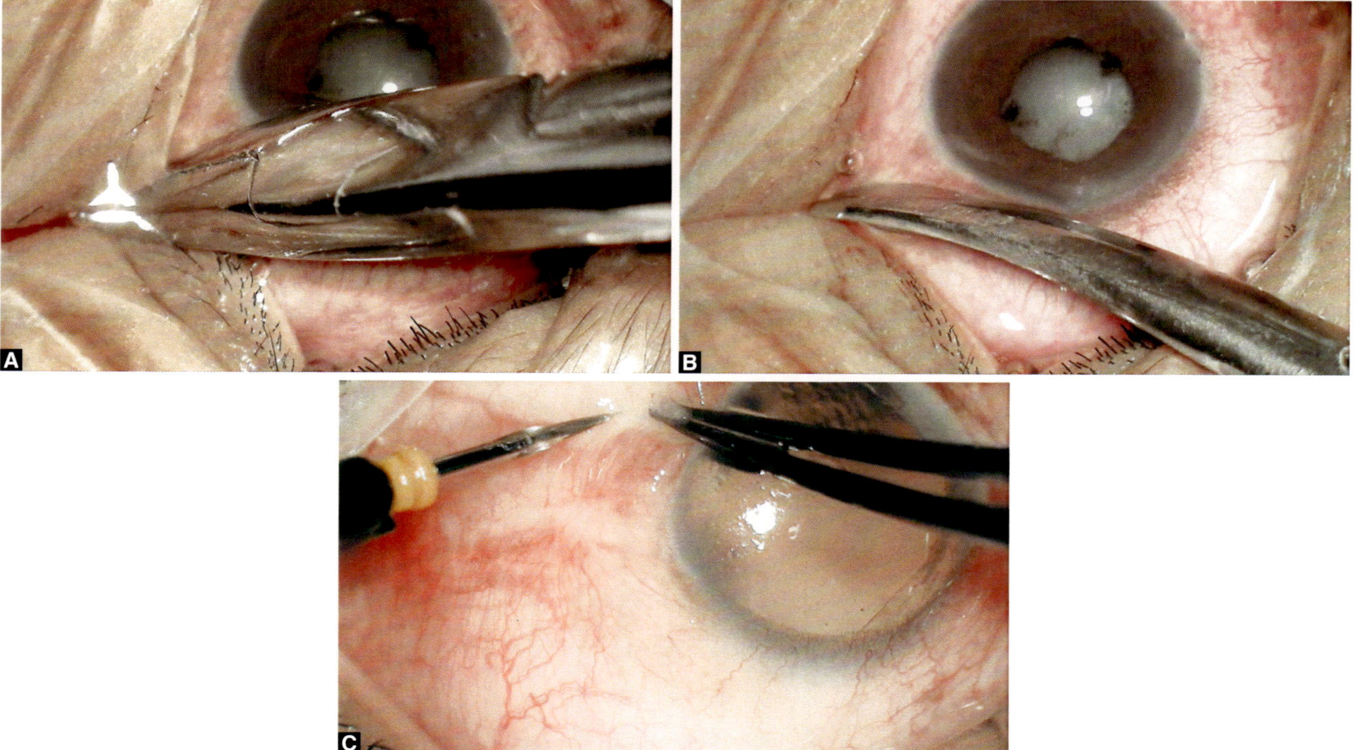

Figs 24.9A to C: (A and B) Technique of canthotomy; (C) Post-vitrectomy scarred conjunctiva

- There was difficulty in introducing trocar-cannula due to soft eye
- Tip of infusion cannula was not visible
- Saline was injected into the vitreous cavity to raise IOP
- Trocar-cannula was introduced for left-handed port and trocar was removed
- Endoilluminator was introduced through the cannula and tip of infusion cannula was seen in suprachoroidal space (Fig. 24.11A)
- Now this endoilluminator tip was used to separate the choroidal layers from the tip of infusion cannula to make it intravitreal (Fig. 24.11B).
- Now infusion was made on
- Right-handed trocar cannula was introduced
- Then vitrectomy was started.

Subretinal Infusion *(Video 10, Chapter 24)*

Case Discussion

- PVD induction was done in a case of bullous RD
- Fluid-air exchange was started for internal drainage of SRF through separate retinotomy
- But tip of 25G infusion cannula was seen in subretinal space (Fig. 24.12A)
- Cutter was used to make it intravitreal and infusion fluid was made on
- Cautery was done for the surrounding retinotomy
- Fluid-air exchange was started again keeping tip of infusion inside the vitreous cavity (Fig. 24.12B)
- Internal drainage of SRF was completed again
- Peripheral breaks were lasered as well as around the retinotomy behind the infusion cannula.

Retinal Incarceration at the Cannula Tip *(Video 11, Chapter 24)*

Case Discussion

- In a case of choroidal coloboma with retinal detachment, during vitreous base excision, retinal incarceration seen at the cannula tip (Fig. 24.13A)
- Incarcerated detached retina separated from the cannula and retinectomy done for the redundant retina at the base of the cannula (Fig. 24.13B)
- Subretinal blood removed. PFCL injected to stabilize posterior pole and for peripheral internal drainage of SRF
- Fluid-air exchange done
- Laser done surrounding the retinal breaks.

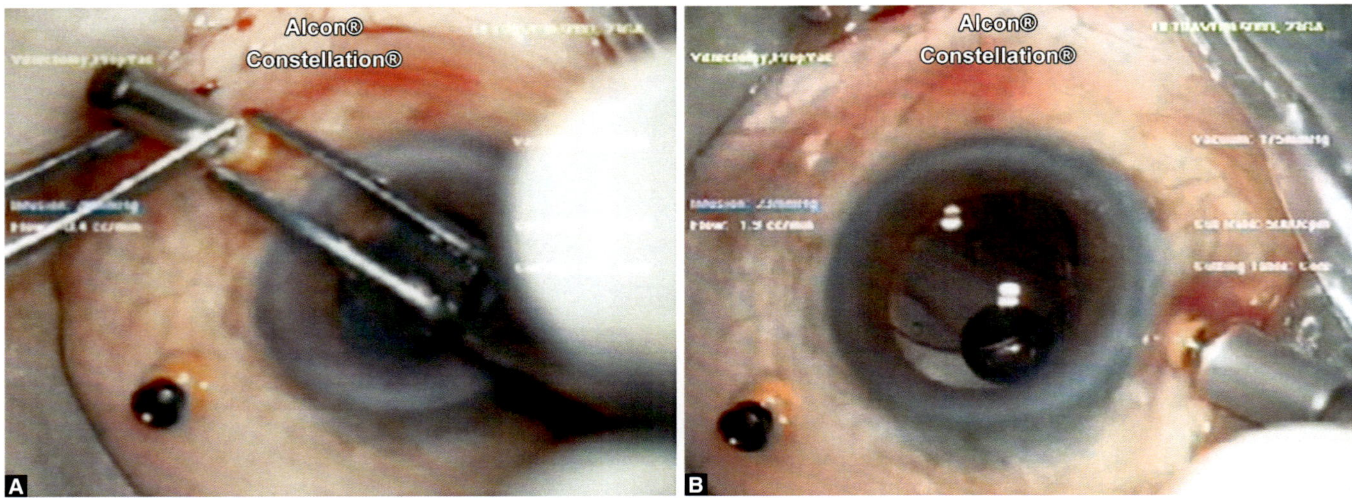

Figs 24.10A and B: Intraoperative steps of surgery managing slippage of infusion cannula

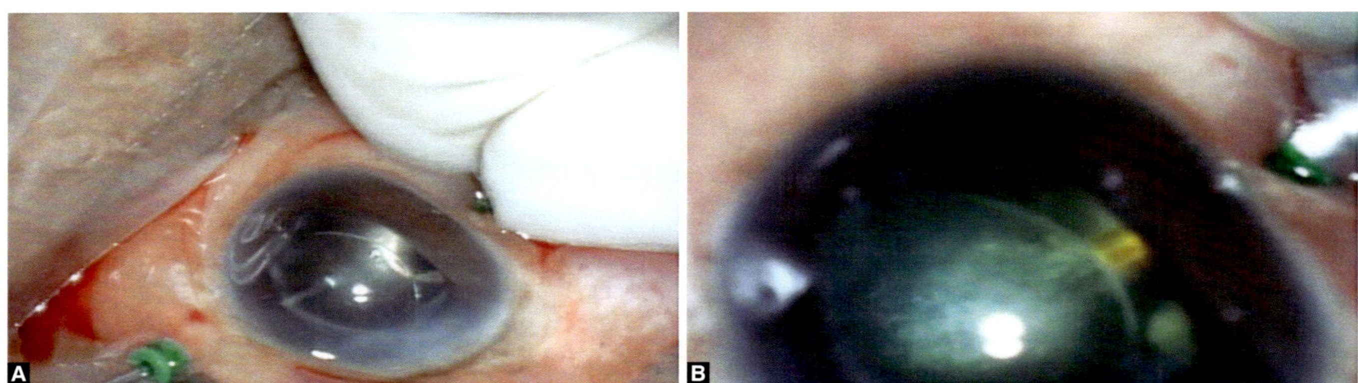

Figs 24.11A and B: Intraoperative steps of surgery managing suprachoroidal infusion tip

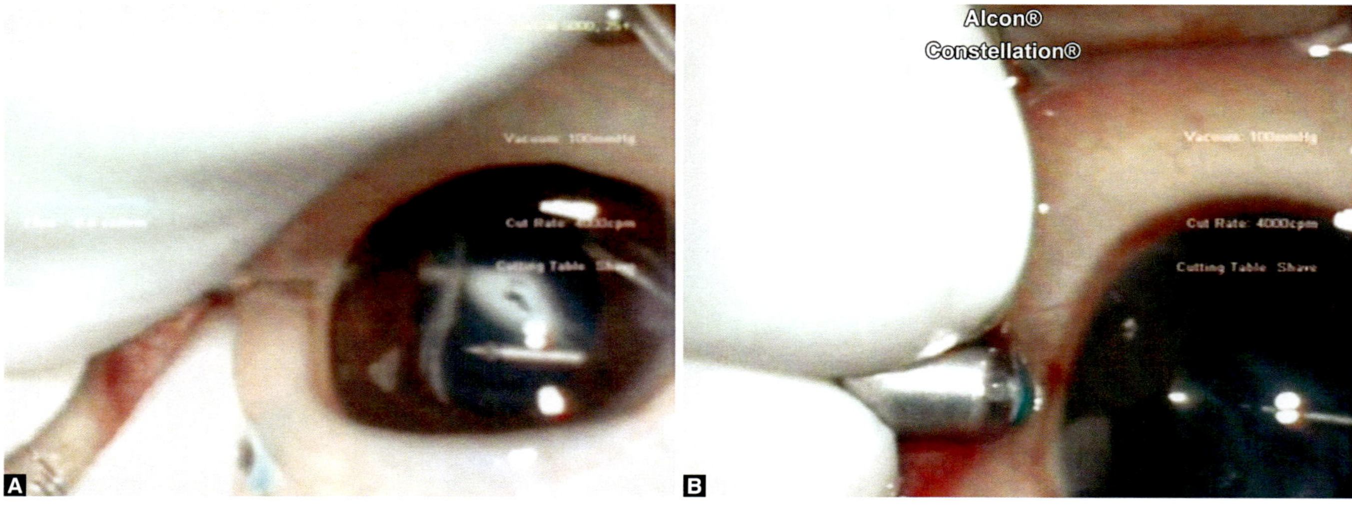

Figs 24.12A and B: Intraoperative steps of surgery managing subretinal infusion

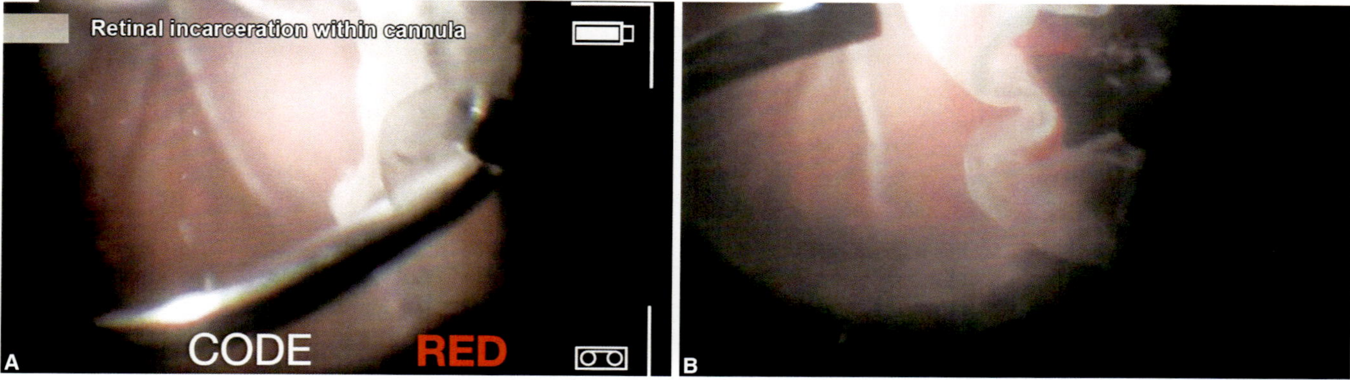

Figs 24.13A and B: Intraoperative steps of surgery managing retinal incarceration at cannula tip

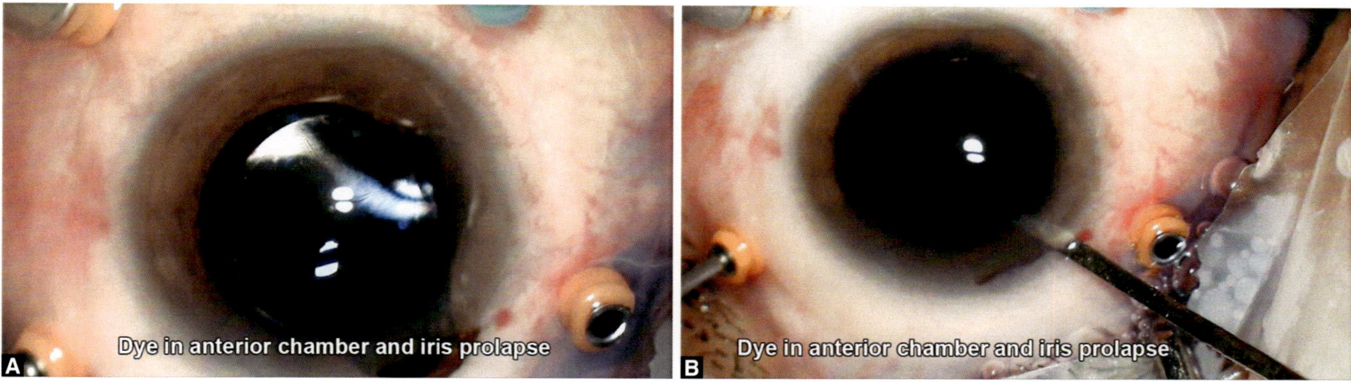

Figs 24.14A and B: Intraoperative steps of surgery managing iris prolapse during dye injection in a case of combined phacoemulsification with ERM removal surgery

Complications during Phacovitrectomy

1. *Extension during capsulorrhexis:* It may happen due to sudden introduction of infusion fluid inside the vitreous cavity, resulting in increase in intravitreal pressure and shallowing of anterior chamber. Limited anterior vitrectomy reduce intravitreal pressure and then injecting more viscoelastic into anterior chamber deepen anterior chamber and flatten convex anterior lens capsule and now surgeon can complete further capsulorrhexis.
2. *Inadvertent posterior capsular tear:* Sudden introduction of multiple air bubbles from infusion port can hamper the visibility. During removal of these retro IOL air bubbles by cutter may damage posterior capsule. Removal of these retro IOL air bubbles should be done by passive suction of silicone tipped flute needle/back-flush needle instead of cutter.
3. *Iris prolapse during dye injection (Video 12, Chapter 24):* It can happen during injection of dye to stain ILM or ERM due to sudden increase in IOP. The other cannula should be open and repositioning of iris tissue with adjustment of IOP solves the problem.

   Case discussion
   - A case of combined phacoemulsification with ERM removal
   - Posterior chamber IOL implanted
   - Trypan blue stain ERM removed
   - But just after injecting Brilliant Blue dye, prolapse of iris tissue seen through the phaco main wound (Fig. 24.14A)
   - Prolapsed iris repositioned again (Fig. 24.14B)
   - And proceeded for peeling ILM.
4. *Sudden influx of air bubbles behind IOL (Video 13, Chapter 24):* Influx of air bubble during vitrectomy may blur the media (Fig. 24.15). Removal of retro IOL air bubbles should be done cautiously as it may cause posterior capsular tear.

Complications during PVD Induction

Complications with Attached Retina

- Inadvertent break formation at the mid-periphery or far periphery may happen during PVD induction when hyaloid face is abnormally thickened and very much sticky and adherent to retina, sometimes happens during operating for a macular surgical pathology like epiretinal membrane

- Especially beyond mid periphery, where retina is thinner and if there is already a thinned-out retina or lattice degeneration is present
- One can due simple laser if no retinal detachment developed.

In case of intraoperative inadvertent retinal break formation with ongoing retinal detachment:

- Use low suction and maximum high cutting rate
- Start cutting vitreous in other areas, otherwise ongoing traction by suction of cutter can increase area of retinal detachment.

Case discussion (Video 14, Chapter 24):

- It was an ERM removal surgery
- During TA-assisted PVD induction, peripheral break formed and shallow subretinal fluid appeared (Fig. 24.16A)
- Vitreous, surrounding the break checked and vitrectomy started in areas away from the break using low suction and maximum high cutting rate
- Break cauterized

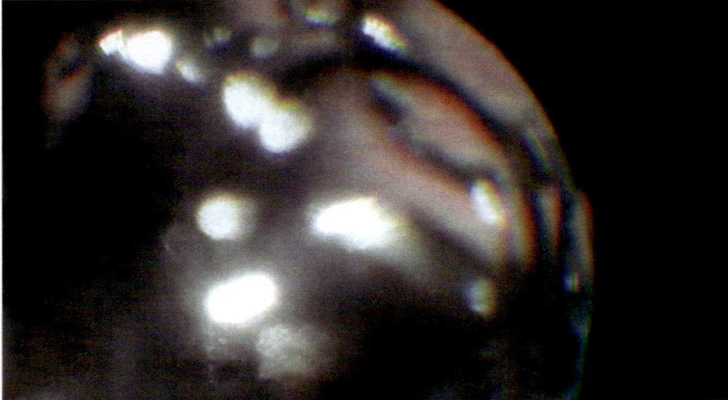

Fig. 24.15: Sudden influx of air bubbles during combined phacovitrectomy

- Peripheral vitrectomy completed
- Trypan blue dye injected under air to stain ERM
- ERM removal done
- Fluid air exchange done and peripheral localized SRF drained through the break
- Barrage laser done around the inadvertent break (Fig. 24.16B)
- Postoperatively retina was stable with improvement in macular anatomy without ERM.

Complications with Detached Retina

Inadvertent break can form because of sudden influx of mobile detached retina inside the cutter port

Case discussion (Video 15, Chapter 24):

Case I: During removal of attached peripheral posterior hyaloid on a detached retina with PFCL-assisted posterior pole stabilization in a case of PDR with combined retinal detachment, accidentally retina is engaged in cutter port (Fig. 24.17A). With the help of proportionate reflux mode of the cutter, detached engaged retina can be separated from the cutter port (Fig. 24.17B) and accidental break marked with cautery. Fluid-air exchange started for internal drainage (Fig. 24.17C) and laser barrage done after settling retina (Fig. 24.17D).

Case II: In an another case of diabetic retinal detachment, during removal of vitreoschisis membrane, detached retina may accidentally engage in cutter port (Fig. 24.17E). Again with the help of proportionate reflux mode of cutter the engaged retina should be separated and the vitreoschisis removal can be carried out with the help of forceps.

Intraoperative Sudden Unplanned Hypotony

Sudden precipitation of fall in IOP due to leakage intraocular fluid or air can cause sudden hypotony and appearance of

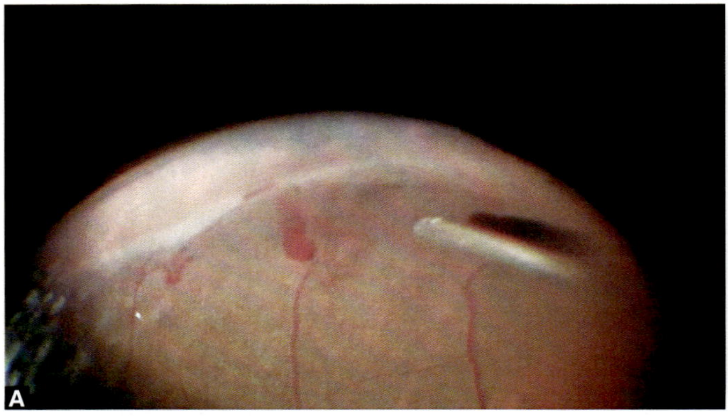

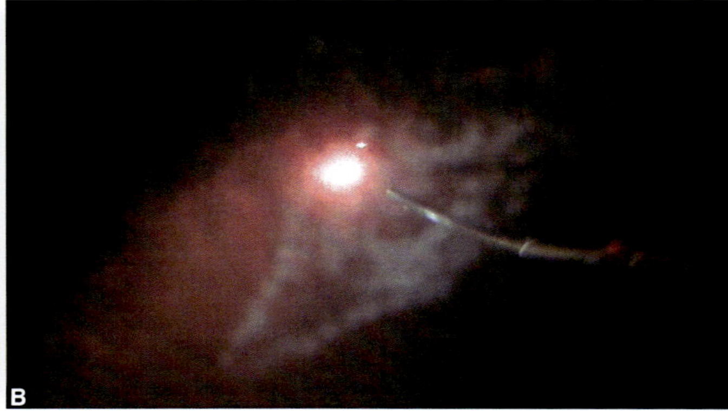

Figs 24.16A and B: Intraoperative steps of surgery managing inadvertent break formation at the periphery during PVD induction with attached retina

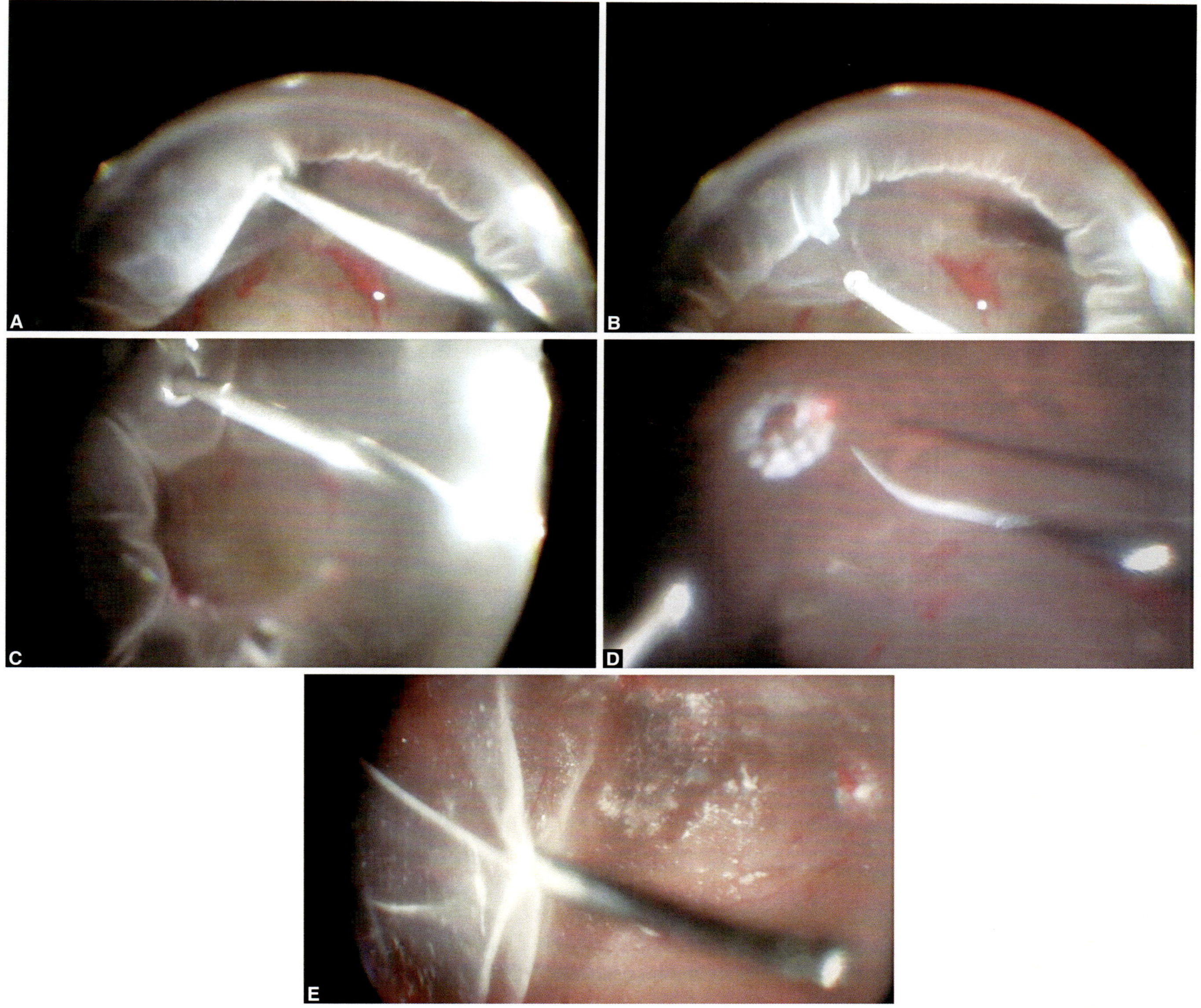

Figs 24.17A to E: Intraoperative steps of surgery managing inadvertent retinal break formation during PVD induction in detached retina

choroidals. It occurs during increase in suction or sudden stoppage of infusion due to lack of gas in the cylinder which may induce choroidal detachment intraoperatively.

Diagnosis: By sudden appearance of choroidals

How to Manage?

- Avoid aggravating hypotony, especially rapid changes in IOP
- Change of fluid
- Start fluid-air exchange
- *Evaluation infusion tip:* Suprachoroidal/tissue occlusion
- *Evaluate tubings* to exclude kinging/leak
- Stop active aspiration
- Wait for some time
- Check for peripheral retinal dialysis
- Complete the surgery keeping high IOP
- *Need for drainage of choroidal fluid:* When massive and presence of choroidal hamper subsequent laser.

Case Discussion

Post-boston K Pro intraoperative sudden unplanned hypotony (Video 16, Chapter 24):

- A case of retinal detachment in an eye with Boston Keratoprosthesis 1 with thin sclera, recurrent choroidal detachment appeared at the time of internal drainage of subretinal fluid by fluid-air exchange and laser (Fig. 24.18A)

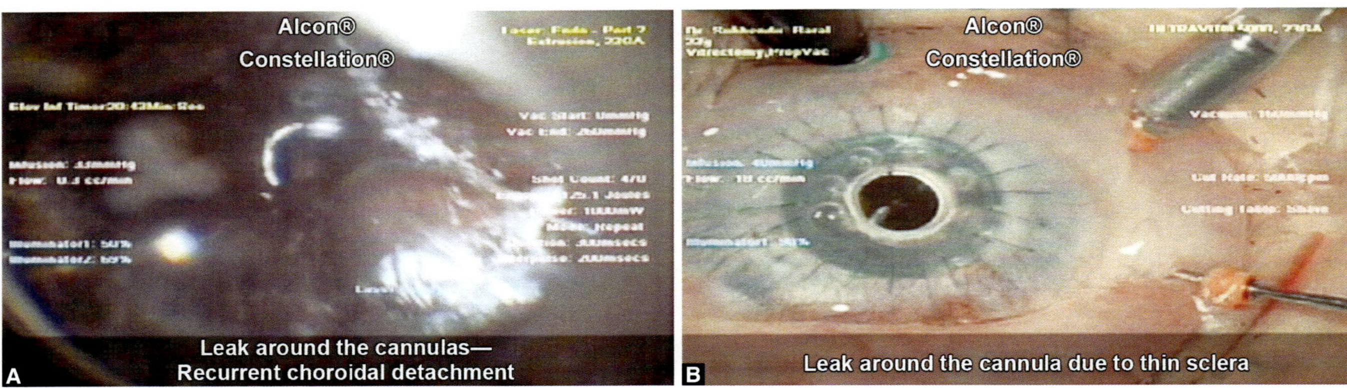

Figs 24.18A and B: Intraoperative steps of surgery managing post Boston KPro retinal detachment with sudden onset recurrent hypotony with choroidal detachment

- The cause of this sudden recurrent choroidal detachment was recurrent fall of intraocular pressure to leakage of air surrounding the cannula due to thin sclera (Fig. 24.18B)
- All scleral ports had to be sutured at the end of surgery to prevent postoperative hypotony.

Intraoperative Media Haziness *(Video 17, Chapter 24)*

Causes

i. *Fogging of visualizing lens:* Presence of fogging of visualizing lens can hamper visibility—changing the visualizing lens can improves visibility (Fig. 24.19A).
ii. *Presence of corneal epithelial edema, especially in case of endophthalmitis:* Removal of edematous corneal epithelium by an iris spatula can improve further visibility to work with more precision (Fig. 24.19B).
iii. While operating in a case of retinal detachment, media becomes hazy just immediate after injection of triamcinolone acetone particles to perform TA-assisted vitrectomy. Thorough wash of all TA particles improves visibility (Fig. 24.19C).
iv. During separation of peripheral vitreous from a detached retina after stabilizing posterior pole with PFCL, media sometimes become cloudy due to presence of pigment dispersion/blood oozing in anterior chamber due to friction of IOL with iris (Fig. 24.19D). Anterior chamber wash improves the media clarity.
v. While performing laser under air, media appeared hazy due to presence of vapor particles in posterior surface of IOL in case of posterior capsular rent (PCR) (Fig. 24.19E) gentle rubbing of soft tip cannula with the vapors on posterior surface of IOL at the area of PCR, improves visibility.
vi. Intraoperative posterior subcapsular cataract formation during fluid-air exchange (Fig. 24.19F). Sometimes while operating under air, media became hazy due to development of posterior subcapsular cataract.
vii. Oozing of blood from bleeders in case of managing fibrovascular proliferations (Fig. 24.19G). Careful adequate cautery of all bleeders can improve media visibility.

Stepwise Approach to Manage Intraocular Bleed

Cautery

Case discussion (Video 18, Chapter 24):

- In a case of full thickness macular hole with tightly adhered ERM, during removal of ERM, suddenly bleeding started because of firm attachment of ERM with blood vessels (Fig. 24.20)
- ERM removal completed in presence of hazy media
- Cautery of the bleeder tried
- Clotted pre retinal blood removed
- True bleeder noted and cauterised
- BBG dye injected in saline
- ILM peeling started
- Again bleeding started from capillaries due to traction during ILM removal
- IOP kept high
- ILM removal completed with the suction of cutter
- Fluid-air exchange done and fluid removed from the base of macular hole.

Use of Valved Cannula and Raising IOP

Case discussion (Video 19, Chapter 24):

- In a case of tightly adhered ERM using 27 G vitrectomy system, while removing ERM, bleeding started from capillaries due to traction from ERM removal (Fig. 24.21A)

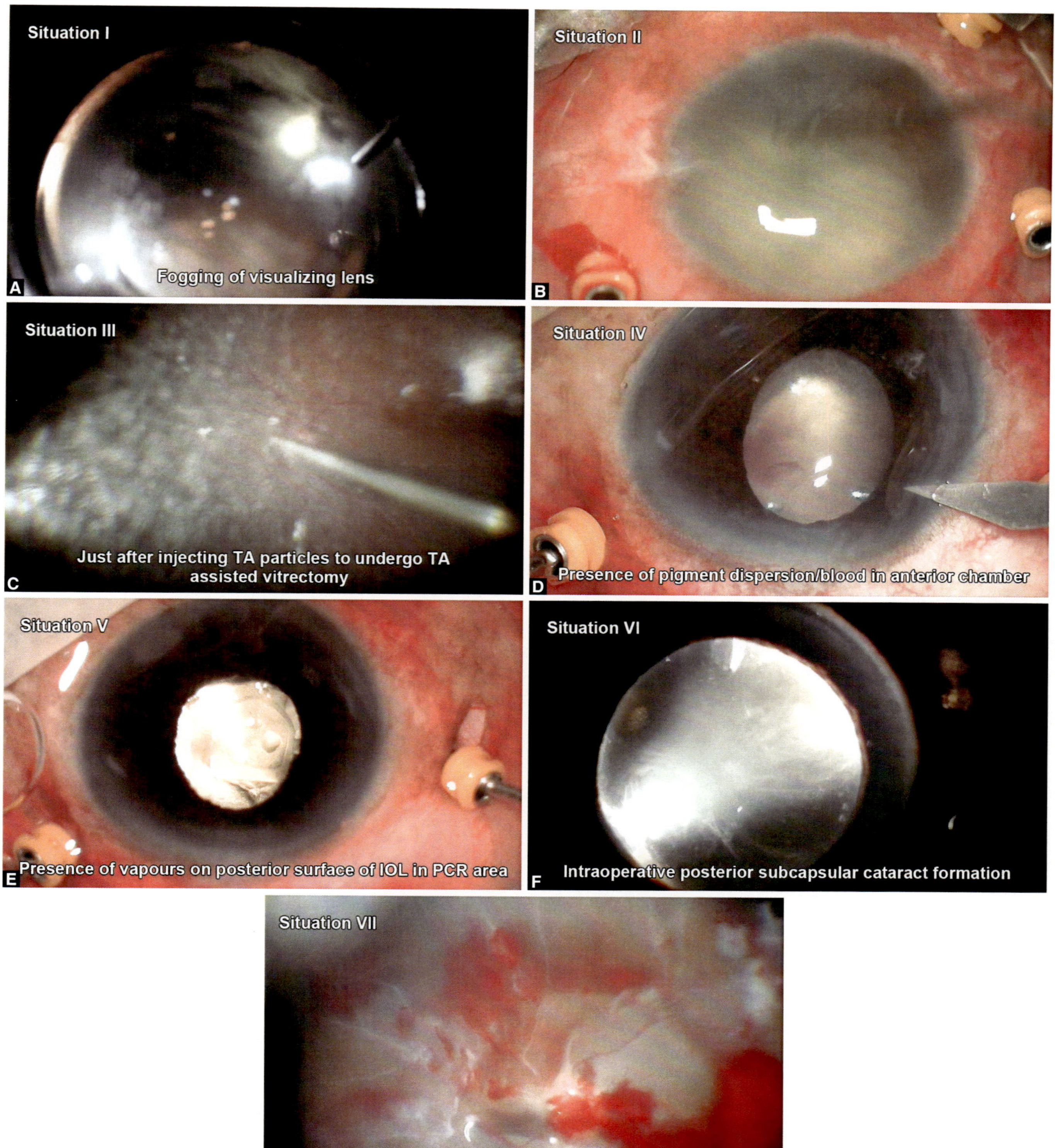

Figs 24.19A to G: Reasons for intraoperative media haziness

- Rest of the ERM removed with the help of suction of cutter only in a very controlled way as the cutter can go very close to the retina (Fig. 24.21B)
- 27 G valved cannula system maintained the closed chamber environment, high IOP was set and bleeding stopped (Fig. 24.21C)
- Mild cautery at the base and laser around that ended the case safely (Fig. 24.21D).

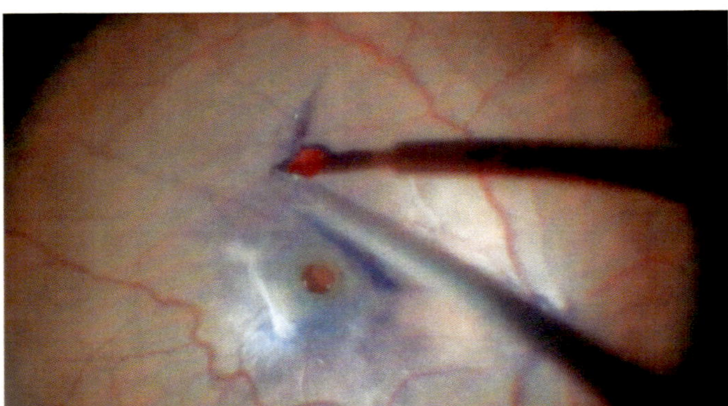

Fig. 24.20: Bleeding from capillaries during removal of tightly adhered ERM in a case of macular hole surgery

Start Fluid-Air Exchange in High IOP

Case discussion (Video 20, Chapter 24):

- Removal of large elevated papillovitreal neovascular polyp is necessary to prevent recurrent vitreous hemorrhage (Fig. 24.22A)
- Oozing from the disk after removal of neovascular polyp is sometimes uncontrollable (Fig. 24.22B)
- Fluid-air exchange followed by keeping IOP high, stop the disc hemorrhage (Figs 24.22C and D)
- It is always better not to remove the blood clot from the disk to prevent reappearance of bleeding from the disk (Fig. 24.22E).

Application of Triamcinolone Acetonide over the Bleeders

Case discussion (Video 21, Chapter 24):

- Sometimes bleeding from the optic nerve head, especially after removal of neovascular tissue in PDR (Figs 24.23A and B), can be stopped by applying triamcinolone particles over the disk directly (Figs 24.23C and D) or under air
- Case ended up after FAX (Fig. 24.23E). Postoperatively TA mixed blood clot resolves slowly (Figs 24.23F to H).

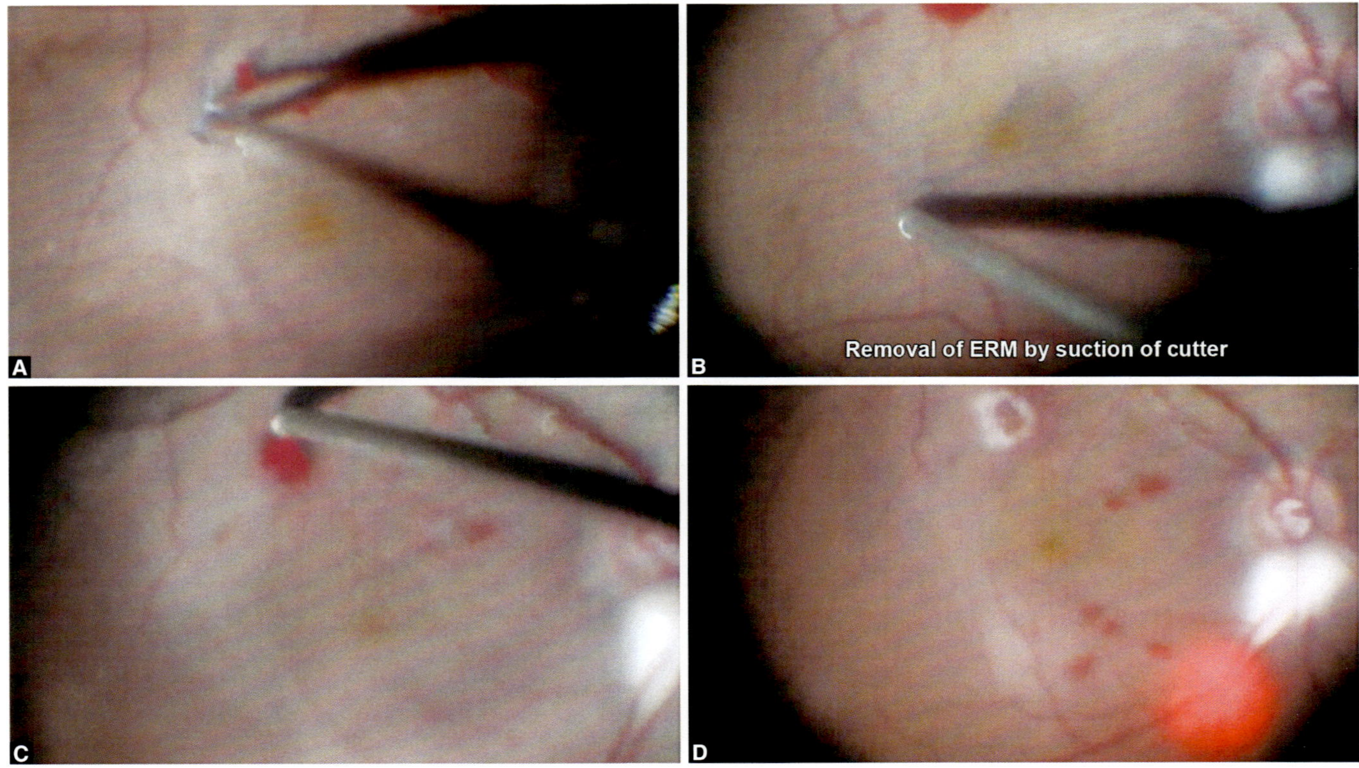

Figs 24.21A to D: Intraoperative steps of stoppage of bleeding from capillaries during removal of tightly adhered ERM by raising IOP with 27G+ valved cannula system in a case of ERM removal surgery

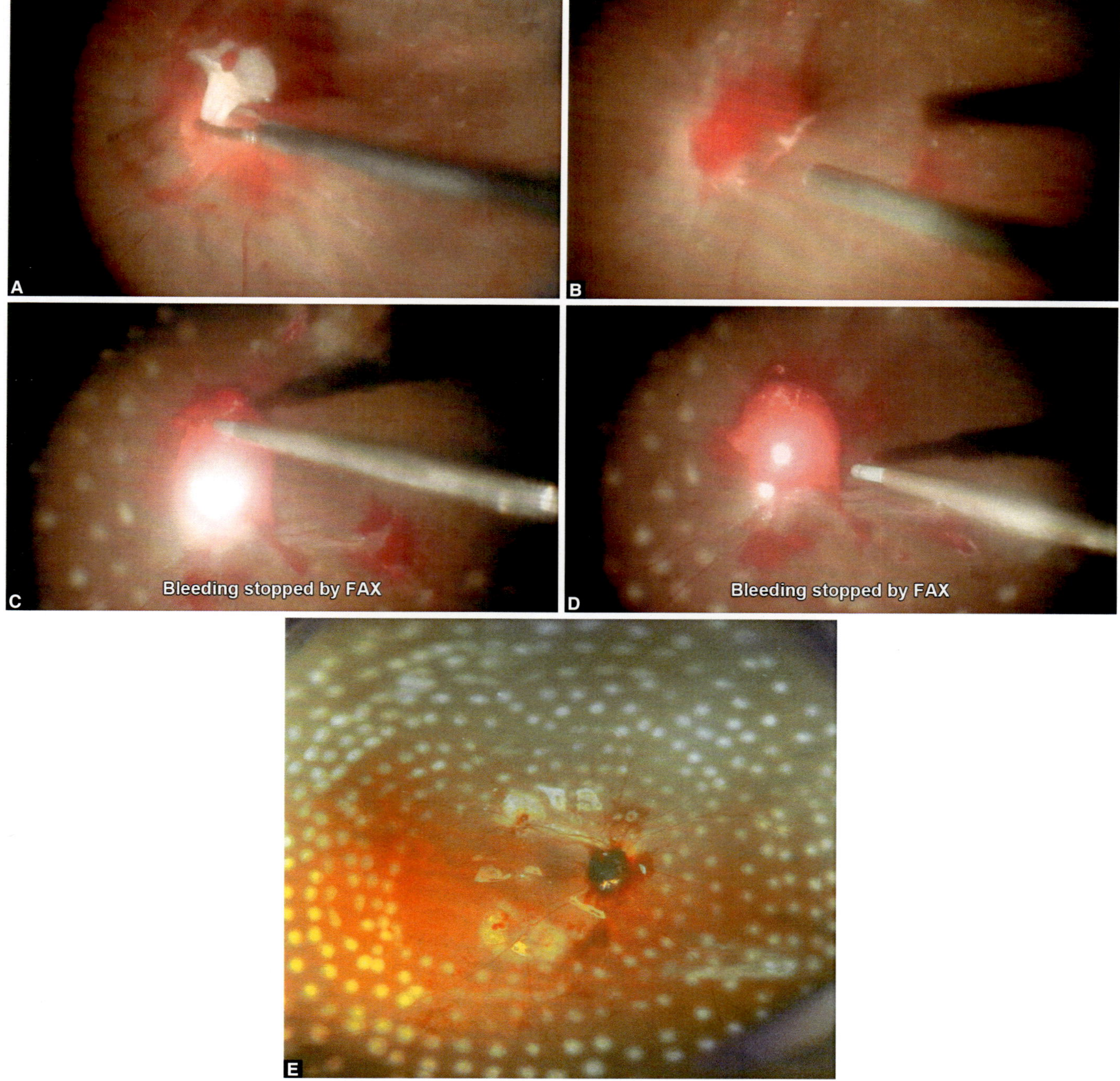

Figs 24.22A to E: (A to D) Stoppage of disk hemorrhage after completion of FAX in high IOP settings; (E) Postoperative clotted blood over the disk of the same patient after control of bleeding by raising IOP after FAX

Using Heavy Fluid PFCL

- Use of heavy fluid PFCL over the posterior pole can decrease the bleeding due to mechanical pressure over the bleeders.

Case discussion (Video 22, Chapter 24):

- While managing a case of advanced PDR, after removal of fibrovascular proliferations, disc hemorrhage was quiet significant even in high IOP due to active bleeders (Fig. 24.24A)
- Heavy liquid PFCL injected over the posterior pole to decrease the bleeding due to mechanical pressure over the bleeders (Fig. 24.24B)
- PRP completed and bleeding stopped.

Use of Silicone Oil

Sometimes one can use silicone oil over the bleeders and blood clot under silicone oil in a fluid-filled eye, help to remove premacular blood clot membrane with the help of suction of a cutter.

Intraoperative Supracoroidals

The incidence of suprachoroidal hemorrhage during vitrectomy surgery has been estimated to be 0.17–1.9%.

Risk factors for a suprachoroidal hemorrhage during vitreoretinal surgery are:

- Advanced age
- Elevated preoperative IOP

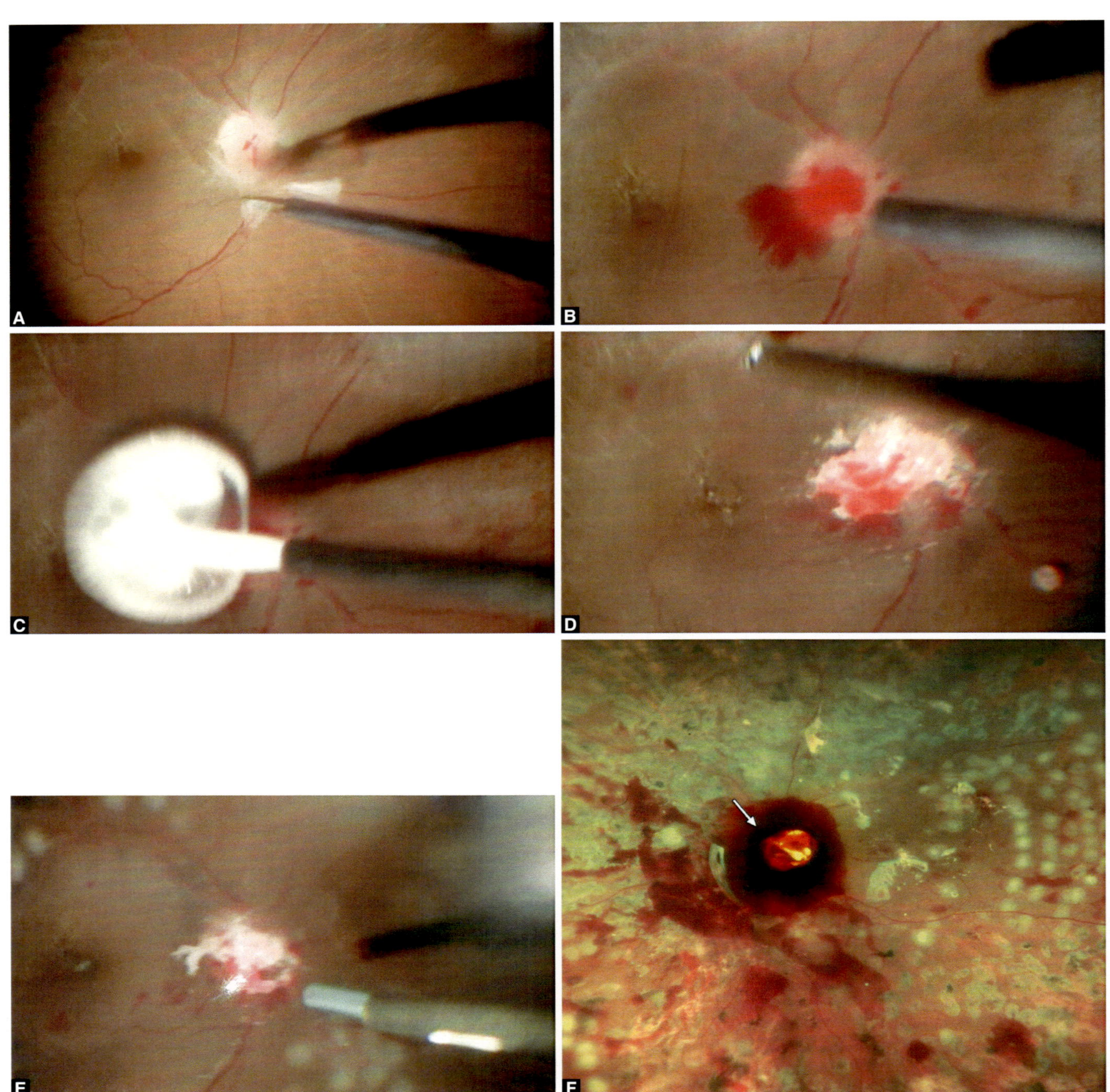

Figs 24.23A to F

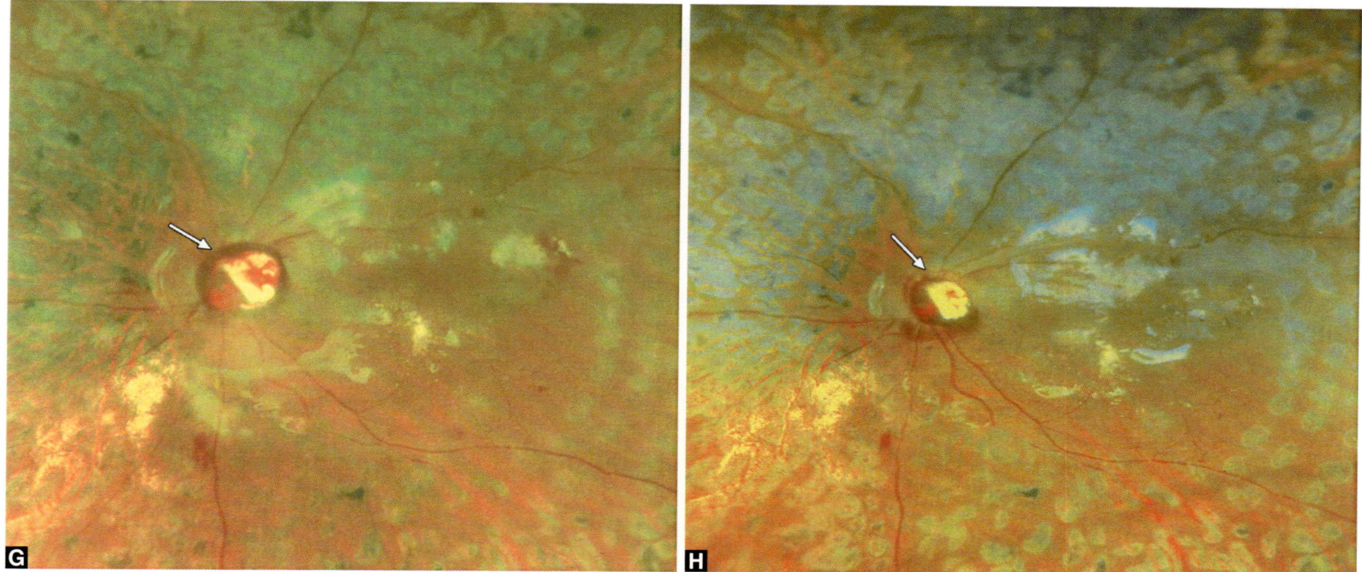

Figs 24.23A to H: (A to D) Stoppage of disk hemorrhage after removal of neovascular tissue with application triamcinolone acetonide particles over the disk directly; (F to H) Clotted blood with TA particles over the disk (white arrows) on first postoperative day; after two weeks (G) and one month (H) of surgery in a case of proliferative diabetic retinopathy with fibrovascular proliferation

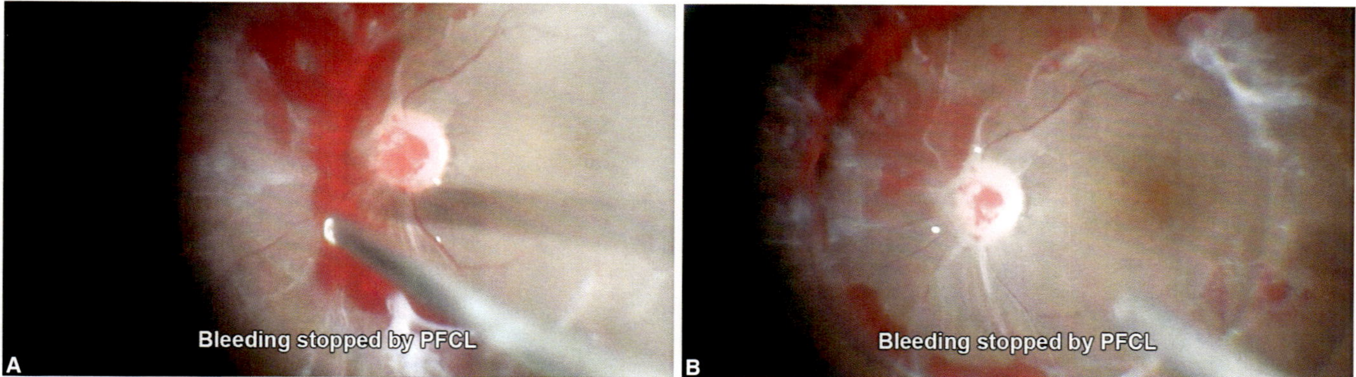

Figs 24.24A and B: Shows stoppage of disk hemorrhage after removal of neovascular tissue with application of heavy fluid PFCL

- Aphakia/pseudophakia
- Scleral buckling
- High myopia
- External drainage of subretinal fluid
- Cryotherapy
- Coughing or "bucking" on the endotracheal tube during general anesthesia
- Intraoperative systemic hypertension.

The underlying pathophysiologic mechanism causing massive suprachoroidal hemorrhage is likely secondary to acute intraoperative ocular hypotony. If the IOP is significantly lowered in a short period of time, especially if it is initially elevated (like just after silicone oil removal before starting FAX), the short or long posterior arteries may rupture, giving rise to a severe suprachoroidal hemorrhage. This can lead to even more bleeding as the forced separation of the choroid away from the sclera will avulse more blood vessels.

While changing the instrument just after completion of PFCL assisted internal drainage of SRF by fluid air exchange, suddenly suprachoroidals may precipitate (Fig. 24.25).

Management of Intraoperative SCH

1. *Keeping IOP at a higher level:* Preferably 40–60 mm Hg
2. Ending the case with a noncompressible endotamponade like silicone oil (gas is better to avoid).

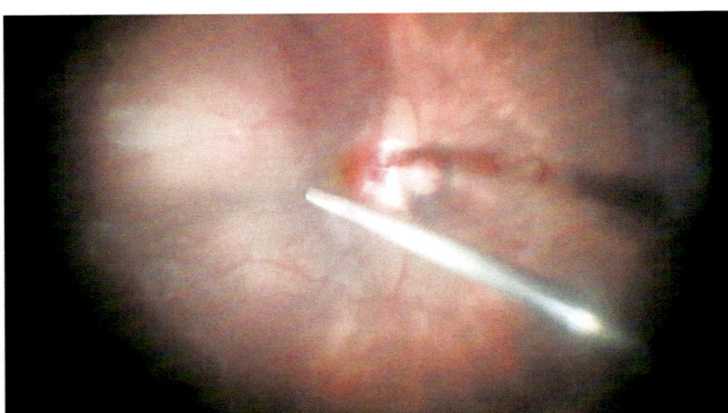

Fig. 24.25: Intraoperative suprachoroidal hematomas during vitreous surgery

3. *If significant bulging or macula threatening:* One can drain it by either radial sclerotomy or by 23 G cannula.

Intraoperative Retinal Break with Retinal Detachment

In case of accidental intraoperative retinal break formation with retinal detachment, one should remember the following points:

- Find out the causative break
- Check tip of infusion cannula, whether it is subretinal or not. Also check vitreous base to rule out dialysis
- Stop ongoing traction
- Remove all traction
- *Location:* Superior—only air/FAX/Gas
- *Inferior:* Gas/silicone oil.

Case Discussion (Video 23, Chapter 24)

A case of macular ERM.

- After PVD induction, trypan blue dye injected under air
- But macula appeared boggy (Fig. 24.26A) and a fluid tract noticed extending towards inferotemporal periphery (Fig. 24.26B)
- The whole appearance was assessed again
- ERM removed from the boggy macula (Fig. 24.26C)
- Suddenly bullous retinal detachment appeared
- Inferior temporal peripheral breaks noticed (Fig. 24.26D)
- The detached retina advanced rapidly and became retrolental (Fig. 24.26E)
- PFCL injected to settle retina
- Peripheral vitrectomy done
- Fluid-air exchange done to settle retina (Fig. 24.26F) and barrage laser done all around (Fig. 24.26G)
- Silicone oil injected
- At the end of surgery, the infusion cannula was realised to be subretinal.

Fluid-air Exchange (FAX) Complications

FAX means fluid in the vitreous cavity is replaced by air. Though this is a simple step to complete vitrectomy, few rare complications can arise like:

i. *Retinal damage with air infusion and fluid infusion:* In presence of raised IOP immediately preceding the infusion of air (sometimes iatrogenically with the vitrectomy foot pedal), the pressure of the air infusion can be high enough to cause damage to the retina just opposite to the infusion cannula. With the infusion cannula placed inferotemporally, damage to the retina from air infusion is usually seen as whitening of the retina in the superonasal quadrant.
   - After FAX, sometimes infusion fluid may have to be started again. A raised IOP, just after making infusion fluid on after FAX in this kind of situation, can cause jet of infusion fluid which can hit contralateral retina and can result in retinal break formation (Fig. 24.27A). Interruption of jet of infusion flow by any instrument (like silicone tip flute needle) or keeping the IOP low while making infusion fluid on after FAX, can prevent direct retinal injury (Fig. 24.27B).

ii. *Mechanical trauma to the optic nerve head during aspiration with the extrusion instrument:* A rare complication and presented with disk pallor with permanent peripheral temporal visual field defects.A soft-tip extrusion cannula is to be used under clear visualisation during air-fluid exchange to minimize mechanical trauma.

iii. *Air embolism and death:* In presence of choroidal detachment or suprachoroidal hemorrhage, while working under fluid-air exchange with high IOP, sometimes high FAX can strip vortex vein and air in high pressure can enter bloodstream, resulted in air embolism. As a consequence, cases of death due to air embolism have been reported. One should start FAX with low IOP and then gradually raise it to avoid sudden stripping of vortex vein, if IOP raised rapidly.

Subretinal Migration of PFCL Bubbles

- During the instrument change, sudden increase in intravitreal turbulence can form multiple 'fish egg' PFCL bubbles. As PFCL is to be filled-up just posterior to the edge of the breaks, these bubbles are in immediate vicinity of break margin and can access to enter in subretinal space. Careful removal of all PFCL bubbles from the subretinal space can prevent postoperative 'subretinal PFCL' situation

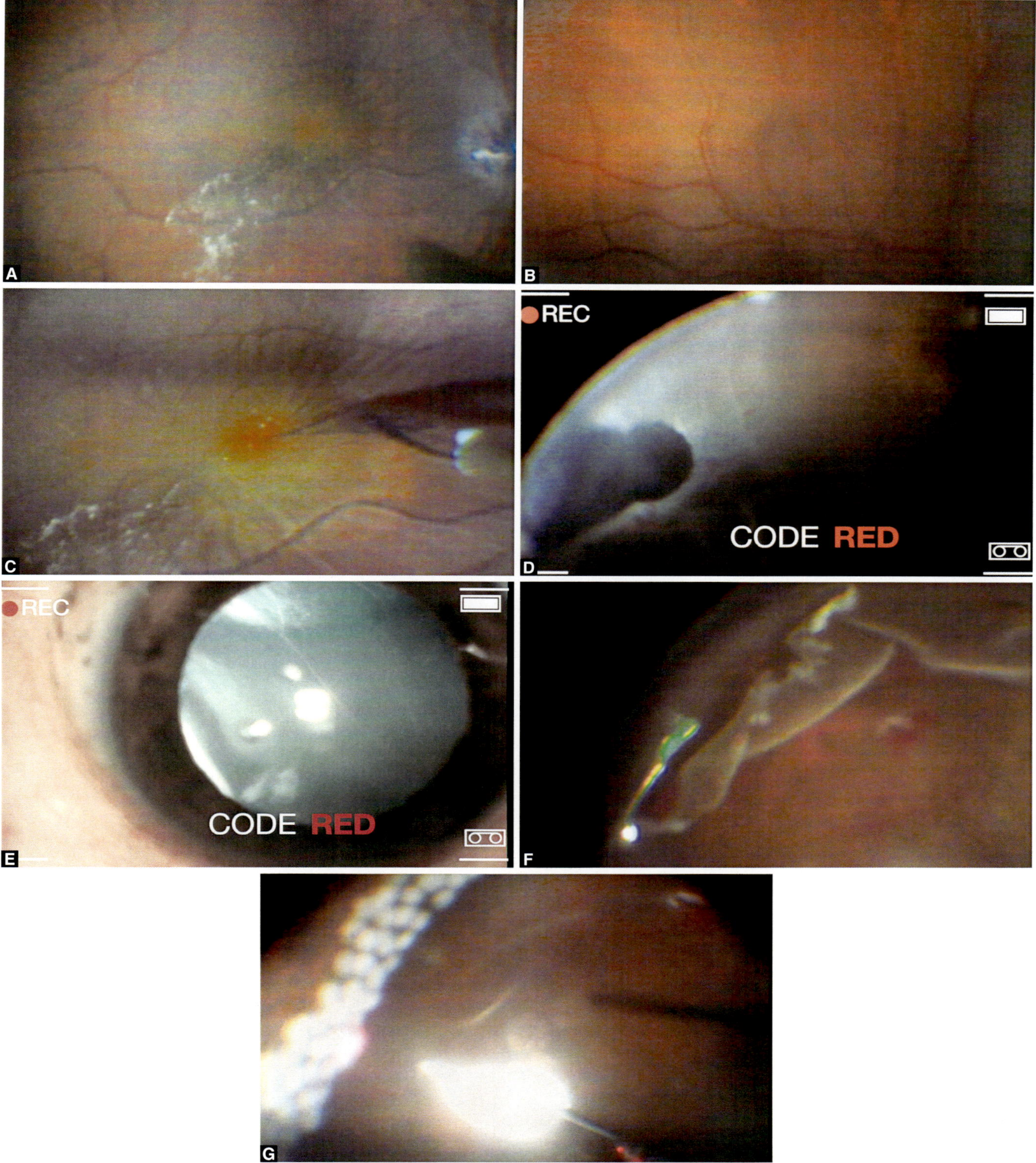

Figs 24.26A to G: Intraoperative steps of surgery managing accidental intraoperative retinal break formation with retinal detachment

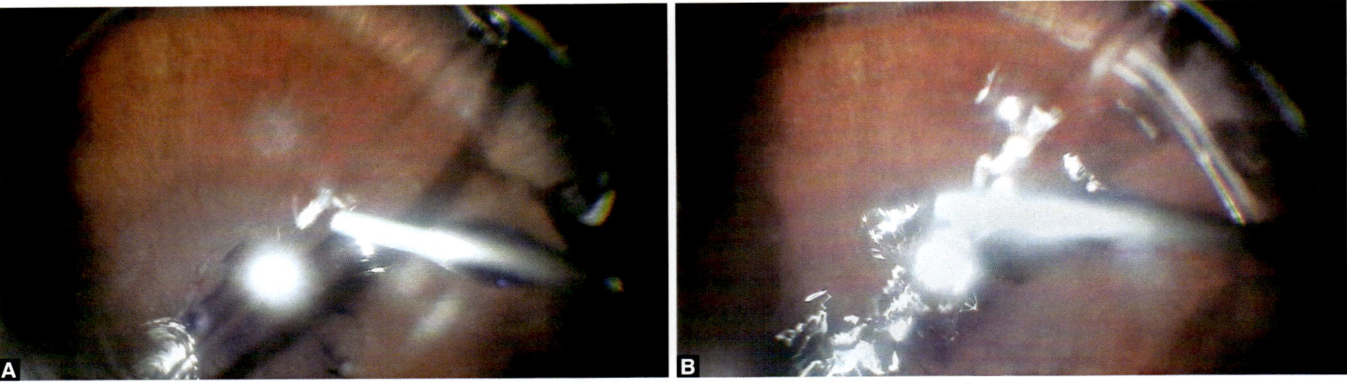

Figs 24.27A and B: (A) A jet of infusion fluid, just after making infusion fluid after FAX, can injure contralateral retina; (B) Interruption of jet of infusion flow by any instrument (like silicone tip flute needle) while making infusion fluid on after FAX, can prevent direct retinal injury

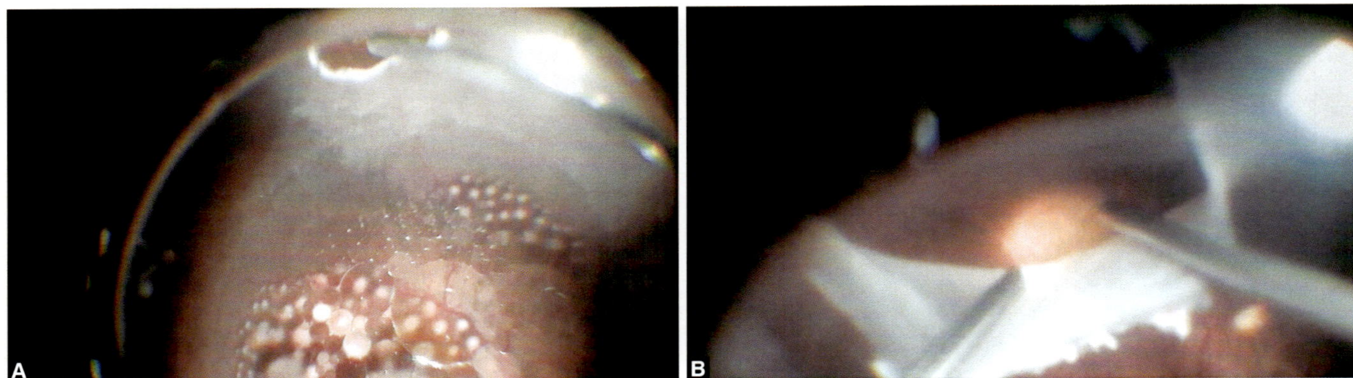

Figs 24.28A and B: (A) Formation of multiple PFCL bubbles near the margin of inferior break; (B) Removal of subretinal migrated PFCL bubbles through the inferior break

- Use of all-time closed environment system like valved cannula can stop sudden high intravitreal turbulence; thus prevents fish-egging of the PFCL globule
- Meticulous search for the subretinal PFCL bubble is necessary intraoperatively.

Case Discussion (Video 24, Chapter 24)

- Just after stabilization of posterior pole by PFCL, during change of instruments, multiple PFCL bubbles can form (Fig. 24.28A)
- Care should always be taken to note subretinal presence of PFCL bubbles
- All the migrated PFCL bubbles from the subretinal space should be removed carefully (Fig. 24.28B) and fluid-air exchange started to drain anterior SRF followed by laser.

POSTOPERATIVE COMPLICATIONS

Corneal Erosion

In diabetics, incidence of postvitrectomy corneal problem is very high and varies from 28–52%. Corneal erosion leading to persistent epithelial defect is very frequent because diabetic eyes have abnormal basement membranes and attachments

- Mild erosion often heal with lubricants and patching
- If persistent, bandage contact lens or rarely tarsorrhaphy is necessary for reepithelialization (Figs 24.29A and B).

Postvitrectomy Cataract

Types of cataract: PSC in young patient and nuclear sclerosis in both young and older patients (Fig. 24.30).

Problems with Postvitrectomy Cataract

i. *Weak zonules:* Vitrectomy may also weaken the zonules.
ii. *Subluxated cataract:* Unfortunately, it is difficult to identify this as they do not exhibit phacodenesis preoperatively.
iii. *Dehiscent posterior capsule:* May also have occult tears and a cataract developing within few weeks of the vitrectomy, this should raise suspicion for damage to the posterior capsule during surgery.

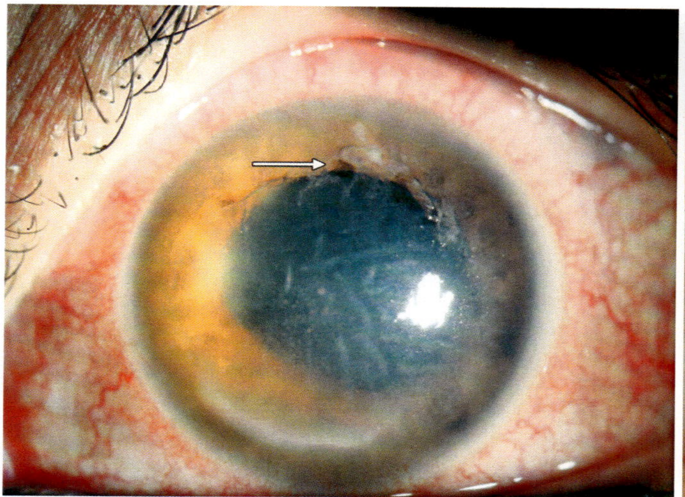
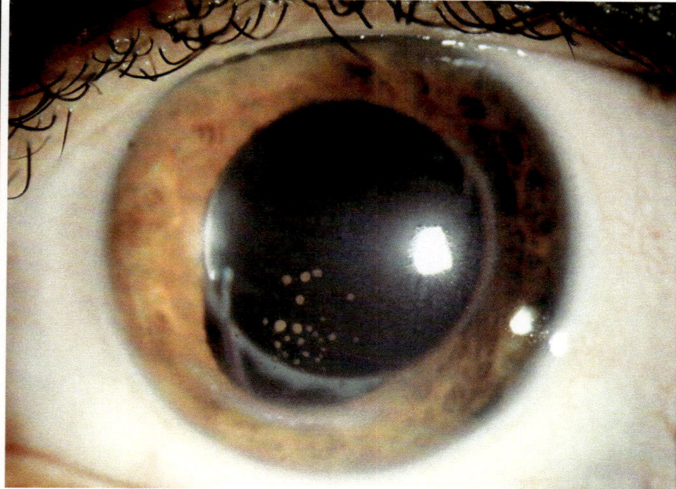

Figs 24.29A and B: (A) Corneal epithelial defect, two weeks after diabetic vitrectomy; (B) Healed corneal epithelial defect after seven days of medical management

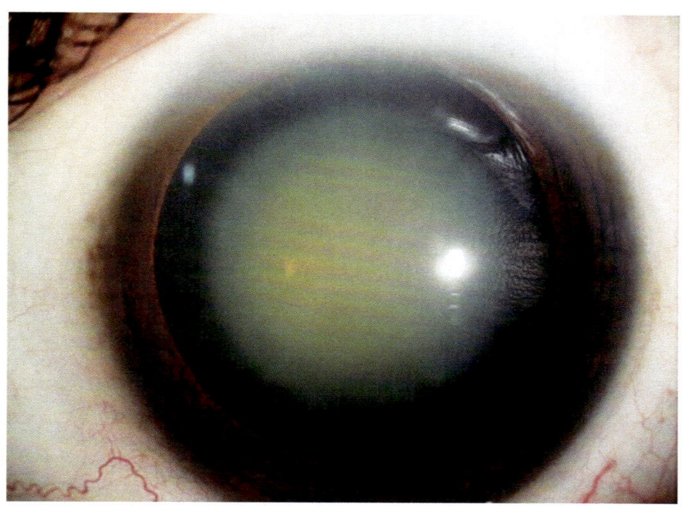

Fig. 24.30: Postvitrectomy cataract

iv. Loss of vitreous support results in an unstable posterior capsule that is unusually mobile and flaccid.
v. Flaccid posterior capsule, in combination of weak zonules, may allow the lens-iris diaphragm to move excessively. Fluctuation of the anterior-chamber depth can make surgical maneuvers during phacoemulsification difficult and can increase the risk of complications.
vi. As these are fluid-filled eyes, chance of intraoperative hypotony is there.
vii. Abnormal corticocapsular and corticoepinuclear adhesion
viii. Poor mydriasis is also not uncommon and sometimes necessitating the use of iris hooks or pupil-expander ring.
ix. Posterior capsule plaques are also not uncommon and their removal may damage the posterior capsule.
x. The increased energy needed to phacoemulsify denser nuclear sclerosis and it results in intraoperative and postoperative corneal edema, as well as inflammation.
xi. *Fluid misdirection syndrome:* Due to weak zonules, anterior chamber fluid may go beneath the iris or even vitreous cavity, resulting in ballooning of iris and shallow anterior chamber. Posterior capsular tear by tip of phaco probe may happen accidentally in this situation.

Case Discussion (Video 25, Chapter 24)

A case of postvitrectomy cataract.

- Capsulorrhexis completed
- While doing hydrodissection, hypotony precipitated (Fig. 24.31A)
- Viscoelastic injected to build up IOP
- Nuclear rotation done
- Trenching started and the nucleus was divided into two halves
- Separation of nuclear halves was difficult due to cortico-nuclear adhesions (Fig. 24.31B).
- Inferior half of nucleus again divided into two halves by direct chop and each small half emulsified
- Superior half again divided into two small halves by direct chop (Fig. 24.31C) and each fragments emulsified
- Cortical aspiration done bimanually carefully as there was inferior zonular dialysis (Fig. 24.31D)
- Foldable multi-piece posterior chamber IOL implanted in the bag and positioned such a way so that one haptic should support inferior zonular dehiscent area.

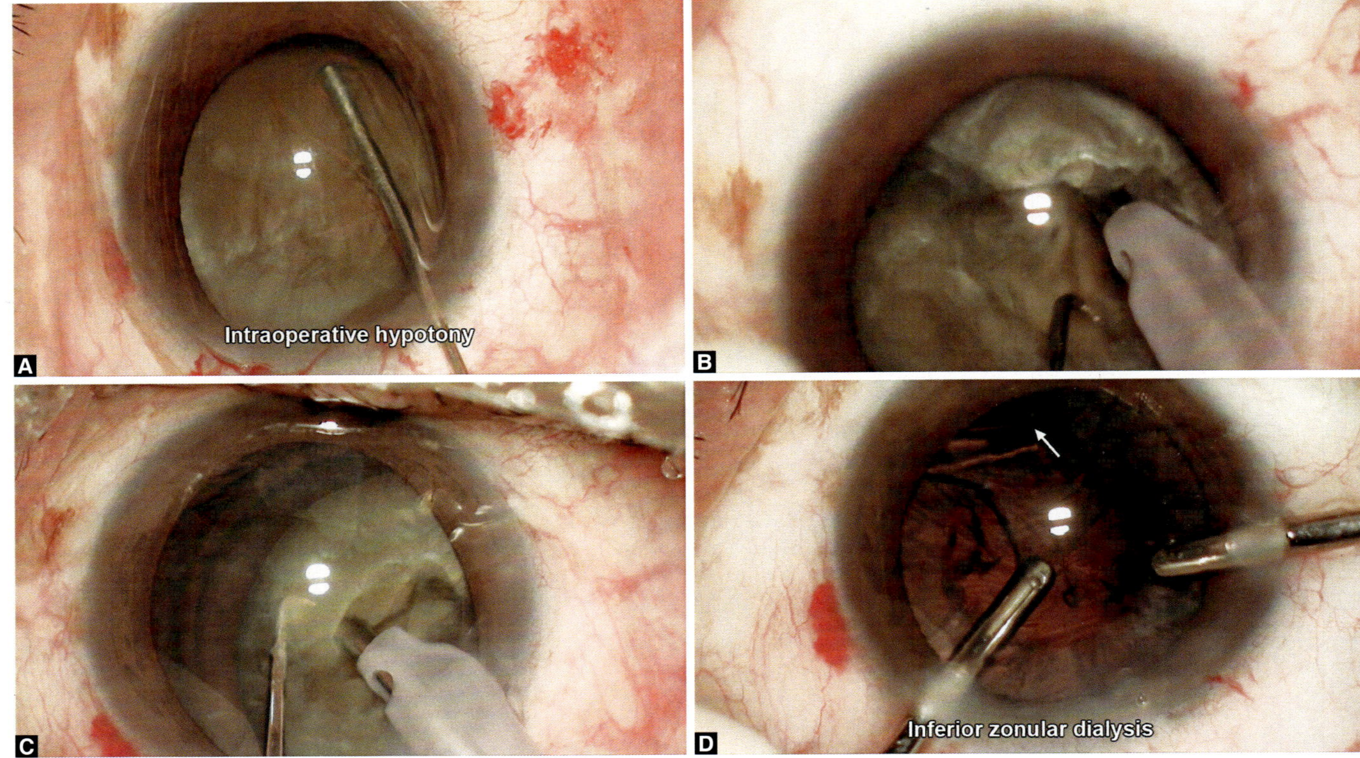

Figs 24.31A to D: Intraoperative steps of surgery managing postvitrectomy cataract

Intraocular Fibrin Deposition and Pupillary Block

Vitrectomy in diabetics often lead to breakdown of blood-retinal barrier and resulting in intracameral fibrin deposition and pupillary block in first two weeks. Frequent topical steroid with cycloplegics are sufficient in most of the situation or sub-tenon's steroid injection is required in chronic cases.

Secondary Glaucoma

Commonly encountered by retina surgeon, in following situations:

1. *Post-cataract surgery secondary glaucoma:* This situation may arise from—
   - Dropped nucleus/lens fragments during cataract extraction
   - Lens induced uveitis—inflammatory cause
   - *Preoperative management*
     - Systemic and topical steroid
     - Systemic and topical antiglaucoma
   - *Treatment:* Vitrectomy + Nucleus/lens frag removal (by cutter/phacofragmentor)
   - Postoperative treatment—topical and systemic anti-glaucoma
   - Do not ignore even a small dropped lens fragment if it is nucleus in origin as it may lead to chronic IOP elevation which can damage optic nerve.
2. *Postscleral buckling surgery:*
   - *Anterior movement of lens:* Iris diaphragm can induce formation of peripheral anterior synechia formation. Buckle sutures have to be loosen
   - Use of buckle/encirclage can cause vortex vein compression which can cause chronic IOP elevation and this necessitates buckle removal/encirclage
   - Malignant glaucoma may occur due to aqueous misdirection (aqueous pockets in vitreous cavity on USG). Urgently core vitrectomy to reduce vitreous volume decrease IOP.
3. *Postvitreoretinal surgery:*
   - Expansile gas (C_3F_8) → Adequate antiglaucoma coverage and proper prone positioning is required. Gas in nonexpansile form (14–18%) may decrease the chance of IOP rise
   - Silicone oil—
     - Inferior PI is mandatory where lens is spared
     - Avoid overfilling
     - Maintain positioning
   - Postoperative SO emulsification can cause blockade of trabecular meshwork
   - IOP remains elevated sometimes even after silicone oil removal (Fig. 24.32) and this necessitates long term antiglaucoma treatment

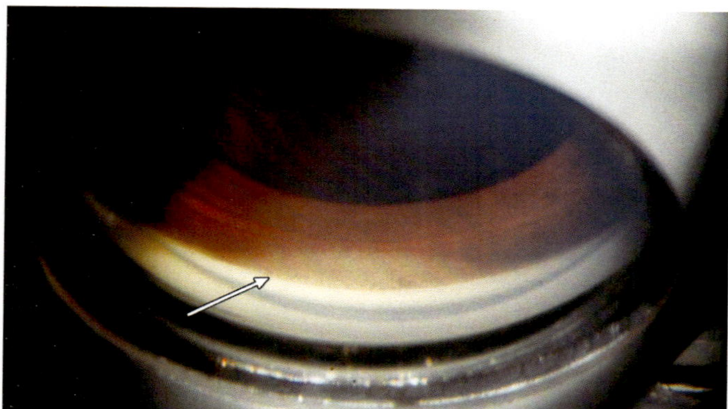

Fig. 24.32: Post-silicone oil removal residual emulsified silicone oil particles (white arrow) at superior angle on gonioscopy cause blockade of trabecular meshwork

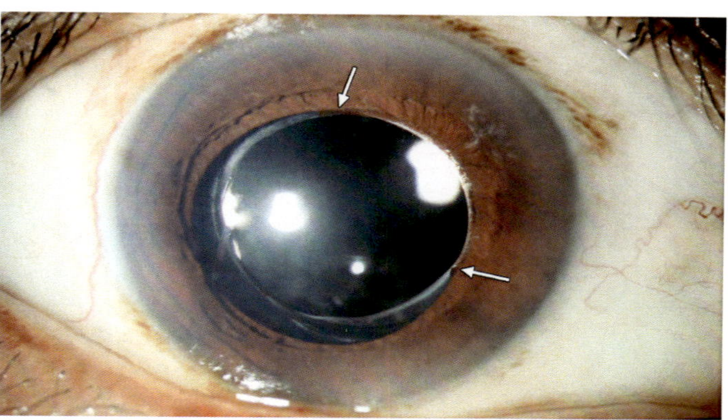

Fig. 24.33: Early posterior synechia (white arrows) after combined phacovitrectomy

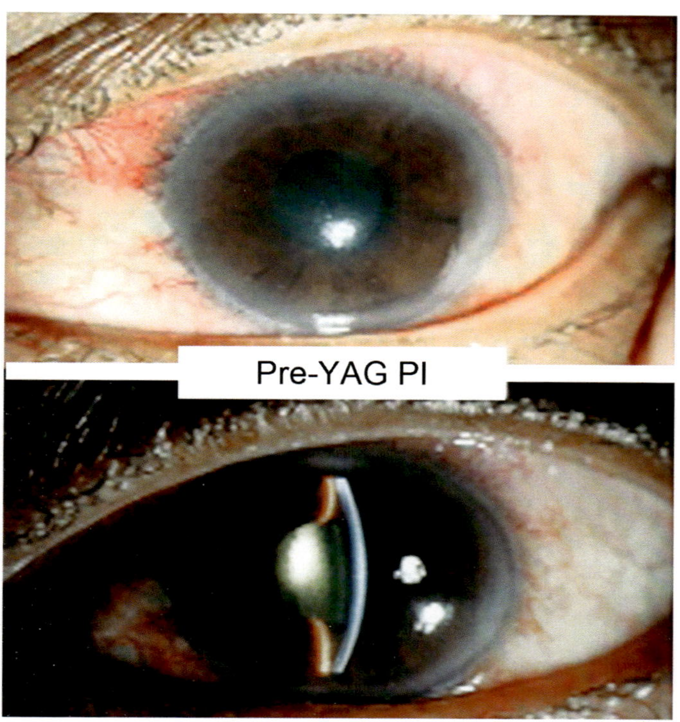

Fig. 24.34: Shows pre-YAG CAP ASP with 360° iris bombe

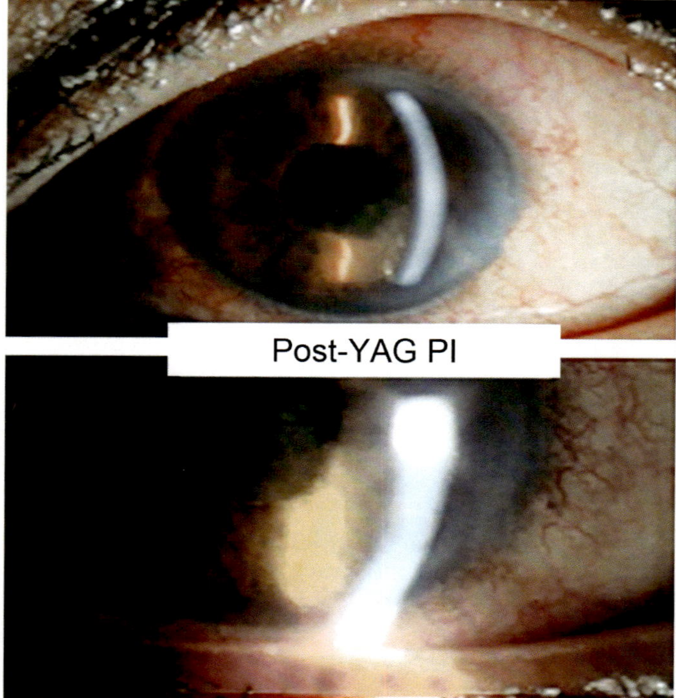

Fig. 24.35: Shows post-YAG Cap ASP with patent PI and deep anterior chamber

- It may warrant meticulous removal of emulsified silicone oil particles from the anterior chamber angle
- Endolaser destruction of ciliary process
- Cyclodestructive procedure/implant surgery.

4. *Postcombined phacoemulsification + vitrectomy:* Post-synechia between iris and capsulorrhexis margin—it occurs especially in cases with intravirtual gas tamponade (C_3F_8).

   Prevention: Use of short-acting dilator to keep pupil mobile, site may prevent posterior synechia formation.

Treatment:

i. *Early posterior synechia (Fig. 24.33):* Need no treatment.
ii. 360 degree posterior synechia between iris and capsulorrhexis margin can result in situation with high IOP with flat anterior chamber and iris bombe (Fig. 24.34). Laser YAG peripheral iridotomy immidiately form anterior chamber and normalizes IOP (Fig. 24.35).

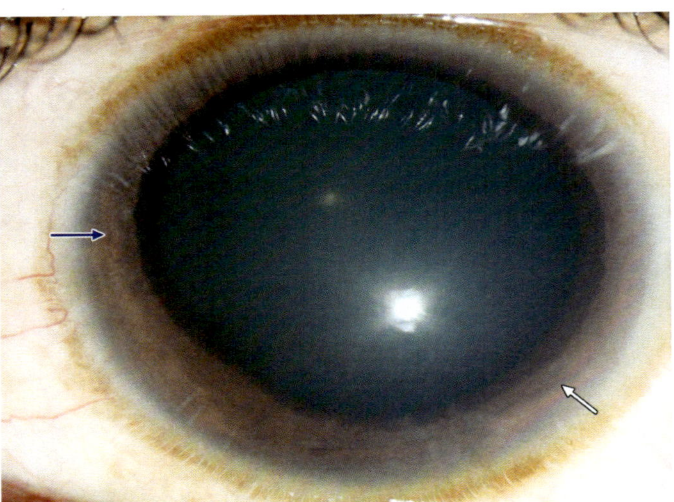

Fig. 24.36: Postvitrectomy neovascular glaucoma with NVI (blue arrow) and ectropion uveae (white arrow)

5. *Rubeosis iridis and neovascular glaucoma*
   - It is common in diabetics
   - Iris neovascularization is 2–3 times more common in aphakic diabetic eyes than phakic eyes (Fig. 24.36)
   - Incidence of postvitrectomy NVG is 8–11% in diabetics
   - Initially with conservative antiglaucoma treatment, anterior PRP, anti-VEGF therapy
   - Cyclodestructive procedure in advanced situation is necessary.

Silicone Oil in Anterior Chamber

It occurs more often in aphakic, phakic or pseudophakic eyes with compromised zonular or capsular support. It appears as a single globule through the pupil or as a corneal ghost image along with loss of the aqueous-silicone oil interface at the pupil which is suggestive of total filling of silicone oil in anterior chamber.

- *Early postoperative period (within 6 months after primary surgery):* Hypotony in early postoperative period induces silicone oil bubble to migrate into anterior chamber. Normalization of IOP and miotic agent in anterior chamber to keep pupil in miotic phase is thus important to prevent this occurrence.
  - If there is a small nonemulsified silicone oil bubble with normal IOP, without any anterior chamber reaction and on retina, it can be simply observed for 3-4 month as the oil-endothelial contact is negligible (Fig. 24.37A)
  - If large silicone oil bubble or total anterior chamber with normal IOP, without any anterior chamber reaction and on retina, it should be removed replacing it by viscoelastic as the oil-endothelial contact is large to prevent keratopathy (Fig. 24.37B)
  - If there is any evidence of inflammation (as silicone oil is proinflammatory) or blocked inferior peripheral iridectomy (in aphakics) due to inflammation or secondary glaucoma, intense anti-inflammatory agents topically with antiglaucoma treatments is to be started and if it fails to control inflammation or IOP, silicone oil bubble is to be removed from anterior chamber irrespective of it's size (Fig. 24.37C)
  - In presence of recurrent retinal detachment, silicone oil bubble in anterior chamber is to be removed along with management of recurrent retinal detachment.

  In late postoperative period (after 6 months primary surgery): It can appear in anterior chamber in emulsified form. Emulsified silicone oil appears as multiple droplets layering out in the superior angle and IOP may be chronically elevated (Fig. 24.37D)
  - Silicone removal is to be advocated. Simple silicone oil removal with proper washing of all oil droplets from anterior chamber many a times normalize IOP. Rarely oil removal should be accompanied by trabeculectomy or tube shunt or transcleral cyclophotocoagulation, but there is risk of post operative hypotony after these added procedures.

Subconjunctival Silicone Oil (Fig. 24.37E)

Sometimes mild leakage of silicone oil bubbles through the suture less ports have access to the sub conjunctival space and appear as bleb or cyst like elevations. It may present asymptomatically or with cosmetic problems which warrants drainage of silicone oil bubbles by needle.

Retained PFCL Bubbles

- PFCL bubbles can remain intraocularly and may be revealed incidentally even after meticulous removal of all PFCL bubbles.
  - *Retained PFCL bubble in anterior chamber (Figs 24.38A and B):* After a long complicated vitreoretinal procedure, PFCL droplets may stay in the vitreous cavity, which may come to anterior chamber later on and revealed in the postoperative visits
  - *Subsilicone oil PFCL bubbles:* May remain at macula (Fig. 24.38C) or elsewhere (Fig. 24.38D).
  - *Submacular PFCL bubbles (Fig. 24.38E):* Subfoveal PFCL bubble many times detected before or at the time of silicone oil removal.

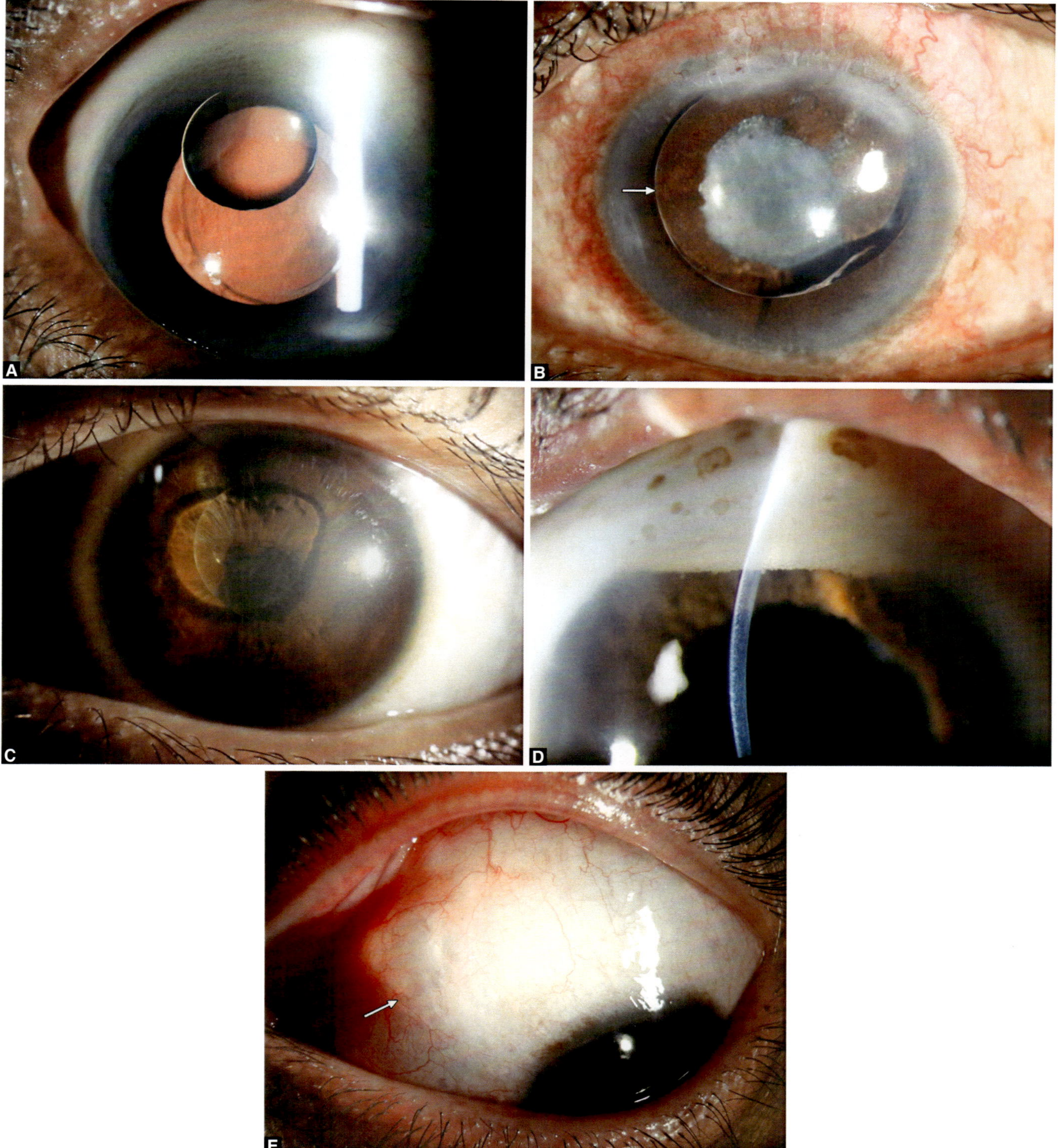

Figs 24.37A to E: (A) Small silicone oil bubble in anterior chamber; (B) Anterior chamber full of silicone oil bubble; (C) Silicone oil in anterior chamber with inflammatory iris bombe after a combined surgery; (D) Emulsified silicone oil appears as multiple droplets layering out in the superior angle; (E) Postvitrectomy subconjunctival silicone oil bubble (white arrow)

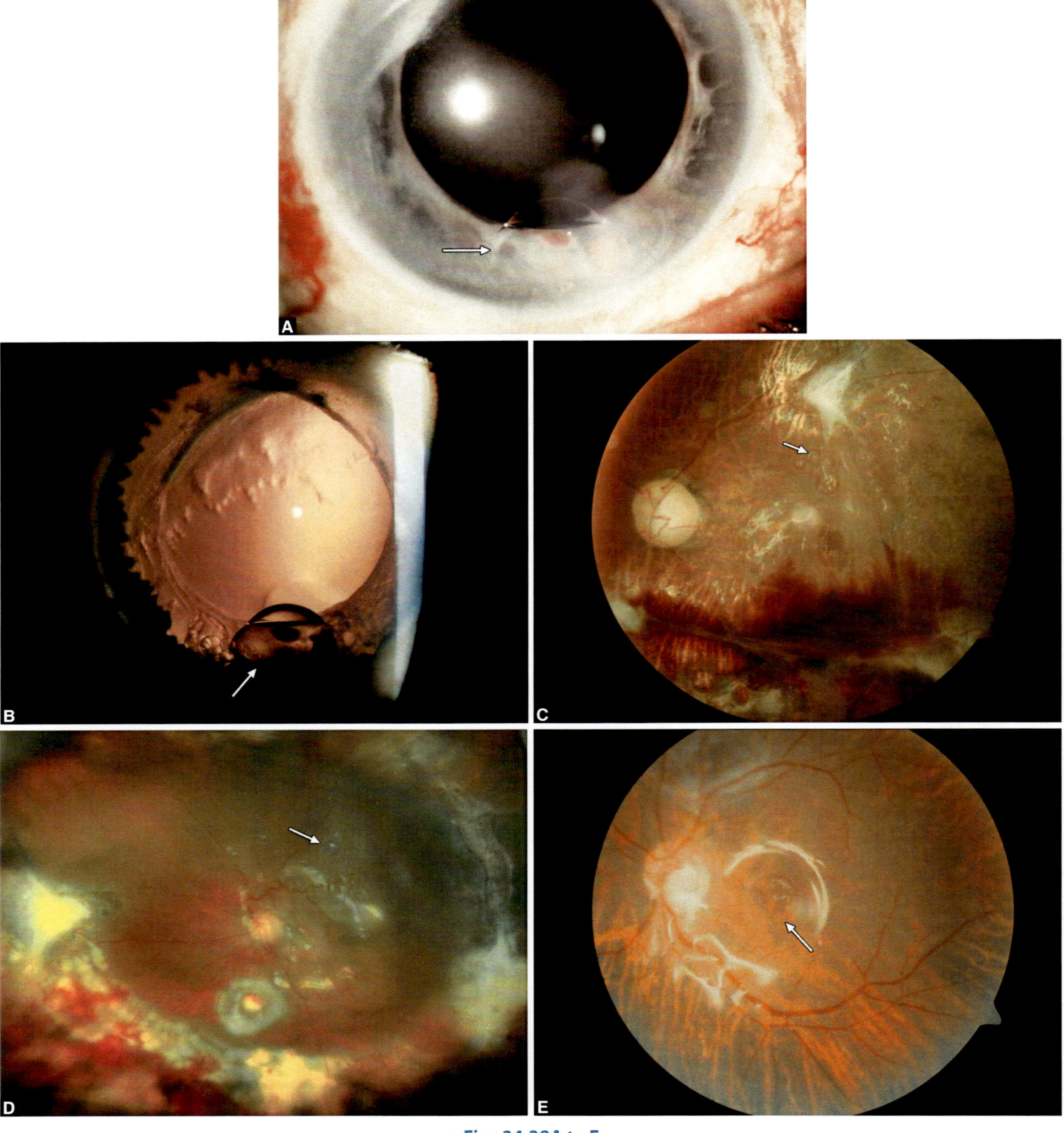

Figs 24.38A to E

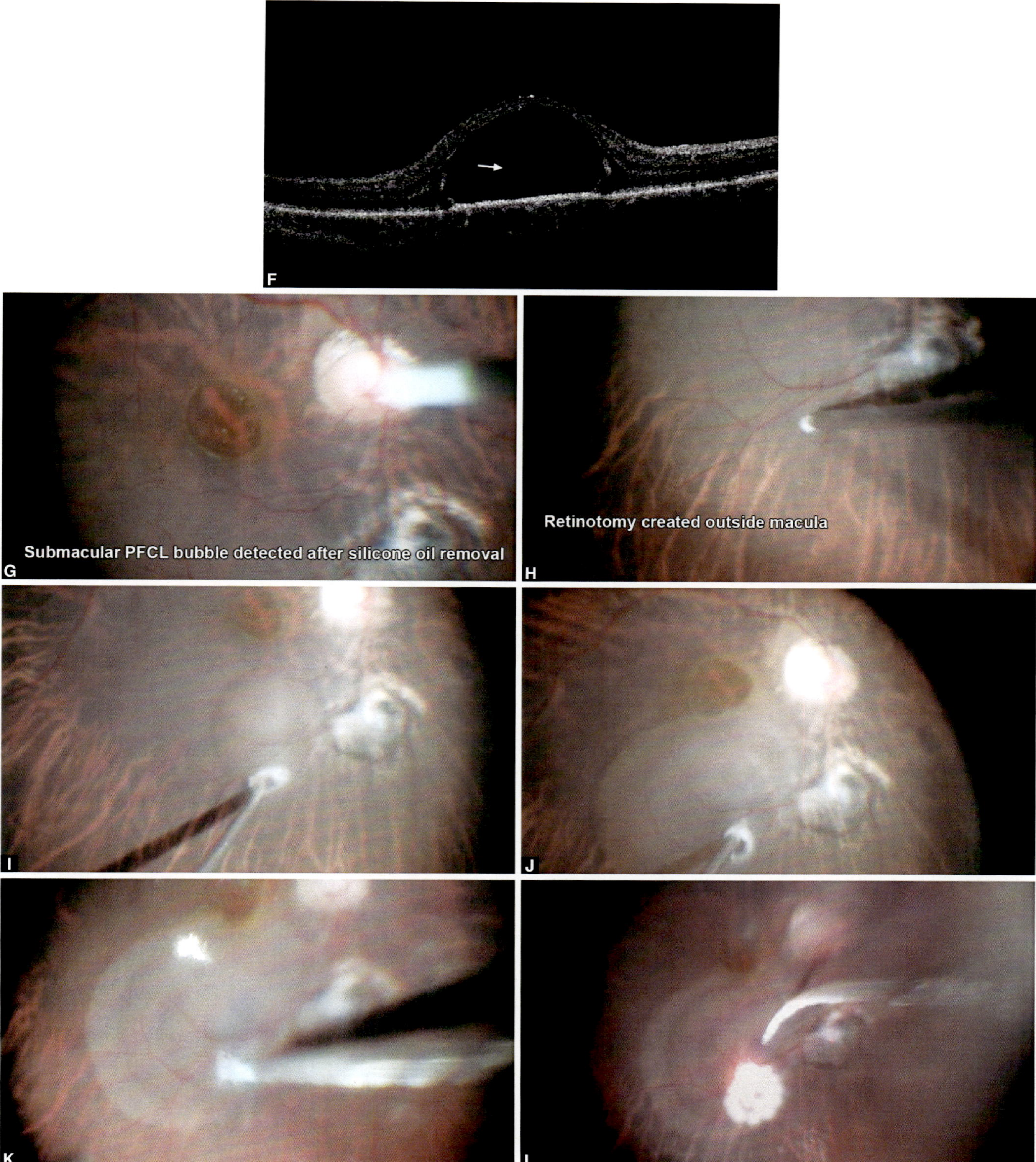

Figs 24.38F to L

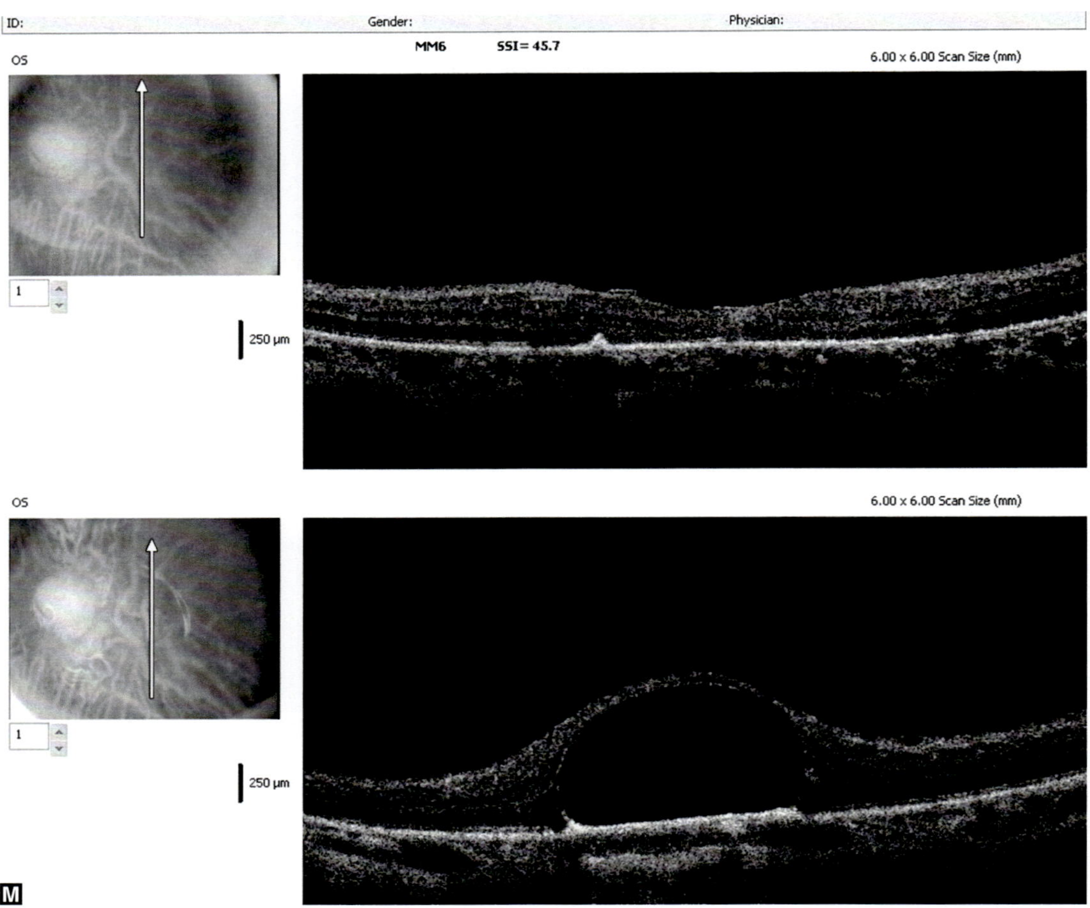

Figs 24.38A to M: (A) Postvitrectomy retained PFCL bubble in anterior chamber after managing a case of suprachoroidal hemorrhage; (B) Postvitrectomy retained PFCL bubble in anterior chamber (in retroillumination); (C) Subsilicone oil PFCL bubble (white arrow) at macula; (D) Sub silicone oil PFCL bubble (white arrow) elsewhere; (E) Subfoveal PFCL bubbles (white arrow); (F) Submacular PFCL on OCT (white arrow); (G and L) Intraoperative steps of surgery managing submacular PFCL bubble; (M) Preoperative and three week postoperative OCT after subfoveal PFCL removal surgery

- On OCT it appear as classical 'omega sign' with overlying neurosensory retinal atrophy (Fig. 24.38F). Retina adapts to the shape of the PFCL bubble, resembling a Greek letter omega. Thus, the angle between the RPE and neurosensory retina at the base of PFCL is acute.

Reason

1. Due to fish egging phenomenon while taking instrument out of the vitreous cavity. High turbulence inside the vitreous cavity in standard 23G/25G MIVS system can occur while taking out the instruments from the vitreous cavity with PFCL bubble inside or during external scleral indentation at the time of vitreous base excision or laser. It can cause fish egg bubble formation of PFCL fluid. This occurs when infusion fluid impacts on the surface of PFCL. These PFCL bubbles can enter the subretinal space through the existing peripheral breaks.
2. Retinal traction at the edge of retinal break can cause entry of PFCL bubbles inside the subretinal space. All tractions surrounding the retinal break should be released before raising the height of PFCL bubble.
   - All PFCL droplets should be removed around the retinotomies and break before or at the time of fluid air exchange.

Effect of submacular PFCL bubble: In postoperative period, only subfoveal PFCL bubbles have to be removed as these can cause visual field defect, scotomas, due to underlying RPE atrophy and overlying neurosensory retinal atrophy.

Extramacular subretinal PFCL can be observed carefully. Laser barrage around the subretinal PFCL can prevent its submacular migration.

Surgery for removal of subfoveal PFCL *(Video 26, Chapter 24)* (Figs 24.38G to M):

- Subfoveal PFCL bubble detected after removal of silicone oil (Fig. 24.38G)
- Removal of sub foveal PFCL is done by creating a extra-macular small retinotomy by either 41 G cannula or by

a bent tip 24 G needle (Fig. 24.38H), creating macular retinal detachment (Fig. 24.38I)

- And then displacing the PFCL bubble from subfoveal space to that retinotomy site (Fig. 24.38J)
- Then PFCL has to to be injected over the macula to displace submacular PFCL bubble
- Settled the induced RD by performing FAX (Fig. 24.38K) and then laser around the retinotomy site (Fig. 24.38L)
- Long-acting gas C3F8 injected.

Several techniques for removing submacular or sub-foveal PFCL bubbles:

- Direct aspiration of sub-macular PFCL bubble manually by 23G silicone tipped flute needle (Pan Q et al.).... *It creates retinal micro-tears or retinal incarceration*
- Direct active aspiration by 41G needle, attached with VFC (Viscous Fluid Control) after inducing an artificial RD by injecting BSS (Falavarjani KG et al)... *can cause the sudden collapse of subretinal space due to high aspiration pressure an risk of a foveal blowout tear.*
- Direct removal through a therapeutic macular hole (Kim JM et al)...*may also complicate visual recovery.*

Micro-VFC

We have developed a simple homemade micro-viscous fluid control to gain access to subretinal space in a controlled way. The rubber cap of the plunger of a 1-mL syringe was cut; this cut rubber cap of the plunger was fitted inside an empty 1-mL tuberculin syringe, and its end was fitted with the tubings of viscous fluid control of the vitrectomy machine. Now, viscous fluid control mode was activated by attaching a 38-G/41-G subretinal needle for extracting submacular PFCL bubbles (vide Video 27, Chapter 24). [*Boral SK, Dan S, Mitra S. "Micro-Viscous Fluid Control": A Simple Homemade New Tool to Access Subretinal Space in a Controlled Way. Retina. 2025;45(2):358-62. doi: 10.1097/IAE.0000000000004137. PMID: 39836928.*]

Advantages of Micro-VFC for extraction of submacular PFCL

i. If we consider aspirating the same volume of fluid by standard VFC and micro-VFC, then much more force has to be applied for a standard VFC syringe with a greater diameter in comparison with the micro-VFC syringe with a smaller diameter to exert the same pressure in both cases.
ii. For extraction of subfoveal or submacular PFCL bubble, we have used low aspiration pressure (300–400 mm Hg), thus avoiding high aspiration force, which prevents sudden collapse of subretinal space or any occurrence of retinal incarceration or retinal micro-tear formation.
iii. The standard VFC theoretically exerts more force for aspiration purposes even at low-pressure settings.
iv. The traumatic effects of our gentle transretinal aspiration would have applied forces to the retina in the inner-to-outer layer direction, and we did not detect any inner neurosensory retinal damage during the following OCT examinations.

Managing Failed Macular Holes

For Failed Macular Holes: More advanced surgical techniques have been used, like

a. Extending area of ILM peeling
b. Complete FAE with gas tamponade—flatten the hole edges without any SRF and completely cover the defect of the neurosensory retina. Vishal MY showed that although anatomical closure was achieved in 89.3% of eyes, functional success was obtained in only 67.9% (19) patients. (Vishal MY, Babu N, Kohli P, Rajendran A, Ramasamy K. *Retrospective study of changes* in ocular coherence tomography characteristics after failed macular hole surgery and outcomes of fluid-*gas exchange for persistent macular holes. Indian J Ophthalmol. 2018;66(8):1130-5. doi: 10.4103/ijo.IJO_1119_17).*
c. Autologous transplantation of free ILM flap—harvesting free ILM flap from a nonpeeled area after staining the ILM with Brilliant blue G dye.
d. Lens capsule transplantation—harvesting a piece of the anterior/posterior lens capsule and placing it into the hole to facilitate hole closure
e. Human amniotic membrane (HAM) graft transplantation—first described by Rizzo S et al. (*A Human Amniotic Membrane Plug to Promote Retinal Break Repair and Recurrent Macular Hole Closure*. Retina. 2019;39 (Suppl 1):S95-S103. doi: 10.1097/IAE.0000000000002320). [The technique described in Chapter 14]
f. Autologous retinal graft transplantation—Grewal and Mahmoud first proposed "autologous retinal free flap transplantation", a surgical technique used when ILM was not available to repair the MH. It means harvesting an autologous neurosensory retinal free flap and positioning it over the FTMH. Studies showed closure rates after autologous retinal graft transplantation ranges from 89 to 100%. The neurosensory retinal free flap serves as a scaffold.

Moreover, it secludes communication between the vitreous and subretinal space and forms a macular plug to seal the macular hole.

Case discussion of Autologous Retinal Graft Transplantation (Video 28, Chapter 24):

- It was an already operated macular hole case, where the macular hole remained open after surgery with a 937-micron diameter and BCVA was 20/200 (Fig. 24.39A).
- Superonasal quadrant was chosen, and two layers of laser were done, barraging the donor site of the harvesting area (Fig. 24.39B).

- Then, a localized blob-like neurosensory detachment was created in the barraged donor site by injecting BSS with a 38-gauge subretinal needle for easy separation of the graft from the underlying RPE-Choroid (Fig. 24.39C).
- Then, PFCL was injected up to beyond the donor area (Fig. 24.39D).
- A finesse flex loop was used to separate the graft from the donor site with minimal use of endo cautery. (Fig. 24.39E).
- Then, the graft was transferred under the PFCL to cover the macular hole using a Finesse flex loop (Fig. 24.39F).
- The graft was aligned to cover the macular hole fully (Fig. 24.39G).
- Then, fluid-air exchange was started, first removing the BSS around the PFCL bubble from the periphery (Fig. 24.39H).
- Then, direct PFCL-silicone oil exchange was performed under the Chandelier's light (Fig. 24.39I).

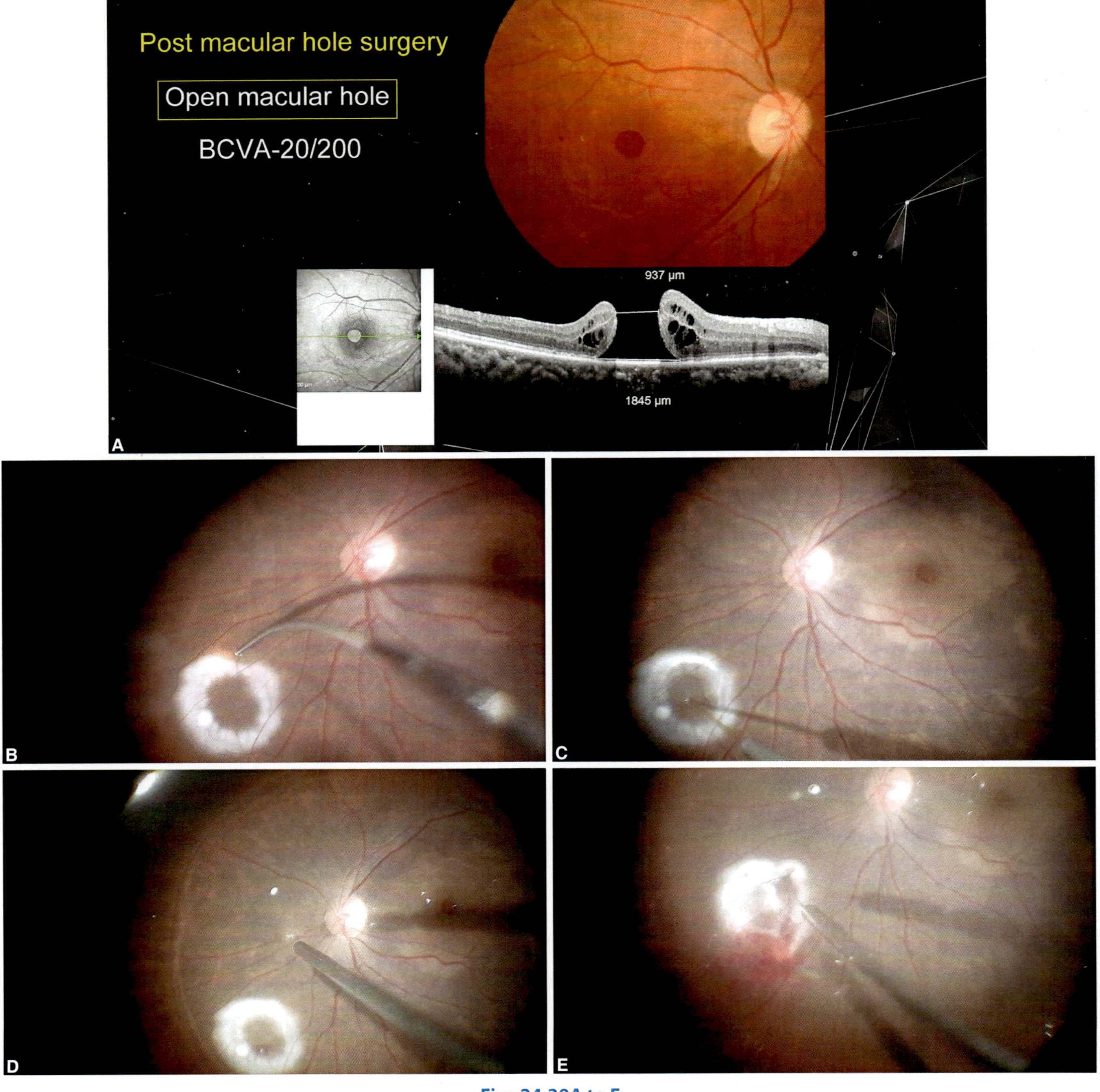

Figs 24.39A to E

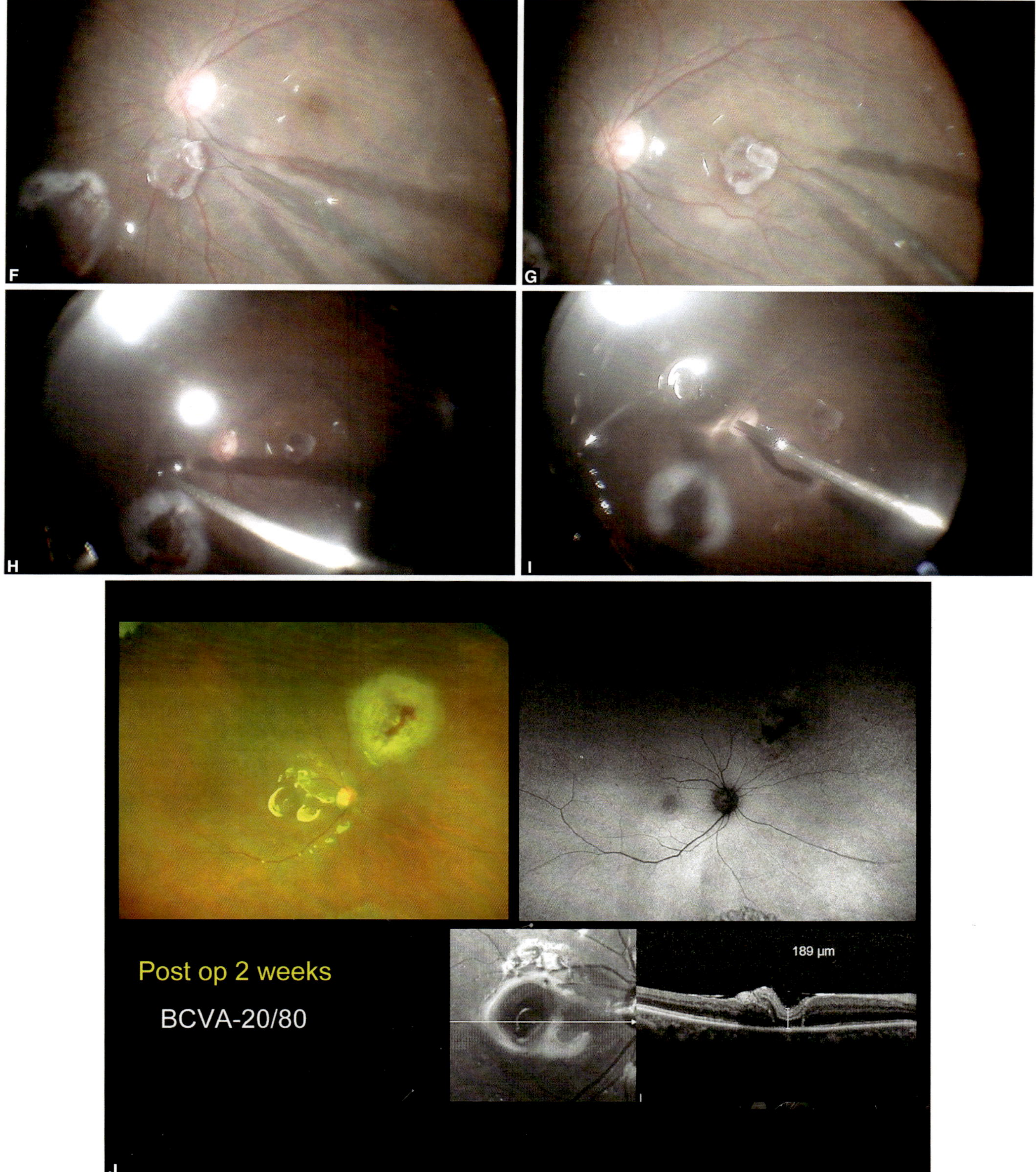

Figs 24.39A to J: Shows steps of surgery with autologous retinal graft transplantation done for a failed open macular hole case.

- After the surgery, OCT was conducted 3 hours later, and the hole was observed to be effectively sealed with the graft (Fig. 24.39J).
- The patient gained 20/80 vision after 3 months with closure of the macular hole (Fig. 24.39J).

Complications Following Phacovitrectomy

- Postoperative posterior capsular opacification
- IOL decentration/subluxation
- Synechia
- Iris bombe with secondary glaucoma to be treated by YAG laser posterior iridotomy.

Postvitrectomy Photopsia and Retinal Detachment

Symptoms of photopsia or flashes of light after vitrectomy with or without tamponade are not uncommon. The reason for this is progressive condensation and contraction of peripheral uncut vitreous skirt (Fig. 24.40). In extreme situation, break may form at the margin or base of uncut vitreous attachment.

Retinal detachment is also recognized to occur as a result of excessive wound healing at the incision site; thus, it can occur at any time after the primary vitrectomy.

- Rates of break formation in macular hole surgery vary from 0% to 14.6%, with retinal detachment occurring in 1.1% to 14%.
- Reported rates for epiretinal membrane surgery range from 0.6% to 6.9% for peripheral retinal breaks and from 1.4% to 6% for retinal detachment.
- The reported incidence of post-vitrectomy retinal detachment for retained intravitreal lens material after phacoemulsification is 4%.

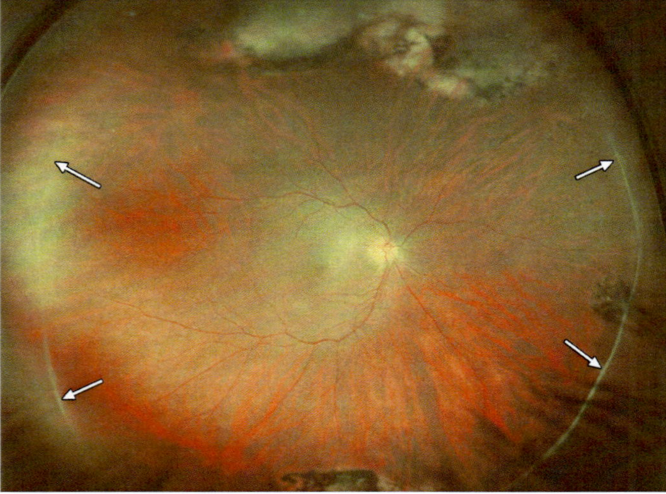

Fig. 24.40: Postvitrectomy (after one year) uncut condensed peripheral vitreous skirt (white arrows)

Failed/Recurrent Retinal Detachment

Common causes of failure after primary repair of RD are:

1. Missed break.
2. New break formation.
3. Absence of 360 degrees endolaser.
4. Absence of encirclage.
5. *Proliferative vitreoretinopathy (PVR):* It is the most common cause of failure after successful retinal detachment (RD) surgery in 5% to 12% of all cases . PVR is a process of fibrovascular scar tissue formation which complicates rhegmatogenous retinal detachments. Study showed PVR was responsible for recurrent RD in 82.2% of the cases.

Case Discussions

- *Case of missed break (Video 29, Chapter 24):*
  - A referred case of recurrent retinal detachment after silicone oil removal
  - Primary case was a 20G surgery
  - We introduced 23G ports
  - Triamcinolone assisted residual vitrectomy was done
  - Small holes (missed breaks) were detected in supero temporal periphery and they were marked with cautery (Fig. 24.41A)
  - FAX performed
  - Now barrage laser was done all around as well as around the holes
  - Silicone oil was injected at the end of surgery.
- *ERM with new break formation (Video 30, Chapter 24):*
  - A case of status post silicone oil removal with recurrent RD with *extensive ERM formation* with fixed folds with *new breaks* at the posterior pole (Fig. 24.41B)
  - Triamcinolone assisted membrane peeling was started with end gripping forceps
  - All new breaks were marked with cautery
  - There was anterior PVR at nasal periphery
  - PVR membranes were peeled with end gripping forceps
  - Any tiny missed break should always be looked for
  - Fluid-air exchange was done to settle retina
  - Laser barrage was done around all the breaks
  - Silicone oil injection is necessary for adequate tamponade.
- *Case of ERM (Video 31, Chapter 24):*
  - A case of recurrent retinal detachment
  - Silicone oil was removed

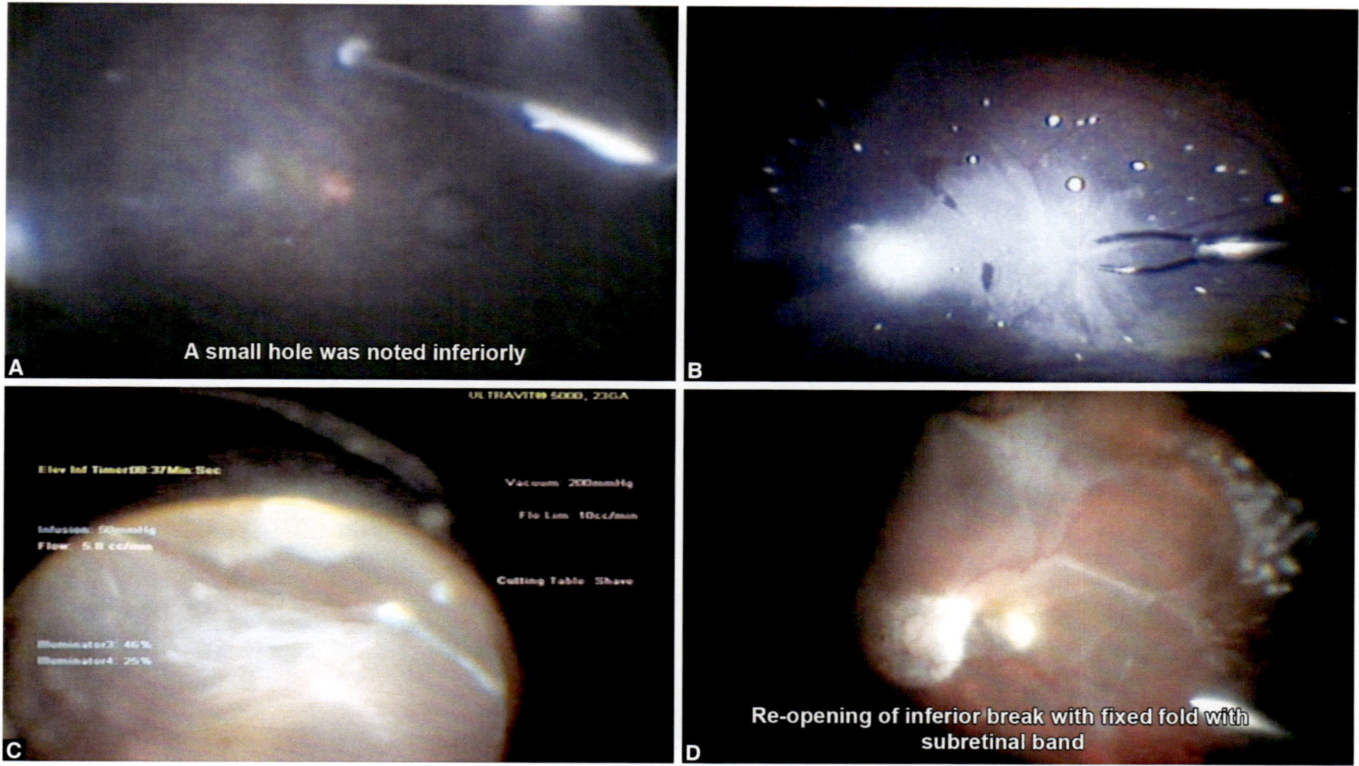

Figs 24.41A to D: (A) Failed RD due to missed break; (B) Failed RD due to new break formation; (C) Failed RD due to ERM formation with reopening of inferior break; (D) Failed RD with reopening of inferior break with inferior fixed fold with subretinal band

- There was ERM formation with reopening of inferior large break (Fig. 24.41C)
- Margin of the break was cauterized
- Membranes from the margins were removed
- Thick ERM from the inferior detached retina was removed
- Fluid-air exchange was performed to settle the retina
- Laser barrage was done at the margin of the break as well as 360° periphery
- Silicone oil was injected at the end of the surgery.

- *Case with reopening of inferior break with inferior fixed fold with sub retinal band (Video 32 , Chapter 24):*
  - Case with reopening of inferior break with inferior fixed fold with sub retinal band (Fig. 24.41D)
  - Cautery to inferior retina done
  - Inferior relaxing retinotomy done
  - Margin of retinotomy cauterized again to stop bleeding
  - Subretinal band with all its extensions removed
  - PFCL injected up to posterior margin of retinotomy
  - Fluid-air exchange completed
  - Inferior barrage laser done
  - PFCL removed
  - Silicone oil injected.
- *Case with incompletely filled silicone oil with extensive ERM with subretinal silicone oil (Video 33, Chapter 24):*
  - Operated case of total retinal detachment with choroidal detachment, where CD had been resolved. However, due to volume deficit, there is recurrent RD with extensive ERM with an inferior open break accompanied by subretinal migration of silicone oil.
  - After the removal of silicone oil, we meticulously removed the ERM (Fig. 24.42A).
  - PFCL was injected (Fig. 24.42B)
  - The inferior open break was enlarged circumferentially to remove subretinal silicone oil (Fig. 24.42C).
  - Retina was settled after the fluid-air exchange (Fig. 24.42D)
  - The laser was done at the break margin (Fig. 24.42E)
  - Silicone oil was injected as tamponade (Fig. 24.42F).

Persistent Hypotony after Silicone Oil Removal

A rare entity, especially in postoperative cases of old retinal detachments with advanced proliferative vitreo-retinopathy

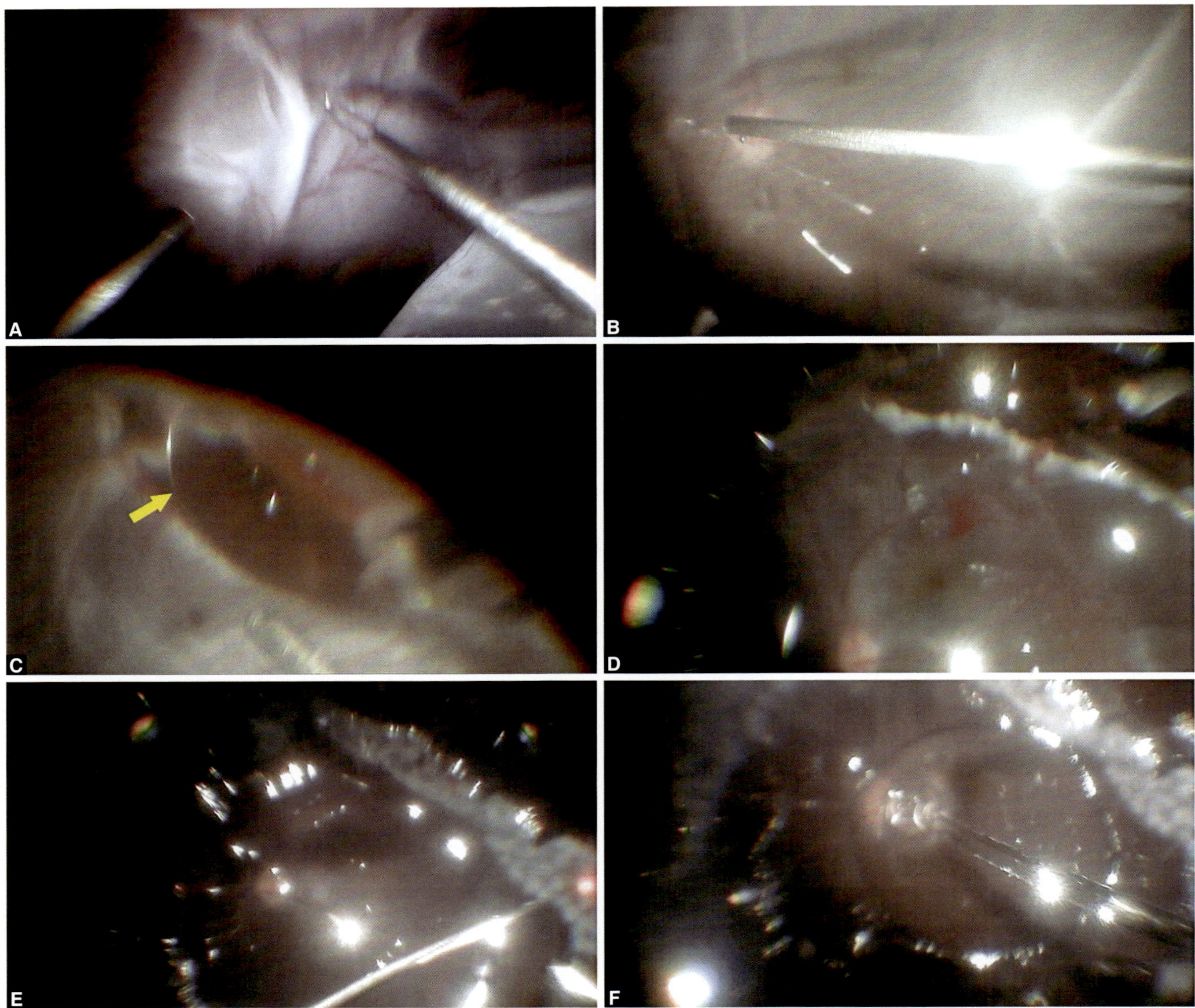

Figs 24.42A to F: Shows intra-operative steps of managing Recurrent retinal detachment with incompletely filled silicone oil with extensive ERM with subretinal silicone oil

changes where large areas of retinectomy had to be performed. Development of cyclitic membrane in early stage, many times are responsible for hypotony in these cases. Persistent low intraocular pressure can lead to soft eye with appearance of a phthisical eye in spite of on retina but with severe choroidal detachments with or without macular fold (Fig. 24.43A). Many times reinjection of silicone oil with higher centi strokes (5000 cst) can maintain the shape and tone of the globe with disappearance of choroidal detachments postoperatively (Fig. 24.43B) along with improvement of vision.

Sympathetic Ophthalmia

Sympathetic ophthalmia, first described by Sir William Mackenzie in his first Textbook of Ophthalmology, is defined as a progressive sight-threatening bilateral diffuse granulomatous intraocular inflammation that occurs in most cases within days or months after surgery or penetrating trauma to one eye. It is probably the first known and the most classic model of an autoimmune-associated disease occurring in humans.

- It is a very unusual complication

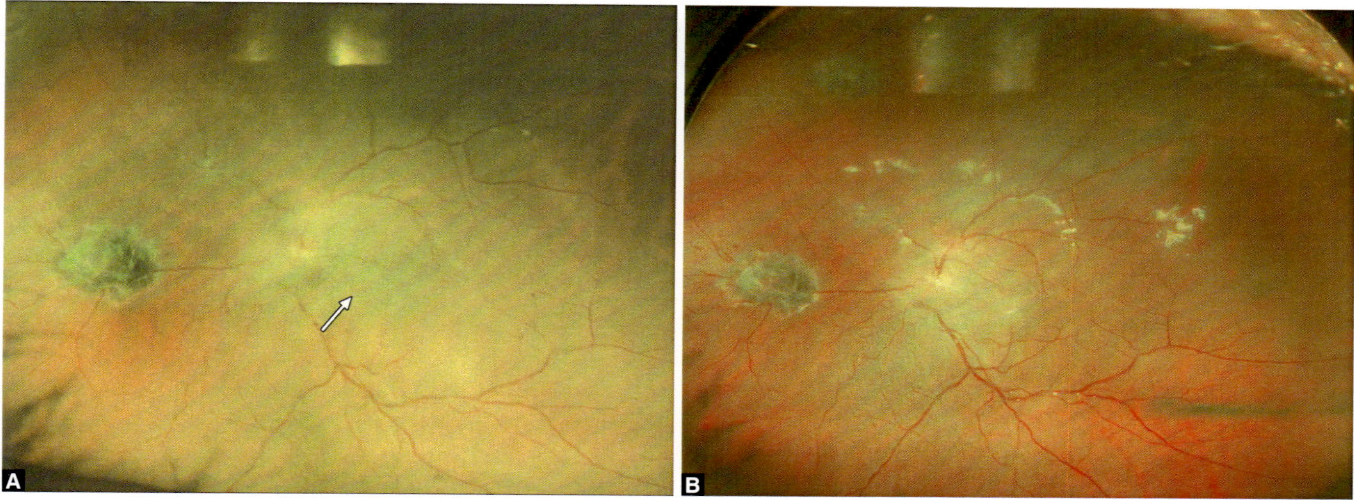

Figs 24.43A and B: (A) Post silicone oil removal (SOR) hypotony with choroidal detachment with macular fold (white arrow); (B) Resolved choroidal detachment and macular fold, after silicone oil (5000 Cst) injection in this case of post-SOR hypotony

- A bilateral diffuse granulomatous uveitis occurring in patients who have sustained previous ocular trauma or surgery persistent
- The incidence of sympathetic ophthalmia following vitrectomy has been estimated to be 0.01%
- Sympathetic ophthalmia tends to occur between 3 weeks and 6 months following vitrectomy and is characterized by bilateral anterior chamber inflammation, vitritis, Dalen-Fuchs nodules and exudative serous retinal detachment. Long-term complications include patchy or diffuse retinal pigment epithelial atrophy and rarely, choroidal neovascularization.

Therapy for sympathetic ophthalmia: Enucleation and immunosuppression.

- *Enucleation:* Some advocate early enucleation, specifically within two weeks after surgery, some say it has no effect on the final visual outcome.
- *Oral prednisone:* Is the first-line agent, but long-term control usually requires use of one or more immunosuppressive agents, such as methotrexate, azothioprine, cyclosporine or chlorambucil.

Vitreoretinal interventions associated with sympathetic ophthalmia are as follows:

a. Multiple surgical procedures
b. Postoperative hypotony
c. Persistent RD with PVR changes
d. Sutureless vitrectomy with leaking sclerotomy

Endophthalmitis after vitrectomy: Although rare, it is the most serious complication after vitrectomy and is often associated with profound vision loss or even blindness, despite proper management.

Incidence: 0.046% after pars plana vitrectomy.

- The diagnosis is often difficult to make because symptoms of endophthalmitis often mimic the normal postoperative pain and intraocular inflammation after vitrectomy.

Predisposing factors in sutureless vitrectomy cases: The unsutured sclerotomy wounds in small-gauge vitrectomy may provide a track for bacterial entry. Even the minimum bacterial inoculum may be enough to initiate endophthalmitis in certain patients, like diabetics. The following are the risk factors for the development of postvitrectomy endophthalmitis:

a. *Hypotony:* Early postoperative hypotony may facilitate the ingress of pathogens through incompletely healed sclerotomies. Conjunctival displacement and longer scleral tunnel formation during oblique insertion of smaller gauge trocar-cannula may reduce the incidence of postoperative leaking sclerotomies. In cases with an obvious leaking sclerotomy, suture closure of the scleral incision has to be considered.
b. *Vitreous wick syndrome:* A more significant risk in sutureless vitrectomies, in which wound stabilization in the early postoperative period may, in some cases, be due to plugging of the wound with vitreous.
c. Diabetic and elderly patients with relative immunocompromised status
d. *Complex cases:* The use of multiple intraocular instruments in more complex cases and the need for vitreous base dissection increases rotations of cannulas, which may damage the valve action of scleral flaps and jeopardize the stability of linear scleral tunnels and thus increase the risk of leaking wounds.

e. Intravitreal adjuvants such as triamcinolone acetonide may also predispose to a higher risk of endophthalmitis, especially of fungal etiology.

The organism responsible: No specific organism has been detected in postvitrectomy endophthalmitis cases, but mostly gram-positive in 75–95% of the reported cases. Reported organisms in cases of postvitrectomy endophthalmitis are *Staphylococcus aureus, Proteus mirabilis, S. epidermidis* and *Pseudomonas aeruginosa* (one case was culture-negative).

Prognosis: The onset is rapidly progressing, and the prognosis of postvitrectomy endophthalmitis is generally worse compared to endophthalmitis after all other intraocular surgeries.

Prevention:

- Preoperative preparation of povidone-iodine with topical antibiotics
- Careful draping to cover lid margins completely to avoid touch with eyelashes
- Intraoperatively, make a proper rigid oblique self-sealing wound, displacing the conjunctiva to create malalignment between conjunctival and scleral incisions.
- Wash out the conjunctival flora with BSS and povidone iodine-iodine before surgery.
- At the end of surgery, proper wound closure and devoid of vitreous wick are to be ensured. A leaky scleral wound should be properly sealed.

Management: The treatment should start at the earliest opportunity. Currently there are no established therapeutic guidelines specifically for postvitrectomy endophthalmitis cases. As these cases of endophthalmitis in vitrectomized eyes are very rapidly progressive and fulminant, urgent intervention is very important.

a. *In no tamponade or gas-filled eye*
   - Prompt culture of vitreous aspirate and intravitreal administration of vancomycin (1 mg/0.1 cc), ceftazidime (2.25 mg/0.1 cc), and optional dexamethasone (400 µg/0.1 cc) should be considered. Intravitreal steroid injection should be avoided in suspected fungal endophthalmitis cases.
   - If a more severe vitreous reaction or membrane formation occurs, early repeat vitrectomy with more extensive removal of residual vitreous along with lavage of the vitreous cavity with broad-spectrum intravitreal antibiotics should be done. However, aggressive removal of exudates and membranes strongly adhered to the fragile retina is not always necessary.

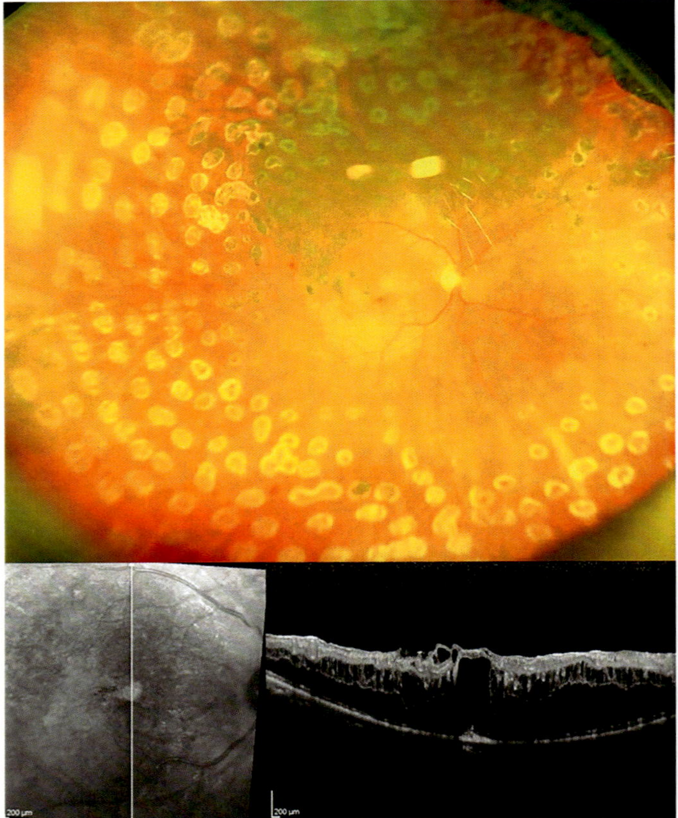

Fig. 24.44: Macular epiretinal formation 3 months postvitrectomy performed to treat diabetic vitreous hemorrhage.

   - Silicone oil can be used as a tamponade to prevent recollection of vitreous debris in severe cases. Silicone oil will compartmentalize the vitreous cavity from the anterior chamber, and help the intravitreal antibiotics present in a thin layer of fluid in the potential space between the silicone oil and retina to act.

b. *In already silicone oil-filled eye:* The course of endophthalmitis is usually indolent and often slowly progressive, mainly presenting with anterior chamber inflammations and sub-silicone oil exudate formation. A tap from the anterior chamber with the initiation of systemic antibiotics and intravitreal antibiotic injection should be considered.

Postoperative epimacular membrane (EMM) formation (Fig. 24.44): Epimacular membrane, also termed epiretinal membrane, premacular fibrosis, epi macular proliferation or macular pucker, may develop after retinal surgery or vitreoretinal intervention. Clinically significant EMMs occur in 3–8.5% of eyes after successful primary retinal detachment surgery. These secondary EMMs usually have mixed cellular composition, mainly macrophages, fibrocytes, fibrous astrocytes and occasionally RPE cells.

EMM following retinal detachment surgery with long-standing tamponade-like silicone oil has architectural features more like those of PVR membranes, such as mixed fibrocellular components like glial cells, fibroblast, RPE and myofibroblast-like cells (which explains the contractile property).

Risk factors:

1. *Time of onset:* Typically, the epi macular membrane develops after 1–6 months of retinal detachment surgery.
2. *Age of the patient:* Aged patients have a higher chance of postoperative EMM formation.
3. *Preoperative proliferative vitreoretinopathy (PVR):* Preoperative PVR changes like star folds, rolled-out edges of retinal breaks, etc. indicate higher chances of postoperative EMM formation.
4. *Number and size of breaks:* Multiple breaks and large-sized breaks, GRT have a higher chance of postoperative EMM formation. Silicone Oil Study Report 8 did find a 1.4 times increased incidence of EMM formation with longer radial relaxing retinotomies but did not find this increased association of EMM formation with posterior retinotomies.
5. *Preoperative vitreous hemorrhage:* It increases the risk of postoperative EMM formation.
6. Extensive cryoretinopexy during scleral buckling or endolaser during vitrectomy increases further EMM formation as they induce inflammation and release of RPE and inflammatory cells. Cryotherapy also causes the breakdown of the blood-retinal barrier, but diathermy and laser do not.
7. *Drainage of subretinal fluid:* A study shows SRF drainage during scleral buckling has a higher chance of postoperative EMM formation than non-drainage procedure.
8. *Duration of retinal detachment and macular involvement:* Long-standing RD increases postoperative EMM formation.

Preventive measures: Some factors cannot be modified, like the age of the patient, number and size of the breaks, duration of RD, pre-existing vitreous hemorrhage and PVR. But the following factors can be taken care of like–

1. A complete vitrectomy with complete removal of the posterior hyaloid face is necessary. Triamcinolone acetone particles-assisted vitrectomy ensures complete vitreous removal and removal of posterior hyaloid face and vitreoschisis components. Intraoperative use of triamcinolone acetone particles stain vitreous fibrils as well as stabilizes the blood-retinal barrier.
2. The use of endophotocoagulation rather than cryotherapy may reduce the postoperative EMM formation due to less dispersion of pigments.
3. Drainage of subretinal fluid may increase the risk of EMM formation after scleral buckling surgeries. Care should be taken to drain in selected cases like bulbous RD, chronic inferior RD or sometimes in total RD. Care should also be taken during suture placement to prevent inadvertent scleral perforation.

Management: Secondary EMMs are often stable, showing no significant increase in macular thickness on OCT or decrease in vision. However, if they cause substantial vision limitation with an associated increase in neurosensory retinal thickness, their removal is necessary. In cases of EMM formation in a silicone oil-filled eye, removing the silicone oil along with the EMM enhances visual outcomes.

Postvitrectomy macular edema

Postoperative macular edema was first described by Irvine in 1953 following cataract surgery. Postvitrectomy cystoid macular edema (CME) was defined as the postoperative observation of intraretinal cysts on optical coherence tomography, which prevents improvement or causes a reduction in vision compared to the preoperative value (Fig. 24.45). Macular edema arising de novo after pars plana vitrectomy is uncommon, probably due to the absence of traction and absence of vitreous, a depot of inflammatory medium.

Persistent or new CME is often identified after PPV for idiopathic ERM removal. Studies have suggested that

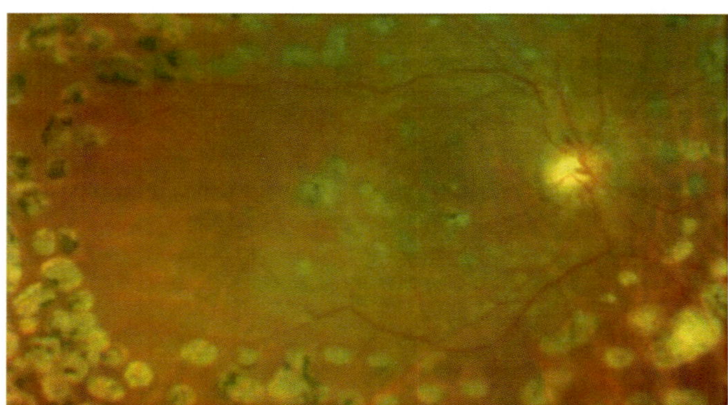

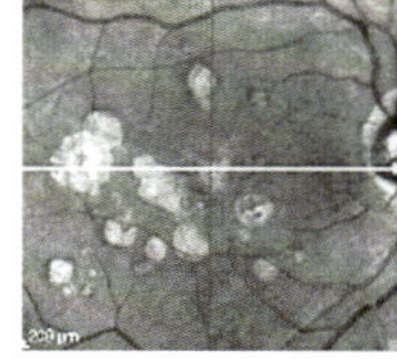

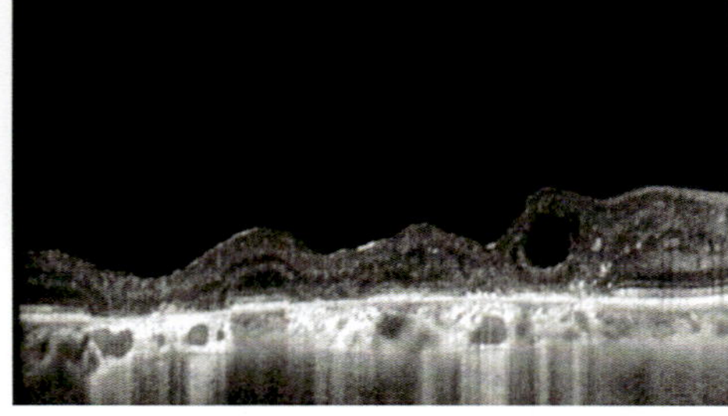

Fig. 24.45: Shows post-vitrectomy (done for diabetic vitreous hemorrhage) fundus photograph with CME on OCT

intraretinal cysts and increased preoperative central foveal thickness (CFT) are associated with reduced visual acuity after surgery.

CME may also develop after PPV for retained lens fragments after 3 to 4 months of surgery, and it may recur.

Risk factors and mechanism:

i. Postvitrectomy macular edema often results from an increase in microvascular permeability due to the postoperative release of inflammatory mediators like cytokines and vasoproliferative factors.
ii. Often, pre-existing macular edema can persist or increase after vitreoretinal surgery
iii. In cases of retinal vascular occlusion or diabetic maculopathy, the primary disease persists and many times progressive. Persistence or recurrence of macular edema can occur after surgery.
iv. In the case of the epiretinal membrane with vitreomacular traction, macular edema may persist, even if traction is successfully relieved during surgery. It has been seen that the incidence of OCT-proven macular edema after 1 month of epiretinal membrane removal is 64%.
v. Although the associated macular edema usually resolves to a great extent after successful reattachment of retinal detachment, macular edema may be observed postoperatively.
vi. In the case of postoperative or endogenous endophthalmitis, there is often severe inflammation of the posterior segment, which may give rise to cystoid macular edema with damage in macular function. This macular edema many times can persist after vitrectomy and last longer even after the resolution of the infection and inflammatory process.
vii. *Other risk factors:* Associated pre-existing uveitis, increased duration of surgery, surgical techniques (20G vs minimally invasive surgery).

Management for postvitrectomy macular edema:

1. Medical -
   i. Topical NSAID
      - Ketorolac (0.4%)—they act by lowering prostaglandin production in the anterior segment.
      - Nepafenac (0.1%)—a prodrug form. It is metabolized to amfenac, which is a potent COX-2 inhibitor. It has a significantly better posterior segment permeation than Ketorolac.
   ii. *Topical corticosteroid (Prednisolone acetate 0.5% or 1%, Dexamethasone 0.1%):* It is the mainstay treatment as an anti-inflammatory drug in postoperative patients. It inhibits the arachidonic acid by phospholipase A2, reducing the prostaglandin/leukotriene synthesis. If postoperative macular edema is secondary to anterior segment inflammation, topical steroid works better.
   iii. *Periocular steroid administration:* Depot injection of triamcinolone acetonide in the posterior sub-Tenon's space often works well in postvitrectomy macular edema cases. Periocular steroid diffuses through the sclera, especially in inflamed eyes.
   iv. *Intravitreal steroid:* Either triamcinolone acetonide injection (IVTA) or 0.7 mg sustained release dexamethasone implant (Ozurdex). Intravitreal steroid implant has special value in postvitrectomy macular edema as IVTA stays intravitreally only for very few days.
   v. *Surgical treatment:* If postoperative OCT shows a thickened neurosensory retina along with residual ERM or residual vitreomacular traction, further surgical removal of residual ERM or traction is necessary.

Postoperative macular hole

Postoperative macular hole characterized by partial or full thickness defect in the foveal neurosensory retina with visual disturbances, ranging from mild distortion to frank central scotoma.

Macular hole formation as a sequel of vitreoretinal surgery is a rare but well-recognized complication.

Mechanism: Although not well understood, residual traction plays an important role

1. *Residual cortical vitreous:* This can be only detected during macular hole surgery. Further surgery with ILM peeling ensures complete removal of cortical vitreous and then successful closure of the macular hole.
2. *Persistent cystoid macular edema or vitreomacular traction with thin ILM band:* ILM peeling in eyes with persistent CME may result in rapture or de-roofing of the cysts and formation of partial thickness or full thickness macular hole formation.
3. *Unusual postoperative inflammation:* It may result in CME formation and subsequent rupture of cysts or ERM formation with puckering effect or foveal necrosis in endophthalmitis cases.

Prevention and management:

- Proper identification of residual vitreous cortex or vitreoschisis layer by repeated staining with triamcinolone acetone particles.
- Proper planning before surgery, especially in cases with persistent CME with a thin ILM band where there is always the risk of de-roofing of the cysts, is required. ILM peeling should be carried out sparing fovea.
- If a partial-thickness macular hole forms, the removal of macular membranes and peeling of ILM is enough to heal the foveal defect.

- If there is full-thickness macular hole formation, gentle ILM peeling, taking care of boggy, cystoid macula.
- Many times, gentle manipulation of the edges of holes by soft-tipped cannula or Tanno's scraper to approximate them is necessary, especially with large macular holes.
- The inverted ILM flap technique is helpful in large-sized full-thickness defects in the foveal neurosensory retina.
- An inverted ILM flap is also very helpful if there is an associated elevated neurosensory retina with localized serous retinal detachment.

Postoperative macular fold

Macular folds after vitreoretinal surgery form when the detached retina fails to return to its original topographic position following retinal reattachment and take the shape of a fold of redundant retina.

This excess of the redundant retina at the folded area becomes possible as a result of stretching of the retina elsewhere. They are different from the folding of the retina due to ERM or PVR.

Clinical features:

- When macular folds are across the fovea it causes poor vision with severe metamorphopsia.
- But when it is far below the fovea, caused by marked downward shifting or translocation of the whole macula, vision may be good with little metamorphopsia but significant incyclotorsion or tilting of the image and resultant diplopia.

This metamorphopsia or incyclotorsion is the main reason for the severe dissatisfaction of the patients despite their good visual acuity.

Management: The Postoperative macular fold under silicone oil may settle without any further intervention. Sometimes, re-surgery is required if the fold does not settle with time. [Management of macular fold is discussed in detail in Chapter 25]

Subretinal migration of silicone oil: It may occur during direct PFCL-silicone exchange or after PFCL-air exchange, utilizing both standard and heavy silicone oils (Oxane HD, Densiron 68), particularly in complicated retinal detachment cases. The silicone oil can access the subretinal space through breaks or retinotomies with elevated margins due to persistent retinal traction. [This case has already been discussed in Chapter 24 (Video 33, Chapter 24)]

Risk factors:

a. Persistent retinal traction along the edges of a break or retinotomy in cases of retinal detachment with advanced PVR changes
b. Large break with taut retina around
c. Postoperative migration of silicone oil in cases of recurrent retinal detachments with reopening of old break or retinotomy with or without elevated margins.

Management

- The presence of silicone oil under the fovea can lead to retinal degeneration and poor visual outcomes
- It is crucial to exclude any intraoperative traction before inserting silicone oil. Fluid-air exchange is a useful test to confirm whether breaks and retinotomies are free of residual traction and that the retina around them is flattened before injecting silicone oil.
- Complete removal of subretinal silicone oil should be done under endoillumination via pars plana approach, as well as it is important to remove all the residual traction to flatten the retina and the edges of retinal breaks.
- In the case of removing heavy silicone oil, a prewarmed balanced salt solution is used as the infusion to reduce its viscosity and facilitate aspiration. The oil is aspirated through a 20G intravenous plastic cannula cut obliquely to maximize the surface area for aspiration.

Kindly scan the QR code below to access the online Video.

CHAPTER 25

How to Set-up a Good Vitreoretinal Operation Theater and Recording System?

On setting up a well-equipped vitreoretinal surgery theater, the following requirements are to be considered:

1. *Ideal dimensions of operating theater*—It should not be less than 16 feet/16 feet and if possible 20 feet/20 feet.
2. *Two types of operating theaters should be there:*
   - *Aseptic OT:* Ideally there should be twin OTs to allow the surgeon to use the second OT if he faces a suspicious infected case in the primary OT.
   - *Septic OT:* For cases with open globe injuries, penetrating injuries or endophthalmitis.

BASIC REQUIREMENTS

1. Good vitrectomy machine with high speed cutter.
2. Endolaser console with flexible curved probe.
3. Cryo unit, comprising of cryoprobe, cryomachine and nitrous oxide gas cylinder.
4. Gas (nitrogen gas cylinder) or air compressor. Nitrogen gas/compressor (ideally should be present outside the OT and connected to the vitrectomy machine via a pipeline) should feed the vitrectomy machine.
5. Wide angle visualization system—either BIOM or ROLs.
6. Illumination system with xenon or mercury vapor or LED light source. One can use in-built or additional light sources for dual illumination.
7. Disposable or reusable instruments like end grasping forceps, ILM forceps, serrated forceps, intravitreal scissor, flute needle, backflush needle, soft-tip needle, Tanoscraper, etc.
8. Good microscope with X-Y movement with respect to the patient's eye, foot switch controlled zoom, on-off and fine focus and it should be fitted with the laser filter and image inverting systems.

ADVANCED REQUIREMENTS

1. Laser indirect ophthalmoscope (LIO) to deliver laser where endolaser is not possible.
2. Auxiliary lighting—required during scleral buckling surgery.
3. Heavy fluid perfluorocarbon liquid (PFCL)
4. Vitreous substitute:
   - Perfluoropropane (C_3F_8) and sulfur hexafluoride (SF_6) gas, available in cylinder/pouch. Care should be taken to check the presence of gas inside the cylinder/pouch
   - *Silicone oil (SO):* At least two varieties of silicone oil should be available—SO with lower viscosity (1000 or 1300 cst) and SO with higher viscosity (5000 cst). Heavy silicone oil can be arranged as per planning to use it
   - *Intraocular magnet:* Two types of magnets—external magnets to create powerful magnetic field to the IOFB when applied on the outside of the eye and internal, rare earth magnets, which exert relatively less magnetism, are for intraocular use and for precise delivery of the IOFB.
   - *Intraocular lens:* For combined phacovitrectomy or to deal post-vitrectomy cataract or to plan for glue-assisted scleral fixation of IOL, a foldable multi-piece IOL with large optic is preferable
   - *Sitting arrangement for the surgeon:* The surgeon's chair should be adjustable with adjustable hand rest.
   - Standing/sitting arrangement for the assistant.
   - Instrument trays, what needs to be in the room.
5. *Ocular anesthesias for vitreoretinal surgeries:* Previously, retina surgeons used to do almost all major retinal procedures under general anesthesia, but nowadays everybody prefers peribulbar or retrobulbar anesthesia with long-acting local anesthetic agents. For children and young teenagers, there is no choice other than general anesthesia. Infusion-pump system for controlled general anesthesia can also be used.

RECORDING SYSTEM IN THE OPERATING THEATER

It is better to install a recording system with a camera and a recorder in the operating theater to document a surgery for medicolegal purpose as well as for academic purpose to present a surgical step.

Recording of a surgical video can be done by two options:

1. *By a single CCD (charged couple device) or a three chip CCD camera (for better quality) as analog signal*: Recording stored in a DVD recorder in MPEG2/VOB [(Video Object)] format. One should take the recorded file in a DVD. The next step is to convert the VOB file into avi format by a software (canopus procoder 2/any converter software) and then edit it in Adobe premiere 6.5 or any version timeline. A charge-coupled device (CCD) is a light-sensitive integrated circuit that stores and displays the data for an image in such a way that each pixel (picture element) in the image is converted into an electrical charge, the intensity of which is related to a color in the color spectrum. A three-CCD camera is a camera whose imaging system uses three separate CCDs, each one taking a separate measurement of the primary colors, red, green or blue light. Three-CCD cameras generally provide superior image quality through enhance resolution and lower noise. By taking separate readings of red, green and blue values for each pixel, three-CCD cameras achieve much better precision than single-CCD cameras. Three-CCD cameras are generally more expensive than single-CCD cameras. Nowadays, the CCD image sensor has been replaced by CMOS (Complementary Metal Oxide Semiconductor) imaging system.
2. *Single chip or three chip high definition camera:* Wide range of options starting from game capture HD to high end HD camera with recorder. CMOS imaging system is very much useful for high speed, HD cameras at a very low price with great improvement in image quality. All the recordings will be stored in 1TB/2TB/4TB external hard disc in HD or in a blue-ray recorder in MPEG4 format. Now, one should edit this MPEG4 file directly in Final cut pro (FCP) timeline in Mac or Adobe premiere higher version in windows.

One should remember the followings during recording a surgical video:

1. *Settings:* Match color temperature of the camera with the endoilluminator to get the most natural color of the surgical field. For monochromatic light (LED), match 6400 degree kelvin temperature of endoilluminator with the color temperature. Pure xenon have a color temperature of about 6200 K. For mixed light (Halogen), match 3200 kelvin temperature of endoilluminator with the camera color temperature.
2. White balance adjustment should be done before starting a surgery.
3. Adjust the surgical field of view (FOV).
4. Always concentrate on the last three basic points in all kinds of surgeries, i.e fine focussing, proper centration of the most active area of the surgical field and ideal zoomed field. For all these a television panel (LED or LCD), just in front of the surgeon is required and surgeon or an OT personal has to check the surgical field repeatedly to check centration.

Kindly scan the QR code below to access the online Video.

Index

Page numbers followed by *f* refer to figure and *t* refer to table.

D

E

K

L

M

R

S

T

U

V

W

X

Y